METHODS IN
DIABETES RESEARCH

METHODS IN DIABETES RESEARCH

Volume I: Laboratory Methods

Part C

Edited by

JOSEPH LARNER
STEPHEN L. POHL

University of Virginia Diabetes Research and Training Center
School of Medicine
Charlottesville, Virginia

A Wiley-Interscience Publication

JOHN WILEY & SONS

New York / Chichester / Brisbane / Toronto / Singapore

Library of Congress Cataloging in Publication Data:

Main entry under title:
Methods in diabetes research.

"A Wiley-Interscience publication."
Includes indexes.
Contents: v. 1. Laboratory methods (3 v.)
1. Diabetes. 2. Diabetes—Research. I. Larner,
Joseph, 1921– . II. Pohl, Stephen L. [DNLM:
1. Diabetes mellitus. 2. Research design. WK 810 M592]

RC660.M49 1984   616.4′62′0072   84-3714
ISBN 0-471-80971-3 (v. 1., pt. C)

Printed in the United States of America

10 9 8 7 6 5 4 3 2 1

PREFACE

Diabetes Mellitus is a complex disorder which involves multiple etiologic factors and produces many clinical outcomes. The past 10 years have seen a major expansion in research related to diabetes. A notable feature is the remarkable interdisciplinary nature of the investigations. Techniques currently in use for diabetes research run the entire spectrum from genetic engineering to psychological testing. The diabetes researcher in pursuit of the solution to a problem must often move about among scientific fields employing a diversity of methodologies. The purpose of *Methods in Diabetes Research* is to provide ready access to a wide array of investigative techniques. These techniques are broadly classified in the areas of basic, clinical, and behavioral/educational research. As the search for discovery of the causes and cures of diabetes progresses and intensifies, we hope to update and expand this resource through future volumes.

We have decided to launch the series with three volumes to be subtitled *Laboratory Methods*, *Clinical Methods*, and *Behavioral and Educational Methods*. We believe that these volumes will fill a needed void in the diabetes research area. This void exists because of pressure in referred journals to cut down on the experimental details with the result that it is now difficult if not virtually impossible to repeat a preparation procedure from a journal article. In fact, we conceived these volumes as "cookbooks," where methods are described in detail, including perhaps a review of procedures employed in validating a method or critical review of alternative methods. Presentation or review of results, however, was deemed less important. The six broad areas addressed in each of the three parts of Volume I, *Laboratory Methods*, are Receptors; Mediators and Metabolic Methods; Immunological and Immunochemical Investigations; Tissue, Cell, and Culture Preparations; Etiology, Complications, and Animal Models; and Hormone Synthesis and Degradation.

This book is the result of the outstanding interest and cooperation of investigators who were requested to contribute chapters. We hope these volumes will enhance the ease with which both experienced and new investigators will be able to set up research protocols in order to carry out experiments in diabetes research—for the sake of the many patients suffering with this disease.

Joseph Larner
Stephen L. Pohl

Charlottesville, Virginia
November 1984

ACKNOWLEDGMENT

The timely publication of this volume would not have been possible without the superb assistance of Karen Carter, Research Administrator of the University of Virginia Diabetes Research and Training Center, and her staff: Mary Ann B. McMahon and Mary Anne Inglis. We are also indebted to the following members of our Diabetes Center for their assistance in reviewing and editing manuscripts: Joanne Scott, Ph.D., Kevin R. Lynch, Ph.D., Jay W. Fox, Ph.D., Robert E. Dubler, Ph.D., Thomas Sturgill, M.D., Ph.D., R. Leslie Shelton, B.S., Randall T. Curnow, M.D., Michael J. Peach, Ph.D., Joseph Messina, Ph.D., Shinri Tamura, M.D., Carl Malchoff, M.D., Ph.D., Robert G. Langdon, M.D., Ph.D., Joyce L. Hamlin, Ph.D., Thomas W. Tillack, M.D., Alan D. Rogol, M.D., Ph.D., Michael J. Cronin, Ph.D., Erik Hewlett, M.D., Arthur E. Freedlender, Ph.D., Carl E. Creutz, Ph.D., David E. Normansell, Ph.D., Kang Cheng, Ph.D., and Charles Schwartz, Ph.D. Research at our Diabetes Center is funded primarily by USPHS Grant #AM22125.

J. L.
S. L. P.

CONTENTS

I

RECEPTORS

A

RECEPTOR CHARACTERIZATION

GLEN D. ARMSTRONG

Department of Medical Microbiology, University of Alberta, Edmonton, Alberta, Canada

MORLEY D. HOLLENBERG

Endocrine Research Group, Department of Pharmacology and Therapeutics, Faculty of Medicine, University of Calgary, Calgary, Alberta, Canada

1. INTRODUCTION

Over the past decade enormous strides have been made in the characterization
of membrane-localized receptors for a variety of hormones and neurotrans-
mitters. Perhaps the hallmark for such studies can be seen in work with the
nicotinic receptor for acetylcholine (1). Not only has the complex oligomeric
structure of this ligand-regulated ion channel been determined, but the amino
acid sequences of the four distinct receptor polypeptide chains and the sequences
of their corresponding cloned genes are presently being analyzed. This work
represents a remarkable chapter in a story that began with Langley's interest,
at the turn of the century, in the mechanism whereby nicotine contracts striated
muscle (2). Progress of the kind illustrated by work with the nicotinic receptor
has been made possible by the development of a number of biochemical approaches for dealing with membrane receptors. In sum, the key methodologies
for receptor characterization comprise (i) preparation of suitable radioligand
probes; (ii) a selection of suitable detergents for solubilization of the receptor
from a rich membrane source; (iii) development of a rapid, reliable method
for detecting the soluble receptor; (iv) the use of appropriate lectin and ligand-
specific affinity chromatography columns for receptor isolation; (v) cross-link
labeling of receptors, either with photoprobes or with chemical cross-linking
reagents, with concomitant biochemical (chromatographic, electrophoretic,

We are indebted to Heather Mitchell for her skillful typing of the manuscript. This work was
supported in part by funds from the Canadian Medical Research Council and the Alberta Heritage
Foundation for Medical Research.

etc.) analysis; (vi) the analysis of receptor domains by peptide mapping of radiolabeled receptors; and (vii) preparation and use of antireceptor antibodies. Although a number of review articles, including those resulting from some of our own work (3–6), have described many of the methods in general terms, there are few places in which the methods have been described in the detail we will present in this chapter. Our experimental protocols will be drawn from recent work we have done with receptors for insulin, basic-somatomedin (basic-Sm, or insulinlike growth factor I), and epidermal growth factor urogastrone. Our illustrative studies will deal primarily with items (iii)–(vii) listed above. The details for preparing suitable radioligands (Vol. IA-C, Section VI this series) or photoprobes (Yip, Vol. IA, Section IA) are in large part described elsewhere in this volume, as are the methods for detecting soluble receptors and for using insulin-Sepharose columns to isolate the insulin receptor (ref. 6 and Yamaguchi, Vol. IA, Section IB). The uses of antireceptor antibodies for receptor studies, briefly described in this chapter, are also amply illustrated by the work of Kahn and colleagues (Vol. IA, Section IC); as was the case for the nicotinic receptor, antireceptor antibodies will prove invaluable as a tool for receptor assay and for initial mRNA isolation, in connection with studies probing the molecular biology of the insulin receptor gene. Given the methodologies and approaches now on hand, there is reason to hope that in the near future the precise details of the structure and function of many receptors will become available for comparison with the data presently available for this nicotinic receptor.

2. PREPARATION OF RADIOLABELED LIGAND PROBES AND PLACENTA MEMBRANES FOR THE STUDIES

For our studies epidermal growth factor (EGF) and basic-Sm were purified as described previously (7, 8). The insulin was a gift from Eli Lilly. The peptides were iodinated by a modification of the chloramine-T method (3, 9, 10) to specific activities of $100–150$ $\mu Ci/\mu g$ (1 Ci $= 3.70 \times 10^{10}$ becquerels).

A "microsomal" membrane fraction was prepared from fresh term human placenta by a differential centrifugation procedure described earlier (11) with the exception that 200 mg phenylmethylsulfonyl fluoride (PMSF; dissolved in 10 mL dimethylsulfoxide, DMSO) was added to every 1000 mL of placenta homogenization buffer immediately prior to blending. Optimal results were obtained with preparations made from fresh, rather than fresh-frozen tissue.

3. SOLUBILIZATION OF RECEPTORS AND ANALYSIS BY SEPHAROSE 6B CHROMATOGRAPHY

Many detergents are now available which have been found suitable for characterizing hormone receptors. The key initial experiments comprise (i) the selection of a detergent which will solubilize the receptor from its membrane source and (ii) the design of a suitable assay to measure the binding of ligand to soluble receptor. In many cases the concentration of detergent required to solubilize the receptor efficiently from the membrane may be higher than that required to maintain the soluble receptor in solution and to measure ligand binding. Thus, initial experiments are usually performed to determine the optimum detergent concentration for receptor solubilization and for measuring binding. In practice, detergents such as Triton X-100, Lubrol, digitonin, octyl glucoside, and Ammonyx-LO have proved useful for receptor solubilization. For example, in work with the receptor for insulin and basic-Sm, the optimal concentration of Triton X-100 for receptor solubilization was in the range of 1 percent v/v; to measure binding, it was necessary to dilute the detergent concentration to below about 0.1 percent v/v. For peptide hormone receptors it has proved fruitful to measure binding to the soluble receptor by two approaches: (i) by gel filtration in which the receptor-bound ligand is eluted in a volume smaller than that at which the free ligand appears and (ii) by polyethylene glycol precipitation, wherein the receptor ligand complex is precipitated, while the free ligand remains in solution. Both of these approaches for measuring ligand binding are illustrated in Figure 1, where results for the insulin receptor are depicted. For alternative methods to measure the binding of ligands like steroids to soluble receptors, the reader is referred elsewhere (3, 12).

3.1. Gel Filtration Method

Two aliquots (0.1–0.5 mL) of soluble receptor are equilibrated with radiolabeled ligand usually for about 1 hr at 24°C (e.g., for insulin) or up to 17 hr at 4°C (e.g., for basic-Sm) in the absence of or, after preequilibration (10–20 min) with 100- to 1000-fold excess, unlabeled ligand. After equilibration, both aliquots are applied to gel filtration columns (e.g., 90 × 1.5 cm of Sepharose 6B), and are eluted with detergent-containing buffers. Radioactivity in the eluted fractions is monitored. The elution volume of the receptor corresponds to a peak for which the radioactivity is reduced in the sample pretreated with an excess of unlabeled ligand (see Fig. 1).

3.2. Polyethylene Glycol (PEG) Method

This method, adapted from immunoassay procedures (13), has been used successfully for a variety of receptors, including the one for insulin (14). In brief, a concentration of PEG is sought that is sufficient to precipitate the ligand receptor complex, leaving the labeled ligand in solution. The appropriate PEG concentration is arrived at by trial and error. The procedure for the insulin and basic-Sm receptor follows.

For measurement of insulin binding, 5–50 μL of detergent-extracted receptor is added to 0.2 mL Krebs–Ringer bicarbonate buffer, 0.1 percent w/v albumin,

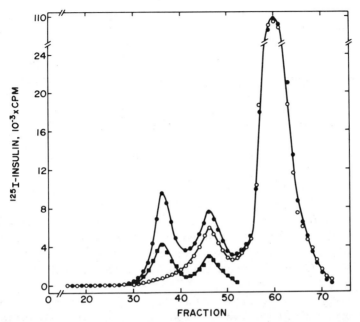

FIGURE 1. Chromatography on Sepharose 6B of crude solubilized insulin-binding material from fibroblasts (SVS AL/N). Samples of the soluble extract from SVS AL/N membranes were analyzed by chromatography on Sepharose 6B. Prior to chromatography two identical aliquots (240 μg of protein in 0.5 mL) were first equilibrated with [^{125}I]-labeled insulin (7.6 × 10^{-10} M) either with (○) or without (●) unlabeled insulin (1.3 × 10^{-5} M); a third sample (540 μg of protein) was chromatographed in the absence of insulin and aliquots (50 μL) of the effluent fractions (2 mL) were assayed for specific insulin binding (■) by the polyethylene glycol method. Two peaks of insulin-binding activity are readily detected. These data are from ref. 31.

pH 7.4, containing [^{125}I]insulin with (control tubes only) or without 25–50 μg of native insulin/mL. Phosphate buffer (0.1 M, pH 7.4) may also be used for the binding assay provided the pH is maintained between pH 7.0–7.4; buffers containing Tris-HCl, however, appear to interfere with the polyethylene glycol precipitation. Equilibration of binding is achieved in about 20–50 min at 24°C, at which time 0.5 mL of ice-cold 0.1 M sodium phosphate buffer (pH 7.4) containing 0.1 percent bovine globulin is added and the tubes are placed in ice. Cold 25 percent w/v polyethylene glycol (0.5 mL) is added (final concentration, 10 percent w/v), and the tubes are thoroughly mixed and placed in ice for 10–15 min. The suspension is then filtered under reduced pressure on cellulose acetate (Millipore EG or EH) filters, and the collected precipitate is washed with 3 mL of 8 percent w/v polyethylene glycol in 0.1 M phosphate buffer (pH 7.4) before measurement of trapped radioactivity by scintillation counting. As for the measurements of binding with cells and membranes, the specific binding is determined by subtracting from the total radioactivity bound that which remains bound in the presence of a high concentration (25–50 μg/

mL) of native insulin. Under the above conditions, less than 0.5 percent of the total free [^{125}I]insulin is precipitated or adsorbed nonspecifically and nearly quantitative precipitation of the insulin receptor complex occurs (14).

Concentrations of polyethylene glycol less than 8 percent (w/v) incompletely precipitate the complex; concentrations higher than 12 percent significantly precipitate free insulin. The presence of γ-globulin is essential as a carrier for the precipitation reaction, but concentrations above 0.1 percent (w/v) cause precipitation of free insulin. If the pH of the buffer containing the γ-globulin is above 8 or below 7, the complex is less effectively precipitated; phosphate buffers (0.1 M, pH 7.4) can be used effectively in the incubation medium. A final concentration of Triton X-100 in the assay mixture in excess of 0.2 percent v/v results in decreased insulin binding. The membrane extracts are therefore diluted before assay so that the final concentration of Triton X-100 is usually less than 0.1 percent and always less than 0.2 percent (v/v). For the estimation of rate data (association/dissociation), it is assumed that the addition of the cold polyethylene glycol-γ-globulin solutions stop the binding reaction at the timed intervals. It is expected that for each hormone studied, different conditions will be necessary to precipitate the maximum amount of hormone receptor complex, leaving most of the free ligand in solution. The procedure that has been used for the insulin receptor may serve as a prototype for other studies. In principal, any analogous method for selective precipitation of hormone receptor complexes (ammonium sulfate or other salting-out agent; trichloroacetic acid; change in pH) should provide a means of assaying soluble receptor, provided the complex is not dissociated by the precipitating agent. For example, salt fractionation has been used to examine the properties of soluble cholinergic receptor proteins. The analysis of soluble receptors for other ligands by a precipitation technique should similarly be possible. It is apparent that if the half-life of the receptor ligand complex is not sufficiently prolonged at low temperatures (4°C), the dilution of the sample (about fivefold in the procedure described above) and the time allowed for precipitation may shift the binding equilibrium appreciably; appropriate corrections of the data will then be necessary. The use of the gel filtration and PEG methods together has led to the detection of soluble receptor forms that might have gone undetected had either assay been used in isolation (e.g., see Fig. 1 and ref. 15).

3.3. Lectin Immobilization Assay

It can often happen (as with the EGF-URO receptor) that the soluble receptor may not be readily detected by either of the above methods. In such instances it has proved useful to aggregate the soluble receptor with an insoluble (6) or soluble (16) lectin (concanavalin A, wheat germ agglutinin) prior to the ligand binding assay. For the immobilization assay (16) the receptor is absorbed from solution on beads of lectin-agarose, and the binding assay is done on the bead-bound receptor.

We have observed that the most readily available and useful lectin for the assay is concanavalin A (ConA). However, other lectins (e.g., wheat germ agglutinin) appear to work equally well, and in principle it should be possible to optimize any assay of interest by an appropriate choice of lectin. ConA-Sepharose 4B CL (approximately 2 mg ConA/mL) is used in 50-μL aliquots for the adsorption of replicate samples of soluble membrane protein (approximately 100 μg protein) in 12 × 75-mm glass tubes (15 min at 24°C; final reaction volume, approximately 300 μL). A variety of detergents (Triton X-100; Ammonyx-LO; Lubrol) do not interfere significantly with the adsorption of protein. The bead-bound protein is then washed by dilution with 5 mL ice-cold buffer, immediately harvested by centrifugation (2 min at 1000 rpm), and is then incubated with radiolabeled ligand either with or without an excess (usually 10- to 100-fold) of unlabeled ligand. After equilibration (usually 1 hr at 24°C), the samples are again washed by suspension in 5 mL ice-cold buffer and harvested by centrifugation (2 min at 2000 rpm) for measurement of bead-bound radioactivity, upon removal of the supernatant solution by aspiration. As in other studies, the "specific" ligand binding is calculated by subtracting from the total radioactivity bound in the absence of unlabeled ligand, the amount of radioactivity bound in the presence of about a 100-fold excess of unlabeled ligand.

The method offers the advantages that the receptor can conveniently be transferred via the beads to a buffer optimized for the measurement of ligand binding and that dilute receptor samples (e.g., column effluent fractions) can be concentrated on the beads for the study of ligand binding.

As a useful variant of this approach (16), the soluble receptor is first equilibrated with soluble ConA. The binding of ligand is then measured by the PEG method, using the usual procedure. The addition of the soluble lectin facilitates the precipitation of the ligand receptor complex and evidently does not appreciably interfere with the binding of ligand to the soluble receptor.

The binding of radiolabeled EGF-URO to its soluble receptor is estimated after 45 min equilibration at 25°C in the presence of 100 μg ConA, 0.1 percent bovine albumin, and 0.2 percent Triton X-100 in 0.5 mL of 20 mM HEPES, pH 7.5 buffer. The [^{125}I]-EGF-URO–receptor complex is precipitated by the addition of 1 mL of 20 mM HEPES buffer, pH 7.5, containing 0.1 percent bovine globulin and 1 mL of 21.3 percent w/v polyethylene glycol 6000 in buffer. The resulting precipitate is collected by centrifugation for the measurement of precipitated radioactivity. Nonspecific binding is determined in replicate tubes containing 1 μg/mL of unlabeled EGF-URO.

4. ANALYSIS OF RECEPTORS BY SEDIMENTATION VELOCITY

In principle, any of the methods of receptor detection described above can be used to measure the sedimentation velocity of receptors in sucrose gradients.

In practice, the receptor has been detected either by the assay of fractions
from the gradient using the PEG method or by monitoring the sedimentation
of radioactive ligand, which is assumed to be bound to the receptor. In the
latter kind of experiment two receptor aliquots are analyzed. Prior to sedimentation analysis each aliquot is equilibrated with radioligand either with or
without an excess (100- to 1000-fold) of unlabeled ligand. As with the gel
filtration experiments outlined above, the peak of radioactivity that is reduced
in the presence of excess unlabeled ligand is assumed to represent the receptor.
The method used to measure the sedimentation velocity of the basic-Sm receptor
is illustrated in Figure 2 (details are recorded in the figure legend).

In both the gel filtration and sedimentation velocity experiments, the properties
of the receptor (Stokes radius; Svedberg constant) are determined with respect
to the properties of well-studied proteins (i.e., see Fig. 2). Both the Stokes
radius and sedimentation constant of the receptor are determined from the
calibration curves. Further, using gradients made with either H_2O or D_2O, it
is possible to estimate the partial specific volume ($\bar{v}$) of the detergent–receptor
complex (e.g., see ref. 17). The hydrodynamic parameters can be used to
calculate the apparent molecular weight of the soluble detergent–receptor
complex, according to the formula

$$Mr = \frac{6\pi N\eta}{1 - \bar{v}\rho} \, aS_{20,w}$$

where a = Stoke's radius, N = Avogadro's number, η = viscosity of water
at 20°C, and ρ = density of water at 20°C. The molecular weights of the
receptor determined in this way can be corrected for the amounts of bound
detergent. It is most instructive to compare the molecular weight of the receptor
observed in detergent solutions with the data obtained by cross-link labeling
and gel electrophoretic analysis, as described below.

5. RECEPTOR STUDIES USING CHEMICAL CROSS-LINKING REAGENTS

Cross-link labeling of receptors with disuccinimidyl suberate (DSS) was performed essentially as described by Pilch and Czech (18). One-milliliter aliquots
of the particulate membrane preparations (2–4 mg membrane protein/mL 50
mM Tris-HCl plus 0.1 percent bovine albumin, pH 7.4) are incubated with
$[^{125}I]$-labeled peptides (1–2 nM final concentration) in the presence or absence
of a 100- to 1000-fold molar excess of unlabeled peptide. Alternately, insulin
and basic-Sm receptors can be selectively cross-link labeled under conditions
whereby $[^{125}I]$insulin is not cross-linked to basic-Sm receptors and vice versa.
This is achieved by cross-link-labeling insulin receptors using 0.5–1.0 nM

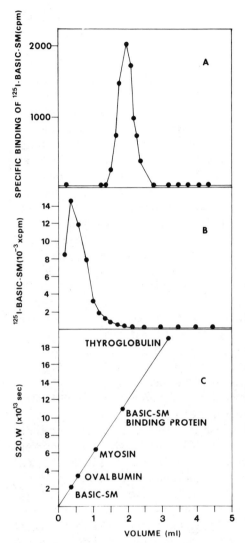

FIGURE 2. Sucrose gradient sedimentation of soluble basic-Sm receptor. (A) Triton X-100 solubilized membrane (300 μL) was layered on the gradient at 4°C and centrifuged at 100,000g for 16 hr. Binding activity was measured by the PEG procedure in 50-μL aliquots of the eluted fractions (200 μL), beginning with material collected from the meniscus. (B) Another sample of buffered sucrose containing [^{125}I]-labeled basic-Sm (about 100,000 cpm) was layered onto the gradient and centrifuged. Radioactivity in the eluted fractions (200 μL) was then measured. (C) The sedimentation coefficient of the basic-Sm receptor was determined from the standard curve for reference proteins. Reference proteins were centrifuged in the gradient simultaneously with the sample of soluble basic-Sm receptor. Radioactivity in the eluted fractions was measured by scintillation counting. These data are from ref. 32.

[^{125}I]insulin in the presence of approximately 10 μg/mL native basic-Sm. Conversely, basic-Sm receptors are cross-link labeled using 2–5 nM [^{125}I]-basic-Sm in the presence of 10 μg/mL native insulin. These conditions are based on our previous measurements of the relative affinities of insulin and basic-Sm for both receptors (19). In the previous work (19) the affinity of basic-Sm for its own receptor, as expressed by the equilibrium dissociation constant (K_D) was observed to be about 300 pM and the affinity of basic-Sm for the insulin receptor (K_i) was observed to be equal to or greater than 2 μM. For insulin the affinity for the insulin receptor (K_D) was estimated at about 800 pM; and for the basic-Sm receptor the affinity for insulin was about 2.8 μM. The peptide affinities for soluble and particulate receptors are equivalent (19, 20). It is often convenient to perform all of the binding reactions in 5-mL polyallomer (Beckman, Palo Alto, CA) ultracentrifuge tubes. EGF and insulin binding is allowed to proceed for 60 min at 22°C. Basic-Sm binding is allowed to equilibrate for 18–24 hr at 4°C. After binding equilibrium is achieved, the membranes are chilled in ice and 4 mL of ice-cold Krebs–Ringer phosphate buffer (KRP, pH 7.4) are added to the tubes. The membranes are sedimented by centrifugation for 20 min at 15,000 rpm (4°C) using a Beckman SW-50.1 rotor. The supernatant solutions are discarded and the pellets are taken up and resuspended in 1 mL KRP using Teflon resin pestles in 10-mL Potter–Elvehjem tissue grinders. Cross-link labeling with disuccinimidyl suberate (DSS) is achieved by adding 10 μL of a freshly prepared solution of DSS (100 mM in dimethylsulfoxide) to the resuspended, washed membranes. The cross-linking reaction is allowed to proceed for 15 min on ice and is then quenched by the addition of 4 mL/reaction of 50 mM Tris-HCl (pH 7.4). The cross-link-labeled membranes are again sedimented by centrifugation and the pellets are resuspended as described above, with the exception that after centrifugation, the resuspension buffer is 1 mL of 10 mM Tris-HCl (pH 7.4). Twenty- to 50-μL aliquots (containing 20–30,000 cpm) of the cross-link-labeled washed membranes are immediately solubilized in 12 × 7.5-mm disposable glass culture tubes using twofold concentrated Laemmli sample buffer (21) and are analyzed by SDS polyacrylamide gel electrophoresis (SDS-PAGE). The SDS-treated samples (100 μL) are heated in a boiling water bath for 5 min in the presence or absence of 50 mM dithiothreitol (DTT) and the entire sample is subjected, within 24 to 48 hr, to SDS-PAGE using linear gradient polyacrylamide separating gels as described by O'Farrell (22). SDS-PAGE samples should be stored at 4°C if they are not used immediately.

SDS-PAGE analysis of the cross-link-labeled, sulfhydryl-reduced EGF receptors resulted in autoradiographic patterns shown in Figure 3 (lane A). Two specifically labeled protein species of 170–180 and 150–160 kilodaltons are generally observed. Work in our laboratory and by others (23–25) suggests that the more rapidly migrating of the two EGF receptor species is a proteolytic product of the native EGF receptor. For the insulin receptor, specifically cross-link labeled in the presence of native basic-Sm, protein species of 300, 130, 100, and 35 kilodaltons are observed (Fig. 4A). For the basic-Sm receptor cross-link labeled in the presence of native insulin, proteins of 300, 130, and 37 kilodaltons are often observed. In the presence of excess native peptides, cross-link labeling of all these receptor species is drastically reduced. In addition, upon SDS-PAGE of unreduced, cross-linked-labeled insulin and basic-Sm receptors, the labeled species migrate with molecular weights greater than 300,000 (data not shown). Therefore, native insulin and basic-Sm receptors appear to exist as sulfhydryl-linked oligomeric structures. On the other hand unreduced,

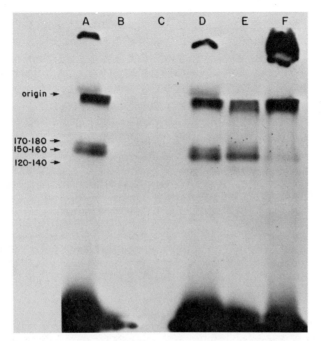

FIGURE 3. SDS–polyacrylamide gel electrophoretic analysis of DSS-cross-linked placental EGF receptors. Placental membranes were cross-linked labeled using [^{125}I]EGF as described in the text. After cross-link labeling, in the absence of excess native EGF, aliquots of the membranes were solubilized directly in SDS sample buffer (lanes A, D). After SDS solubilization, Triton X-100 was added to the sample in lane D to a final concentration of 1 percent (v/v). The remainder of the cross-link-labeled membrane preparation was solubilized for 18–24 hr at 4°C in 1 percent Triton X-100. The Triton-solubilized membranes were centrifuged for 60 min at 150,000g (4°C) and aliquots of the resulting supernatant solution and pellet were solubilized with SDS sample buffer (lane E; Triton supernatant solution, lane F; Triton pellet). Lane B, placental membranes cross-link labeled with [^{125}I]EGF in the presence of 100-fold excess native EGF. All of the samples were reduced with 50 mM DTT prior to electrophoresis. The molecular weights ($\times$ 10^{-3}) of the cross-link-labeled receptor species are shown at the left of lane A. These were calculated using reference proteins as described in the text. Radioactive proteins seen above the origin failed to migrate beyond the stacking gel, whereas those below the origin migrated into the 5–15 percent polyacrylamide separating gel.

cross-link-labeled EGF receptors show a similar SDS-PAGE pattern as reduced receptors. Therefore, the native EGF receptor would not appear to be a sulfhydryl-linked oligomer. The polyacrylamide gels, prepared with "Gel Bond" (Marine Colloids), are 1.5 mm thick and samples, which contain or do not contain DTT, should generally be applied to separate gels. After electrophoresis, the gels are stained in 0.1 percent Coomassie brilliant blue (Bio-Rad) in methanol–acetic acid–water (50:10:40, v/v). Gels are dried under vacuum and exposed at −70°C to Kodak X-Omst R X-ray film using Dupont Cronex Lightening Plus intensifying screens. Molecular weight calibration of the gels is done

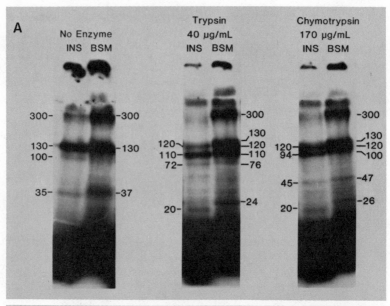

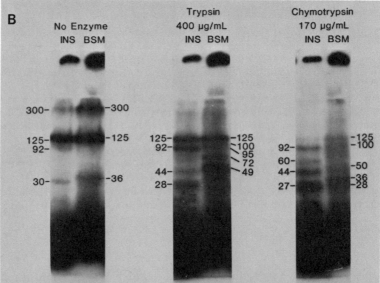

FIGURE 4. Electrophoretic analysis of cross-link-labeled, placental insulin (INS) and basic-Sm (BSM) receptors subjected to tryptic or chymotryptic proteolysis in the (A) membrane-localized or (B) SDS-solubilized state. Insulin receptor was cross-link labeled with [^{125}I]insulin in the presence of excess (10 μg/mL) native basic-Sm using DSS as outlined in the text. Basic-Sm receptor was cross-link labeled with [^{125}I]-basic-Sm in the presence of excess (10 μg/mL) native insulin. (A) 50-μL aliquots of the cross-link-labeled particulate membranes in 50 mM Tris-HCl (pH 7.2) were incubated at room temperature for 15 min with 10 μL Tris-HCl buffer (control) or 2.5 μg trypsin (in 10 μL) or 10 μg chymotrypsin (in 10 μL). Proteolysis was terminated by

using the following markers: human erythrocyte ghosts (26), β-galactosidase, phosphorylase b, bovine serum albumin, carbonic anhydrase, myoglobulin, and soybean trypsin inhibitor.

6. PHOTOAFFINITY LABELING OF EGF RECEPTORS

For receptor purification purposes placental membranes and A431 cell (epidermoid carcinoma; 27) EGF receptors can be labeled by the photoaffinity procedure described by Hock and Hollenberg (11). Briefly, 10–20 μg of EGF is mixed with 100 μL of 0.1 M sodium phosphate buffer (pH 7.5) in acid-washed borosilicate glass tubes precoated with 40 μg of Iodogen (Pierce Chemical Co., Rockford, IL). To coat the tubes, Iodogen is dissolved (2 mg/mL) in chloroform and 20 μL of the solution is added to the tubes. The tubes are shaken using a vortex mixer, and the chloroform is evaporated using a gentle stream of nitrogen. The iodination reaction is initiated by the addition of 0.5–1.0 mCi of ^{125}I (Amersham, Arlington Heights, IL, IMS-300) to the EGF-containing phosphate buffer. After 15 sec, the reaction mixture is removed from the Iodogen tube and filtered through a glass wool-plugged Pasteur pipette into an aluminum foil-covered, 5-mL specimen vial. Aliquots of the reaction mixture are then removed for the determination of peptide-incorporated counts by TCA precipitation. The volume of the reaction mixture is made up to 2 mL with 0.1 M sodium phosphate buffer (pH 7.5), and the solution is gently stirred using a Teflon-coated stir bar and magnetic stirrer. The photoaffinity labeling reagent, SANAH (N-succinimidyl-6(4′-azido-2-nitrophenylamino) hexanoate, Pierce Chemical Co., Rockford, IL) is dissolved (1 mg/mL) in DMSO in a light-protected, screw-top, 2-mL specimen vial. Freshly prepared SANAH solution (200 μL) is added to the iodinated EGF reaction mixture (2 mL). Coupling of SANAH to [^{125}I]EGF is allowed to proceed at room temperature for 30 min, and the reaction is quenched by the addition of 0.5 mL 0.5 M

---

heating the samples for 10 min in a boiling water bath after the addition of 60 μL twofold concentrated sample buffer of Laemmli and 10 μL β-mercaptoethanol. (B) Alternately, 50-μL aliquots of the cross-link-labeled particulate membranes were heated for 2 min in a boiling water bath in the presence of 50 μL twofold concentrated SDS sample buffer as described by Cleveland et al. (28). The samples were chilled on ice, then placed into a 37°C water bath. Samples were incubated for 30 min with control Tris-HCl buffer, trypsin, or chymotrypsin at the indicated concentrations. The reactions were terminated by the addition of 10 μL β-mercaptoethanol followed by heating for 8 min in a boiling water bath. All samples were subjected to SDS–polyacrylamide gel electrophoresis as described previously (22) using 5–20 percent linear separating gels. The molecular weights of the peptides were determined with reference proteins as described in the text. These data are from ref. 29.

lysine-HCl. The [^{125}I]-SANAH-EGF can be stored at 4°C until used for photoaffinity labeling. If not used immediately, the reagent should usually be used within 24 to 48 hr of its production.

To photoaffinity label the EGF receptor in placenta membranes, 100 μL of [^{125}I]-SANAH-EGF reaction mixture is mixed with 1 mL of membranes (2–4 mg/mL membrane protein) in 50 mM Tris-HCl (pH 7.4) containing 0.1 M NaCl. Binding of [^{125}I]-SANAH-EGF is allowed to proceed to equilibrium in the dark, at room temperature, for 60 min. The binding and subsequent steps are conveniently carried out in a 5-mL polyallomer centrifuge tube (Beckman). After binding, the membranes are diluted to 5 mL with ice-cold binding buffer and are sedimented by centrifugation at 15,000 rpm for 20 min (4°C) using a Beckman SW-50.1 rotor. The resulting supernatant solution can be discarded and the pellet resuspended in 1 mL of binding buffer using a Potter–Elvehjem tissue grinder as descibed above. The pellet resuspension step is performed under dim lighting conditions with the tissue grinder immersed in ice. After resuspension, the membranes are transferred back into a 5-mL polyallomer centrifuge tube which is placed in ice. To cross-link-bound, [^{125}I]-SANAH-EGF to the receptor, the membranes are exposed for 10 min to the light from two 200-W incandescent light bulbs placed 10 cm from the mouth of the centrifuge tubes. A shallow, Pyrex baking pan or Petri dish filled with 3–5 cm of water and placed between the lights and the membranes is sufficient to prevent melting of the ice and excessive warming of the sample. After exposure to light, the volume of the mixture is increased to 5 mL with ice-cold 10 mM Tris-HCl buffer and the membranes are again sedimented by centrifugation as described above. The resulting pellet is either resuspended in 1 mL of 10 mM Tris-HCl buffer or dissolved directly in 1 mL of SDS sample buffer prior to SDS-PAGE analysis.

A431 cells are conveniently grown in roller bottles (850 cm^2) at 37°C in minimal essential medium (MEM, with Hanks' buffer, Gibco) containing 10 percent fetal calf serum. When the cell monolayer becomes confluent, the growth medium is decanted and the cells are rapidly but gently washed with ice-cold, 50 mM Tris-HCl buffer containing 0.1 M NaCl. Fifty milliliters of washing buffer is then added to the roller bottle, which has been covered with aluminum foil and placed on ice. Two milliliters of [^{125}I]-SANAH-EGF are added and binding to receptors is allowed to proceed for 20 min while the roller bottle is gently rotated in the ice (by hand if necessary). The binding solution is then decanted and the monolayer is washed with buffer as described above. The aluminum foil is then removed from the roller bottle and the monolayer is exposed, for 10 min, to intense incandescent light as described above. During the exposure period, the roller bottle is rapidly rotated in the ice to prevent excessive warming of the cells. The photoaffinity-labeled A431 cells are then dissolved in 10 mL of SDS sample buffer and the viscous solution is transferred to a 50 × 175-mm test tube and heated for 5 min in a boiling water bath.

7. SOLUBILIZATION OF CROSS-LINK-LABELED RECEPTORS USING TRITON X-100

Cross-link-labeled receptors can be solubilized by diluting the washed membranes 1:1 (v/v) with 2.0 percent Triton X-100 in 50 mM Tris-HCl. The Triton–membrane mixtures are stirred slowly at 4°C for 18–24 hr and then diluted fivefold with 50 mM Tris-HCl buffer. The extracts are clarified by centrifugation at 150,000g for 60 min (4°C) using a Beckman SW-50.1 rotor. The resulting supernatant solutions, which contain solubilized, cross-link-labeled receptors, are retained for the affinity or immunoaffinity isolation procedures which will be described below.

Upon SDS-PAGE the Triton X-100 solubilized, cross-link-labeled insulin and basic-Sm receptors display protein species which are similar to those obtained when the receptors are solubilized directly in SDS sample buffer (see Fig. 4). However, when Triton X-100 solubilized, cross-link-labeled EGF receptor was analyzed by SDS-PAGE, there was a noticeable decrease in the intensity of the 170–180-kilodalton receptor species in the resulting autoradiograms (Fig. 3), which correlated with the faint appearance of a 120–140-kilodalton species. Further, the change in the pattern of cross-link-labeled EGF receptor was not found to be due to the presence of Triton during electrophoresis since SDS solubilized samples to which the appropriate amount of Triton X-100 was added revealed the same protein species observed for receptors solubilized with SDS alone (Fig. 3, lane D). Differential solubilization of the EGF receptor species is ruled out by the equal disappearance of both the 170–180- and 150–160-kilodalton species from the Triton X-100 insoluble, 150,000g pellet (Fig. 3, lane F). Therefore, it would appear that the placenta membranes contain intrinsic proteolytic activity capable of acting on the cross-link-labeled EGF receptors during the Triton solubilization process. Ongoing studies in our laboratory suggest that the intrinsic proteolytic activity may be due to the presence of a calcium-dependent, sulfhydryl protease which could be involved in the cellular processing of the EGF receptor. The presence of such proteases in receptor preparations can often complicate studies of receptor subunit composition.

8. RECEPTOR PURIFICATION BY WHEAT GERM AGGLUTININ AFFINITY CHROMATOGRAPHY

Approximately 3–5 mg of the Triton X-100 solubilized, cross-link-labeled membrane protein in 5 mL 50 mM Tris-HCl buffer containing 0.2 percent v/v Triton X-100 and 0.2 M NaCl is applied to a column of 1.0 mL wheat germ agglutinin–agarose (P&L Biochemicals, Milwaukee, WI) in glass wool-plugged Pasteur pipettes (0.6 cm inside diameter). The absorbed glycoproteins are then washed at 22°C with 40–50 mL of the 0.2 percent Triton X-100-containing buffer and are eluted with aliquots (500 μL) of 0.2 M N-acetyl-D-glucosamine

(NAG) dissolved in the same buffer. The eluted receptor fractions are pooled and up to 100 μL aliquots containing approximately 10^3 cpm can be solubilized in SDS sample buffer and analyzed by SDS-PAGE as described above. Occasionally, the pooled, NAG-eluted fractions may contain too few counts (<1000 cpm) to permit direct analysis of aliquots by SDS-PAGE. In these cases the pooled fractions should be dialyzed for 18 hr at 4°C against 5 mM Tris-HCl buffer (pH 6.3) containing 0.1 percent SDS (see legend to Fig. 5 for procedure).

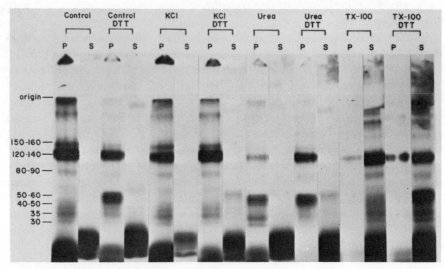

FIGURE 5. Membrane association of trypsin-generated, cross-link labeled EGF receptor peptides. Placenta membranes were cross-link labeled with [^{125}I]EGF using DSS as described in the text. The cross-link labeled membranes were divided into eight 200 μL aliquots which were diluted 1:1 with 50 mM Tris-HCl buffer (pH 7.2) containing or not containing 50 mM DTT (control and control DTT); 6 M KCl ± 50 mM DTT; 8 M urea ± 50 mM DTT; or 2 percent Triton X-100 ± 50 mM DTT. The KCl, urea, or Triton X-100 solutions were prepared in 50 mM Tris-HCl buffer. The samples were incubated for 60 min on ice then centrifuged at 150,000g for 60 min. Centrifugation was carried out using a Beckman SW-50.1 rotor and bucket adaptors for 0.8-mL nitrocellulose centrifuge tubes. The resulting supernatant solutions were dialyzed for 18–24 hr against 5 mM Tris-HCl buffer (pH 6.3) containing 0.1 percent SDS. Dialysis was carried out by placing the supernatant solutions in 12 × 75-mm, disposable, glass culture tubes which were sealed at their open ends with dialysis membrane held in place with elastic bands. The tubes were inserted (membrane-sealed ends down) into holes bored in styrofoam blocks floating in the dialysis buffer. The dialyzed samples were concentrated to approximately 50 μL using a Savant Speed Vac vacuum concentrator. An equivalent volume of twofold concentrated SDS sample buffer was then added to the concentrated samples. The 150,000g pellets were resuspended in SDS sample buffer and 10 μL of β-mercaptoethanol was added to all of the samples which were heated for 10 min in a boiling water bath. The pellet (P) and supernatant (S) solution samples were subjected to SDS-polyacrylamide gel electrophoresis as described previously (22) using 5–15 percent linear gradient gels. Pellet and supernatant solution samples were analyzed on separate gels. Molecular weights of the peptides were determined using standard reference proteins as discussed in the text. The calculated molecular weights (× 10^{-3}) of peptides in the pellets are shown at the left of the figure. Equivalent amounts of radioactivity were not applied to each of the stacking gel sample wells.

The dialyzed fractions can then be concentrated using a centrifuge-vacuum concentrator (Speed vac, Savant, Hicksville, NY). However, care should be taken to ensure that the samples never become totally dry because drying of the samples results in the production of aggregated receptors that cannot be resolubilized completely in SDS sample buffer.

9. RECEPTOR PURIFICATION BY AFFINITY CHROMATOGRAPHY USING ANTIRECEPTOR OR ANTILIGAND ANTIBODY

Purification of selectively cross-link-labeled insulin and basic-Sm receptors by immunoaffinity chromatography utilizes staphylococcal protein A–Sepharose to isolate antibody–antigen complexes. Five milliliter aliquots of the Triton X-100 solubilized, cross-link labeled membranes or the pooled wheat germ agglutinin–agarose-bound fractions are incubated for 24–48 hr at 4°C with 10 μL of anti-rat liver insulin receptor or antiligand antiserum. The polyclonal anti-rat liver insulin receptor antibody (A410) was a gift from Dr. Steve Jacobs (Burrough's Wellcome, Research Triangle Park, NC). Anti-porcine insulin serum was obtained from Miles Biochemicals and anti-basic-Sm was prepared by Bhaumick and Bala (7). Ten milligrams (dry weight) of washed protein A–Sepharose (Pharmacia, Piscataway, NJ) is added and incubation is continued, with gentle stirring, for 1 hr at room temperature. The mixtures are then passed through glass wool-plugged Pasteur pipettes and washed with 10 mL of Tris-HCl–Triton X-100 buffer. Bound antibody–antigen complexes can be eluted into 12 × 75-mm disposable culture tubes using 100 μL SDS-PAGE sample buffer. The entire 100 μL of SDS elution buffer is collected into the culture tubes by applying gentle pressure to the tops of the Pasteur pipettes. The culture tubes are then centrifuged at 2000 rpm for 10 min to reduce the resulting foam. Samples are heated in a boiling water bath for 5 min in the presence of 50 mM DTT and subjected to SDS-PAGE as described above. An identical procedure has been successfully used with anti-EGF antibodies (prepared in our laboratory) to purify EGF receptor complexes.

10. PEPTIDE MAPPING STUDIES OF CROSS-LINK-LABELED RECEPTORS

10.1. Peptide Mapping of Insulin and Basic-Sm Receptors

Aliquots (50 μL) of the cross-link-labeled, particulate membranes in 50 mM Tris-HCl buffer are incubated with 10 μL TPCK-treated trypsin (0.25 mg/mL; Worthington, Freehold, NJ) or 10 μL chymotrypsin (1.0 mg/mL) for 15 min at room temperature. Proteolysis is terminated by heating the samples for 10 min in a boiling water bath after the addition of 60 μL of twofold concentrated SDS sample buffer and 10 μL β-mercaptoethanol. Alternately, 50 μL of cross-link-labeled, particulate membranes are dissolved in 50 μL of twofold concentrated SDS sample buffer and heated for 2 min in a boiling water bath as described previously (28). The samples are transferred to a 37°C water bath and incubated for 30 min with 10 μL TPCK-trypsin (2.5 mg/mL) or 10 μL chymotrypsin (1.0 mg/mL). Proteolysis is terminated by the addition of 10 μL β-mercaptoethanol and heating the samples in a boiling water bath for 8 min. After analysis by SDS-PAGE the peptides are visualized by autoradiography. When particulate membranes are subjected to proteolysis (Fig. 4A), only those receptor domains which are external to the lipid bilayer should be accessable to cleavage by the enzymes. A high degree of peptide domain homology is observed for particulate insulin and basic-Sm receptors. Conversely, peptide map differences which are observed when SDS-solubilized receptors are proteolyzed (Fig. 4B) may reflect differences in receptor domains which are internal to the membrane-lipid bilayer and are responsible for the observed differences in receptor function. The reader is referred to ref. 29 for a complete discussion and possible significance of the results.

10.2.   EGF Receptor: An Approach to Evaluate Its Membrane Topology

Trypsin proteolysis of the cross-link-labeled or unlabeled EGF receptor provides a unique opportunity to study the nature and membrane localization of the resulting peptides. The following results illustrate an approach which can be used for other receptors. Aliquots of 500 μL ($1-2 \times 10^5$ cpm) of cross-link-labeled or unlabeled particulate membranes (2–4 mg/mL membrane protein) in 50 mM Tris-HCl are incubated with 50 μL TPCK-trypsin (see legend to Fig. 5) at 37°C for 2 hr. Proteolysis is terminated by the addition of 5 μL PMSF (10 mg/mL freshly prepared in DMSO) and heating the samples in a boiling water bath for 2 min. The proteolyzed samples can be analyzed by two different approaches. First, to identify trypsin-generated glycopeptides, the samples are solubilized in Triton X-100 and clarified as described above. The resulting receptor-containing supernatant solutions are then subjected to wheat germ agglutinin or concanavalin A (ConA) affinity chromatography as described in Section 7 with the exception that all buffers for ConA affinity chromatography should contain 2 mM Mg^{2+} and Ca^{2+} and the elution sugar is 0.2 M mannose. Second, to identify peptides which are not deeply embedded in the membrane lipid bilayer, the trypsin-treated samples are diluted 1:1 with KCl (3 M final concentration) or urea (4 M final concentration) in 50 mM Tris-HCl buffer in the presence or absence of DTT. Untreated (control) and Triton X-100-solubilized samples are also prepared as described above and all samples are subjected to centrifugation at 150,000g for 60 min at 4°C. The supernatant solutions should be dialyzed for 18–24 hr against 5 mM Tris-HCl buffer (see legend to Fig. 5) and if necessary, concentrated using a vacuum concentrator as described above. Aliquots of the dialyzed supernatant solutions and pellets are then solubilized in SDS sample buffer and analyzed by SDS-PAGE in the presence or absence of β-mercaptoethanol or DTT.

Upon trypsin treatment the membrane-localized 170–180-kilodalton EGF receptor is converted to receptor fragments of 120–140, 80–90, and 25–45 kilodaltons (Fig. 6, lanes F, H). Although the relative amounts of each of the peptides appeared to vary somewhat for each trial, the peptide molecular weights remained within the indicated ranges. Treatment of membrane-localized, cross-link-labeled EGF receptors with chymotrypsin or more vigorous trypsin treatment (longer time and/or trypsin concentration) resulted in the production of peptides with molecular weights similar to those displayed in Figure 6. Therefore, we concluded that the EGF receptor is composed of at least four major domains which are relatively resistant to proteolysis. Moreover, similar trypsin peptides were also observed when membranes were trypsinized prior to cross-link labeling. Therefore, the EGF binding site appears to be resistant to trypsin cleavage, and EGF binding does not seem to affect the molecular size or number of peptides produced.

These findings prompted us to ask which of the trypsin peptides possess carbohydrate and whether any of the peptides were no longer tightly membrane associated. Affinity chromatography using wheat germ agglutinin or ConA-agarose demonstrated that all of the peptides possess carbohydrate moieties (Fig. 6, lanes E, G, I). Alternately, some of the peptides may have been covalently attached to glycopeptides by sulfhydryl bonds. However, the 150–160-, 120–140-, and 80–90-kilodalton peptides were observed when SDS-PAGE was carried out in the presence or absence of sulfhydryl reducing reagents (data not shown) so the latter explanation appears unlikely.

When the trypsin-treated, cross-link-labeled membranes were sedimented by centrifugation in the presence or absence of DTT in 3 M KCl or 4 M urea, all of the peptides remained associated with the membrane pellets (Fig. 6). Urea and KCl are known to be effective for removing peptides associated by ionic or hydrophobic interactions with the periphery of membranes (23, 30). Therefore, we concluded that portions of the trypsin peptides of cross-link-labeled EGF receptors were probably deeply embedded in or even span the membrane-lipid bilayer.

11. PURIFICATION OF PHOTOAFFINITY-LABELED EGF RECEPTORS

Photoaffinity-labeled, SDS-solubilized placental or A431 EGF receptors can be purified by anti-EGF immunoaffinity chromatography after SDS-PAGE. One-milliliter aliquots of the SDS-solubilized cells or membranes are subjected to SDS-PAGE as described above with the exception that a well-forming comb is not employed in the preparation of the stacking gels. The resulting space between the top of the stacking gels and the top of the glass gel forming plates provides a large well into which the 1-mL samples can be added. After electrophoresis the gels are immediately dried (without prior fixation) under vacuum and exposed at −70°C for 1–2 days to X-ray film as described above. Gel

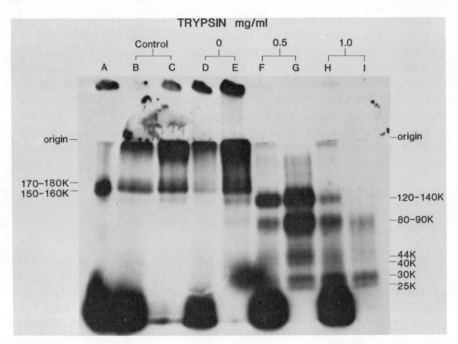

FIGURE 6. Lectin affinity chromatography of trypsin-treated, cross-link labeled placental EGF receptors. EGF receptors were cross-link labeled using DSS and solubilized with Triton X-100 as described in the text. After centrifugation at 150,000g for 60 min, 0.5-mL aliquots of the resulting supernatant solution were incubated for 30 min at 37°C with 50 μL of Tris-HCl buffer (control) or 50 μL of Tris-HCl buffer containing 250 or 1000 μg of TPCK-treated trypsin. Proteolysis was terminated by the addition of 500 μg PMSF (dissolved in 50 μL DMSO) and heating the samples for 2 min in a boiling water bath. Half of each sample was then subjected to wheat germ agglutinin affinity chromatography as described in the text and the washed, wheat germ agglutinin-bound peptides were eluted with 0.2 M NAG. Samples which were not subjected to wheat germ agglutinin affinity chromatography and the pooled, NAG-eluted fractions containing wheat germ agglutinin-bound peptides were dialyzed for 18–24 hrs at 4°C against 5 mM Tris-HCl buffer (pH 6.3) containing 0.1 percent SDS. After dialysis the samples were concentrated to approximately 50 μL using a Savant Speed Vac vacuum concentrator. An equal volume of twofold concentrated SDS sample buffer and 10 μL of β-mercaptoethanol was added and the samples were heated for 10 min in a boiling water bath. The samples were subjected to SDS–polyacrylamide gel electrophoresis as described earlier (22) using 5–20 percent linear polyacrylamide separating gels. Lanes B, D, F, H, samples which were not subjected to wheat germ agglutinin affinity chromatography. Lanes C, E, G, I, wheat germ agglutinin-bound peptides. Lane A, EGF cross-link-labeled receptor solubilized in SDS sample buffer immediately following the cross-link labeling procedure. The molecular weights of the peptides were determined using reference proteins as described in the text. Radioactive proteins observed above the origin failed to migrate out of the stacking gel.

bands containing photoaffinity-labeled EGF receptor species are located by superimposing the developed X-ray films and the dried gels. The bands are cut from the gels with scissors and sliced into 1 mm long pieces which are put into 50 × 175-mm test tubes. The photoaffinity-labeled receptor species are eluted by adding 3 mL of water to rehydrate the dried gel slices. After 18–24 hr at 4°C the rehydrated gel slices are macerated and filtered through glass wool-plugged, 10 mL disposable syringes. The syringe plunger can be used to squeeze as much solution as possible from the gel slices. The filtrate is retained and the elution and filtering steps are repeated two times. The filtrates are pooled and dialyzed for 18–24 hr against 50 mM Tris-HCl buffer containing 0.1 M NaCl and 0.1 percent Triton X-100. The dialyzed samples are incubated for 24–48 hr at 4°C with 10 μL of anti-EGF antiserum and antibody–antigen complexes are isolated using protein A–Sepharose as described above. We have found that this isolation procedure is sufficient for the isolation and separation of the different proteolytic fragments of the EGF receptor. These will prove most useful for determining the exact precursor product relationships of the peptides. Moreover, the purified native receptor will also be useful as a substrate for the subsequent identification and purification of enzymes which are involved in modifying receptor structure and function.

12.   CONCLUDING REMARKS

The techniques outlined in this and other chapters in this volume have been instrumental for developing our current understanding of peptide hormone receptor structure. The challenge now is to correlate structure with receptor function. For instance, it will be of considerable interest to determine the biological significance of receptor processing in terms of cell activation. In addition, the approaches we describe should serve to identify the phosphorylated domains of the EGF, insulin, and basic-Sm receptors; the role of phosphorylation in receptor function is currently the subject of much intensive research. Given the recent advances in receptor purification, the availability of monoclonal receptor antibodies, the availability of tissue culture cell lines which either possess or lack specific receptors, and given the gene cloning and sequencing technologies now available, work in the near future should provide a wealth of information about the structure and function of a wide variety of receptors.

REFERENCES

1.   B. M. Conti-Tronconti and M. A. Raftery, *Ann. Rev. Biochem.* **51**, 491 (1982).

2.   J. N. Langley, *Proc. Roy. Soc. B* **78**, 170 (1906).

3.   P. Cuatrecasas and M. D. Hollenberg, *Adv. Protein Chem.* **30**, 251 (1976).

4.   M. D. Hollenberg and P. Cuatrecasas, in *Methods in Receptor Research*, M. Blecher (ed.), Marcel Dekker, New York, 1976, pp. 429–477.

5.   M. D. Hollenberg and P. Cuatrecasas, in *Methods in Cancer Research* Vol. 12, H. Busch (ed.), 1976, pp. 317–366.

6.   M. D. Hollenberg and E. Nexo, in *Membrane Receptors: Methods for Purification and Characterization, Receptors and Recognition*, Series B, Vol. 1, S. Jacobs and P. Cuatrecasas (eds.), Chapman and Hall, London, 1981, pp. 1–31.

7.   R. M. Bala and B. Bhaumick, *Can. J. Biochem.* **57**, 1289 (1979).

8.   C. R. Savage and S. Cohen, *J. Biol. Chem.* **247**, 7609 (1972).

9.   W. M. Hunter and F. C. Greenwood, *Nature (London)* **194**, 495 (1962).

10. R. M. Bala and B. Bhaumick, *J. Clin. Endocrinol. Metab.* **49**, 770 (1979).

11. R. A. Hock and M. D. Hollenberg, *J. Biol. Chem.* **255**, 10731 (1980).

12. S. G. Korenman, in *Methods in Enzymology*, Vol. 36, part A, B. W. O'Malley and J. G. Hardman (eds.), Academic Press, New York, 1975, p. 49.

13. B. Desbuquois and G. D. Aurbach, *J. Clin. Endocrinol. Metab.* **33**, 732 (1971).

14. P. Cuatrecasas, *Proc. Natl. Acad. Sci. USA* **69**, 318 (1972).

15. J. M. Maturo III and M. D. Hollenberg, *Proc Natl. Acad. Sci. USA* **75**, 3070 (1978).

16. M. N. Krupp, D. T. Connolly, and M. D. Lane, *J. Biol. Chem.* **257**, 11489 (1982).

17. T. W. Siegel, S. Ganguly, S. Jacobs, O. M. Rosen, and C. S. Rubin, *J. Biol. Chem.* **256**, 9266 (1981).

18. P. F. Pilch and M. P. Czech, *J. Biol. Chem.* **254**, 3375 (1979).

19. B. Bhaumick, R. M. Bala, and M. D. Hollenberg, *Proc. Natl. Acad. Sci. USA* **78**, 4279 (1981).

20. J. M. Maturo III, W. H. Shackelford, and M. D. Hollenberg, *Life Sci.* **23**, 2063 (1978).

21. U. K. Laemmli, *Nature (London)* **227**, 680 (1979).

22. P. O'Farrell, *J. Biol. Chem.* **250**, 4007 (1975).

23. E. J. O'Keefe, T. K. Batlin, and U. Bennett, *J. Supra. Struct. Cell. Biochem.* **15**, 15 (1981).

24. P. S. Linsley and C. F. Fox, *J. Supra. Struct. Cell. Biochem.* **14**, 461 (1980).

25. M. D. Hollenberg and G. D. Armstrong, in *Polypeptide Hormone Receptors*, B. Posner (ed.), Marcel Dekker, New York, in press.

26. G. Fairbanks, T. L. Steck, and D. F. H. Wallach, *Biochem.* **10**, 2606 (1971).

27. D. Cassel and L. Glaser, *J. Biol. Chem.* **257**, 9845 (1982).

28. D. W. Cleveland, S. G. Fischer, M. W. Kirschner, and U. K. Laemmli, *J. Biol. Chem.* **252**, 1102 (1977).

29. G. D. Armstrong, M. D. Hollenberg, B. Bhaumick, and R. M. Bala, *J. Cell. Biochem.* **20**, 283 (1982).

30. S. J. Singer, *Ann. Rev. Biochem.* **43**, 805 (1974).

31. J. M. Maturo III and M. D. Hollenberg, *Can. J. Biochem.* **57**, 497 (1979).

32. B. Bhaumick, G. D. Armstrong, M. D. Hollenberg, and R. M. Bala, *Can. J. Biochem.* **60**, 923 (1982).

B

INSULIN INTERNALIZATION, RECEPTOR INTERNALIZATION, AND BIOCHEMICAL CHARACTERIZATION

PAULOS BERHANU
Department of Medicine, University of Colorado Health Sciences Center, Denver, Colorado

ALLAN GREEN
Department of Medicine, University of Florida, Gainesville, Florida

JERROLD M. OLEFSKY
Department of Medicine, University of California at San Diego, La Jolla, California

1. INTRODUCTION

It is now well recognized that following the initial binding of insulin to its cell surface receptors, a proportion of the bound insulin is internalized by adsorptive endocytosis and is subsequently degraded intracellularly, most probably within lysosomes (1, 2). In insulin target cells such as adipocytes and hepatocytes, recent findings show that the insulin receptor is also internalized along with the bound insulin (3–5) and is then degraded at chloroquine-sensitive intracellular sites (3), suggesting lysosomal involvement in the degradation of internalized insulin receptors. Thus, the available data indicate that both ligand and receptor are internalized as insulin receptor complexes and are then degraded at similar, if not the same, intracellular sites. While all of the internalized insulin may be committed to eventual degradation, there is evidence indicating that a proportion of the internalized receptors may be recycled back to the plasma membrane (6).

Internalization of insulin receptor complexes may play an important physiologic role in mediating the well known process of insulin-induced receptor loss or "down-regulation" first demonstrated by Gavin et al. in cultured human

This work was supported in part by grants AM 31072, AM 32880, and AM 25241 from the National Institute of Arthritis, Diabetes and Digestive and Kidney Diseases and in part by grant BRSG-05357 from the Biomedical Research Grant Program, Division of Research Resources, National Institutes of Health.

lymphocytes (7) and subsequently also observed in various other cell types. It has also been suggested that the internalization process may be important in the termination of insulin action by removing it from the cell surface and transporting it to intracellular degradation sites. Furthermore, the demonstration of insulin binding sites in various subcellular organelles (8, 9) has led to the speculation that the intracellular effects of insulin may be mediated through the interaction of these binding sites with internalized insulin. However, direct experimental evidence to support this hypothesis is lacking. It is thus apparent that further work is needed to determine the precise cellular mechanisms subserving the internalization of insulin and its receptors and to identify the physiologic role(s) of the internalization process. In this chapter we describe recent experimental methods that have been used to study the internalization and processing of insulin and insulin receptors in isolated cells.

2. DETERMINATION OF INSULIN INTERNALIZATION USING ACID-BARBITAL EXTRACTION TECHNIQUE

The acid-barbital extraction technique is a modification of the method of Haigler et al. (10) that was originally used in studies of EGF (epidermal growth factor) internalization. Cells are incubated with [^{125}I]insulin at the desired temperature, and following binding equilibration they are exposed to sodium acetate barbital buffer (pH 3.0). With this approach, acid-extractable radioactivity is considered to be surface-bound [^{125}I]insulin and non-acid-extractable radioactivity is taken as intracellular material.

The application of this method to studies of insulin internalization in isolated adipocytes is described below.

2.1. Preparation of Isolated Adipocytes

Isolated adipocytes are prepared by collagenase digestion according to the method of Rodbell (11) as described previously (12), either from epididymal fat pads of male Sprague-Dawley rats weighing 160–225 g or from human adipose tissue specimen obtained by open biopsy from the lower abdominal wall (13).

2.2. Insulin Binding

Adipocytes ($2–5 \times 10^5$ cells/mL) are incubated with 10^{-10} M [^{125}I]insulin (0.6 ng/mL) in the absence or presence of 50 μg of unlabeled insulin in a total volume of 1 mL Tris–bovine serum albumin buffer, pH 7.6, containing 35 mM Tris, 120 mM NaCl, 1.2 mM MgSO$_4$, 2.0 mM CaCl$_2$, 2.5 mM KCl, 10 mM dextrose, 24 mM NaOAc, and 1 percent bovine serum albumin. Incubations are performed at the indicated temperatures in polypropylene tubes (17 × 10 mm) in a rotary water bath. At the indicated times the binding reactions are terminated, and free [^{125}I]insulin separated from cell-bound radioactivity by removing aliquots from the cell suspension and rapidly centrifuging the cells through silicone oil as described previously (12). The cells that layer on top are then removed and the associated radioactivity determined.

2.3. Nonspecific Binding

In these experiments nonspecific binding is defined as the amount of [^{125}I]insulin remaining in the indicated fraction (total cell-associated radioactivity, non-acid-extractable radioactivity, or acid-extractable radioactivity) in the presence of a large excess (50–200 μg/mL) of unlabeled insulin.

2.4. Acid Extraction Procedures

After binding equilibration cell-associated radioactivity is extracted with acid by a modification of the method of Haigler et al. (10) to remove cell-surface-bound insulin. One milliliter of the cell suspension is incubated with 5 mL of sodium acetate barbital buffer, pH 3.0, containing 28 mM Na acetate, 20 mM Na barbital, and 117 mM NaCl at 4°C for 6 min. Control studies demonstrated that this procedure resulted in maximum and complete release of surface-bound radioactivity. The above buffer and incubation conditions were chosen after numerous preliminary studies showed that pure acetic acid buffers, lower pH, or longer incubation times resulted in increased nonextractable nonspecific binding, most likely due to cell membrane damage with nonspecific uptake of [^{125}I]-radioactivity from the buffer into the cells. Following the extraction period the cells are washed in the binding buffer (4°C) and the nonextractable radioactivity remaining with the cells is determined by centrifuging aliquots of cells in microfuge tubes as described for the binding studies.

Figure 1 shows the results obtained when this acid extraction method is applied to studies of the effect of temperature on the internalization of [^{125}I]insulin in isolated rat adipocytes. At 37°C internalization of [^{125}I] insulin is rapid, as shown by the rapid accumulation (after an initial lag of ~2 min) of nonextractable radioactivity. This reached a peak by 30 min and was followed by a slight gradual fall in the amount of nonextractable (intracellular) material over the subsequent 2.5 hr. The time course of accumulation of total cell-associated radioactivity is similar to the time course of nonextractable radioactivity. Cell surface binding, as reflected by extractable radioactivity, reaches a peak between 5 and 12 min, with a plateau until 30 min and then a slight gradual fall. From 30 min on a constant 42–45 percent of the total cell-associated radioactivity is recovered in the nonextractable, or intracellular, compartment. Since endocytotic internalization is inhibited at low temperature (14), it can be seen in Figure 1 that with lowering of the temperature from 37°C to 12°C, the amount of nonextractable radioactivity progressively decreases. Thus, after a 1 hr incubation of adipocytes, 45 percent of cell-associated radioactivity is nonextractable at 37°C, 24 percent at 24°C, 6 percent at 16°C, and 1.5 percent at 12°C. Further studies using the acid extraction technique have shown that

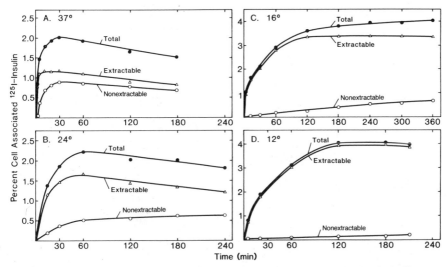

FIGURE 1. Effect of temperature on insulin internalization in adipocytes. Isolated rat adipocytes were incubated with 0.6 ng/mL (10^{-10} M) [^{125}I]insulin at (A) 37°C, (B) 24°C, (C)16°C, or (D) 12°C. At the indicated time points, total (●), acid-extractable (△), and nonextractable (○) cell-associated radioactivity was determined as described in the text. In all cases parallel incubations were conducted in the presence of 200 μg/mL of unlabeled insulin to determine nonspecific cell-associated radioactivity in the total, extractable, and nonextractable fractions. Data represent the mean of three experiments for each temperature.

the internalization of insulin is energy dependent and occurs very slowly in IM-9 lymphocytes (15). Additionally, in the presence of chloroquine, a drug that inhibits lysosomal function (16, 17), a marked increase in the amount of nonextractable (intracellular) radioactivity could be demonstrated (15), indicating that this agent causes intracellular accumulation of insulin by inhibiting its degradation.

3. DETERMINATION OF INSULIN RECEPTOR INTERNALIZATION USING SOLUBLE RECEPTOR ASSAY

Insulin is internalized by a receptor-mediated mechanism, and while the acid extraction method described above provides a useful approach to studies of internalization of the hormone, it provides relatively little information about the fate of the insulin receptor itself. Since the insulin-induced down regulation of its receptors is believed to occur through translocation of the insulin receptor complexes from the cell surface to the cell interior, this premise has been used to devise a method to determine the internalization of insulin receptors in adipocytes. The essential features of this method are outlined in Figure 2. Isolated adipocytes are incubated with insulin ± chloroquine, followed by extensive washing and dissociation procedures to remove all cell-associated

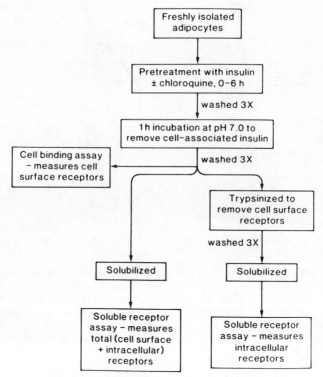

FIGURE 2.   Flow diagram summarizing the methods used for measuring cell surface receptors, and intracellular receptors using soluble receptor assay.

insulin. At this point, an aliquot of cells is taken for measurement of insulin binding at 16°C. At this temperature endocytosis is inhibited and all of the cell-associated insulin is on the cell surface; therefore, this provides a measure of cell surface insulin receptors. Next, an additional aliquot of cells is solubilized in Triton X-100, and insulin binding to solubilized receptors is determined. Since all of the cell's insulin receptors are solubilized by this technique, this assay provides a measure of total cellular (intracellular + cell surface) insulin receptors. Finally, a third aliquot of cells is trypsinized to remove all cell surface insulin-binding activity. These trypsinized cells are then solubilized, and insulin binding to soluble receptors is determined. This provides a measurement of intracellular receptors. The specific procedures used in this overall experimental scheme are described below.

3.1.   Insulin Pretreatment and Dissociation Procedures

Adipocytes $(0.6-1.0 \times 10^6$ cells/mL) suspended in 10 mL of pH 7.6 buffer containing 35 mM Tris, 120 mM NaCl, 1.2 mM MgSO$_4$, 2.0 mM CaCl$_2$, 2.5 mM KCl, 10 mM dextrose, 24 mM NaOAc, and 1 percent bovine serum albumin

(Tris-albumin buffer) are incubated in the absence or presence of various concentrations of insulin in 25-mL polypropylene flasks. Cells are gently agitated in a rotary water bath for the indicated times at 37°C. At the end of the incubation period the cells are transferred to 16 × 125-mm polystyrene tubes and washed three times (by centrifugation at 200 rpm for 2 min) in Tris-albumin buffer (pH 7.0). The cells are then suspended in the Tris-albumin, buffer, pH 7.0, and further incubated for 1 hr at 37°C to allow the dissociation of receptor-bound insulin. It has been demonstrated previously that all receptor-bound insulin and any insulin internalized (including subsequently generated degradation products) is effectively dissociated or released by this procedure (12). After the 1 hr dissociation cells are washed and resuspended in Tris-albumin buffer, pH 7.6, for measurement of cell surface receptors, total (cell surface + intracellular) receptors, and intracellular receptors. Control (insulin-untreated) cells are subjected to similar incubation, dissociation, and washing procedures.

3.2. Trypsinization

Following the insulin pretreatment and dissociation procedures described above, adipocytes are treated with trypsin (200 μg/mL) for 10 min at 37°C. Soybean trypsin inhibitor (400 μg/mL) is then added, and the cells are washed three times in Tris-albumin buffer, pH 7.6.

3.3. Solubilization Procedure

After samples of the cell suspensions have been taken for measurement of intact cell binding, the adipocytes are centrifuged and the buffer is removed. A volume (0.5–2 mL as indicated) of Tris-albumin buffer (pH 7.0) containing Triton X-100 (1 percent) and bacitracin (2 mg/mL to inhibit proteolysis) is added and the cells are agitated at 37°C for 1 hr. The low pH and warm temperature are used to ensure that any remaining intracellular insulin is dissociated from intracellular insulin receptor complexes. At the end of the 1 hr solubilizing step the suspensions are transferred to 1.5-mL centrifuge tubes and centrifuged in a Beckman Microfuge B for 2 min. The aqueous lower layer is removed and transferred to a second centrifuge tube. Talc is added (50 mg for each 1 mL of extract) and the extract is mixed vigorously. The suspension is then centrifuged (10 min, 3000 rpm) and the supernatant is used for measurement of insulin binding (see below). The talc precipitation is used to remove any traces of insulin.

3.4. Solubilized Receptor Binding Studies

Samples (50 μL) of the solubilized cell extracts are added to Tris-albumin, pH 7.6, buffer (final volume, 0.5 mL) with [^{125}I]insulin (0.3 ng/mL) in the presence or absence of unlabeled insulin (50 μg/mL) for determination of nonspecific binding. The tubes are incubated at 4°C for 16 hr, and bound [^{125}I]insulin is precipitated by adding 0.5 mL of Tris buffer (pH 7.6) containing 0.2 percent γ-globulin followed by 1 mL of 20 percent (w/v) polyethylene glycol (18). The assays are performed in triplicate, and the binding data corrected for nonspecific binding.

The results presented in Figure 3 demonstrate the application of the method described above to studies of the insulin-induced internalization of insulin receptors in isolated rat adipocytes. The cells were incubated at 37°C in the presence or absence of insulin (with or without chloroquine) and the total, cell surface, and intracellular receptors were then quantitated. It can be seen in Figure 3 (panel A) that a 4-hr incubation of adipocytes with insulin (100 ng/mL) at 37°C leads to a 62 percent loss of cell surface insulin receptors. When the same experiment was done in the presence of chloroquine (0.2 mM), insulin's ability to bring about a loss of receptors was inhibited, such that only a 35 percent decrease in binding capacity was observed. Incubation of cells with chloroquine alone had no effect on insulin binding (data not shown). It is important to note that the measurements of [^{125}I]insulin binding were performed at 16°C; because internalization is blocked at this low temperature

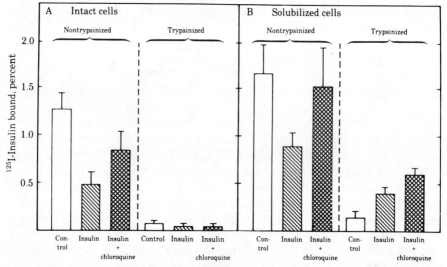

FIGURE 3.   Effect of 4 hr incubation of rat adipocytes with insulin or insulin plus chloroquine on distribution of insulin receptors between the cell surface and the cell interior. Adipocytes ($\sim$ 8 × 10^5 cells/mL) were incubated with no additions (control), insulin (100 ng/mL), or insulin (100 ng/mL) plus chloroquine (0.2 mM) for 4 hr, at 37°C. Cells were then washed, and bound insulin was allowed to dissociate. After further washes, each group of cells was divided into two, and one-half were trypsinized to remove cell surface receptors. Samples ($\sim$ 2 × 10^5 cells) were taken for measurement of intact cell binding. The remaining cells were then solubilized and insulin binding to the soluble extract was measured, using a volume of extract equivalent to the number of cells (i.e., $\sim$ 2 × 10^5 cells) used in the intact cell binding assay. Results are the mean + SEM of three separate experiments performed on different days.

(14, 19), the results reflect binding to cell surface receptors. The cells were then solubilized and the insulin binding capacity of the solubilized extracts were measured (Fig. 3, panel B). This approach provides a measure of the cell surface plus intracellular insulin receptors, that is, the total insulin-binding capacity of the cells. When studied in this way, the insulin treatment of intact cells resulted in only a 46 percent loss of total binding capacity, which is significantly less ($p < .01$) than the 62 percent loss of cell surface receptors (Fig. 3, panel A). The cells treated with insulin in the presence of chloroquine showed no significant loss of total binding capacity. When the results from the intact and solubilized cells are considered together, it is evident that if total binding capacity is measured (solubilized cells), the insulin-induced decrease in insulin binding is smaller than when only cell surface binding (intact cells) is measured. This indicates that insulin treatment induces a loss of receptors from the cell surface and that some of these receptors can be recovered in an intracellular location. These effects are even more pronounced when chloroquine is used. Thus, there is essentially no loss of total cellular insulin-binding capacity when cells are exposed to insulin in the presence of chloroquine. This suggests that when cells are incubated with insulin plus chloroquine, a loss of receptors from the cell surface occurs, and these receptors are essentially quantitatively recovered within the cells.

To more specifically evaluate the intracellular receptor pool, cell surface receptors were removed with trypsin. As seen in Figure 3 (panel A), trypsin destroyed greater than 90 percent of the insulin-binding capacity of control, insulin-treated, or insulin plus chloroquine-treated intact cells. However, when insulin binding was measured using solubilized extracts of trypsinized cells (far right panel of Fig. 3), the insulin-treated cells had a greater binding capacity than control cells, and the cells treated with insulin plus chloroquine showed an even higher binding capacity. Again, chloroquine was without effect when added alone (data not shown). These results show that in the control state almost all of the cells' total binding capacity represents cell surface receptors, with a relatively small intracellular pool. Insulin treatment leads to a decrease in cell surface receptors and an increase in the number of receptors in the intracellular pool. Chloroquine partially inhibits the insulin-induced loss of surface receptors, but these receptors are now quantitatively recovered intracellularly and no net loss of total binding capacity is observed. This suggests that chloroquine inhibits the intracellular processing of internalized insulin receptors.

Additional studies of insulin receptor internalization in the rat adipocytes using the above method have also shown that the internalized receptors are specific for insulin, yield curvilinear Scatchard plots, and have the same relative affinities for various insulin analogues as the cell surface receptors (20). Furthermore, the internalization of the receptors is dependent on the concentration of insulin to which the cells are exposed (half-maximal effect at ~ 2.5 ng/mL and maximal effect at 25 ng/mL), and the time-dependent loss (at 37°C) of receptors from the cell surface is directly and significantly correlated with the intracellular accumulation of the receptors (20).

4. STUDIES OF INSULIN RECEPTOR INTERNALIZATION AND PROCESSING: APPLICATION OF PHOTOAFFINITY LABELING TECHNIQUE

Although the soluble receptor assay method described in the preceding section provides a reasonably good means of studying the internalization of insulin receptors, it offers no insight into the structure of the receptors or the biochemical characteristics of their cellular processing. The technique of photoaffinity labeling affords a highly sensitive and attractive approach by which the biochemical characteristics and the cellular fate of insulin receptors can be studied in living cells. In this approach photoreactive insulin analogues are used for receptor labeling, and these are synthesized by reacting native insulin with heterobifunctional photosensitive cross-linking agents, thereby attaching a photoreactive group, usually a nitrophenyl azide moiety, to one of the three primary amino groups of the insulin molecule. Ideally, the derivatized insulin molecule should retain its receptor binding and biological activities; this is largely achieved by derivatizing the B-1 primary amino group which is farthest from the receptor binding domain of the insulin molecule (21). The synthesis and characterization of various photoreactive insulins and their use in probing insulin receptor structure and function have been described (22–27).

To study the internalization and cellular processing of insulin receptors using photoaffinity labeling techniques, it is obviously necessary that the receptors are photolabeled on intact cells and that the labeling process does not alter cell viability or metabolic function. Cells are incubated in the dark with [125I]-labeled photosensitive insulin derivative, and after the appropriate binding period they are washed and exposed to light of appropriate wavelengths. This activates the photosensitive arylazide moiety by generating highly reactive arylnitrene intermediates which can readily form covalent bonds with nearby C–C or C–H bonds. The net result is the covalent attachment of the cell-bound [125I]insulin to insulin receptors on the cell surface. The cells are then solubilized either directly at the end of the labeling period or after incubations under different conditions so that the cellular processing of the receptors can be followed. The solubilized labeled receptors and their processing products are then analyzed by polyacrylamide gel electrophoresis and autoradiography. The procedures for applying this technique for studies of the internalization and processing of insulin receptors in isolated adipocytes are described below.

4.1. Photoreactive Insulin Derivative

The photosensitive insulin analogue used in our studies is B2(2-nitro-4-azido-phenylacetyl)-des-Phe[B1]-insulin (NAPA-DP-insulin), which has been well characterized and retains almost all of the biological activity and receptor binding affinity of native porcine insulin (5, 28, 29). This derivative was synthesized (23, 24) and kindly provided by Dr. Dietrich Brandenburg's group from Aachen, W. Germany. Other investigators have also successfully used different photosensitive insulin derivatives for similar studies (30).

4.2. Iodination of the Photoreactive Insulin

NAPA-DP-insulin is iodinated in a darkroom under photographic safelight to a specific activity of 100–200 cpm/pg by using the water-insoluble oxidizing agent, 1,3,4,6-tetrachloro-3,6-diphenylglycoluril (IODO-GEN; Pierce, Rockford, IL) essentially as we have described previously (3). The IODO-GEN is coated as a thin film (40 µg in 20 µL of chloroform) to the bottom of 12 × 75-mm glass test tubes. Ten micrograms of NAPA-DP-insulin in 0.01 M HCl are reacted for 3 min with 2-3 mCi of Na^{125}I in 200 µL of 0.1 M phosphate buffer (pH 7.5) in the IODO-GEN tube. The reaction mixture is then transferred to a clean test tube, and 50 µL of 10 percent bovine serum albumin is added and the volume adjusted to 2.5 ml with 0.1 M phosphate buffer. This mixture is dialyzed at 4°C against 0.1 M phosphate buffer (pH 7.5) containing 0.2 percent BSA to remove free ^{125}I, and the iodinated product is stored in the dark at 4°C and used within 1–2 weeks.

4.3. Binding and Photolysis of [^{125}I]-NAPA-DP-Insulin

Suspensions of isolated human or rat adipocytes ($\sim 2.5 \times 10^5$ cells/mL) are incubated with various concentrations of [^{125}I]-NAPA-DP-insulin in minimal essential medium containing 10 mM HEPES (pH 7.5) and 1 percent bovine serum albumin (BSA). The incubations are carried out at 16°C in aluminum-foil-covered plastic scintillation vials. Native porcine insulin, 20 µg/mL, is included where appropriate to determine nonspecific labeling. At the concentrations of [^{125}I]-NAPA-DP-insulin (40–80 ng/mL) usually used in our photolabeling studies, binding equilibrium is reached within 30 min at 16°C. Following this, the cells are transferred to 60 × 15-mm plastic Petri dishes and photolysis is carried out for 3 min by exposure to a long-wave (366 nm) UV lamp (Blak-Ray; Ultraviolet Products, San Gabrieli, CA) placed 10 cm from the cell samples. It is important to use long-wave UV light and short photolysis periods in order to avoid damage to the cells. After the photolysis step the cells are transferred to polypropylene tubes, centrifuged at 400 rpm for 2 min, and the infranatant-containing unbound hormone is removed. The cells are then washed two additional times at 16°C with minimal essential medium per 10 mM HEPES per 1 percent BSA, pH 7.5. After a final wash with the same medium from which the BSA is omitted (to avoid its appearance as a broad dense band on SDS gels), the cells are solubilized with 3 percent sodium dodecyl sulfate (SDS) containing 1 mM N-ethylmaleimide (NEM) and 2 mM phenylmethylsulfonylfluoride (PMSF) to inhibit *in vitro* proteolysis. In experiments that are designed to study the cellular fate of labeled insulin receptor complexes, the photolabeled cells are washed at 16°C, resuspended in the incubation medium, and then incubated at 37°C for various periods. At selected times the cells are washed and solubilized.

4.4. Polyacrylamide Gel Electrophoresis and Autoradiography

The solubilized samples from the photoaffinity-labeled cells are centrifuged at 1400g for 20 min at 4°C. The resulting infranatant containing the solubilized cellular proteins is separated and analyzed by SDS polyacrylamide gel electrophoresis according to the method of Laemmli (31). The samples are boiled for 2 min in Laemmli's sample buffer in the presence or absence of 25 mM dithiothreitol before application to the gels. Molecular weight standard proteins are also included for molecular weight calibration. The gels are stained with Coomassie brilliant blue, destained, dried, and autoradiographed at −70°C using Kodak X-Omat AR film and Cronex Lightning Plus (Dupont, Wilmington, DE) intensifying screen.

The procedures described above have been used to photolabel and characterize insulin receptors on viable isolated human adipocytes and also to study the

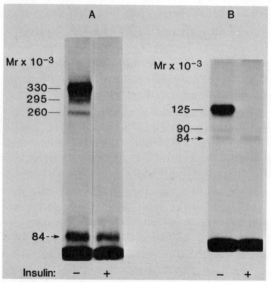

FIGURE 4. *In situ* photoaffinity labeling of insulin receptors on intact human adipocytes. Isolated adipocytes (~ 2.5 × 10^5 cells/mL) were incubated in the dark (16°C; 30 min) with 80 ng/mL [125I]-NAPA-DP-insulin in the absence (−) or presence (+) of excess unlabeled native insulin. The cells were then washed and subjected to photolysis as described in the text. After further washing, the adipocytes were solubilized with 1 percent SDS containing 1 mM NEM and 2 mM PMSF. Aliquots of the solubilized samples were then either electrophoresced under nonreducing conditions on a 5 percent porous acrylamide gel with acrylamide–bisacrylamide ratio of 100:1 (A), or were reduced with dithiothreitol and electrophoresced on a 7.5 percent acrylamide gel (B). Autoradiograms of the dried gels are shown. The arrows indicate the nonspecifically labeled band.

intracellular translocation of the labeled receptors in these cells. As shown in Figure 4 (panel A), three unreduced forms of the insulin receptor are specifically labeled by [^{125}I]-NAPA-DP-insulin on intact human adipocytes. These proteins have apparent molecular weights of 330,000, 295,000, and 260,000 daltons when electrophoresis is performed in the absence of disulfide reductants. In this experiment the photolabeled cells were solubilized using a 1 percent solution of the denaturing ionic detergent, SDS, containing 1 mM NEM and 2 mM PMSF, and under such conditions, the Mr 330,000 species appears as the major labeled nonreduced form of the insulin receptor while the Mr 295,000 and 260,000 species are labeled less intensely. The Mr values of the unreduced forms of the insulin receptor shown in this experiment should be considered only as estimates since they are obtained by extrapolation of the standard molecular weight calibration curve above Mr 200,000 (highest molecular weight protein used was myosin with Mr 200,000), and also because of the known anomalous mobility of glycoproteins in SDS–polyacrylamide gels.

When the solubilized proteins from the photolabeled adipocytes were treated with dithiothreitol and then electrophoresced, all of the nonreduced forms of the insulin receptor were converted into only two specifically labeled bands of Mr 125,000 and 90,000 (Fig. 4, panel B). In the reduced form of the receptor, almost all of the radioactive label is in the Mr 125,000 band indicating

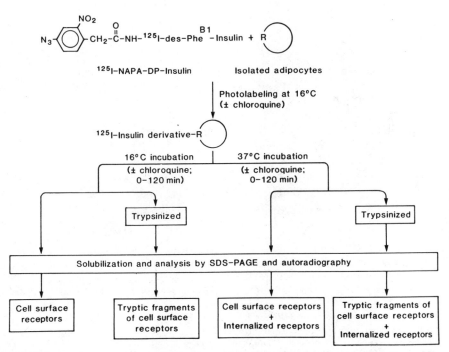

FIGURE 5. Experimental protocol used for studying the internalization and cellular processing of photolabeled insulin receptor complexes in isolated adipocytes.

that this subunit contains essentially all of the insulin binding site(s) of the receptor. The specific labeling of this binding subunit could be observed at $[^{125}I]$-NAPA-DP-insulin concentrations as low as 5 ng/mL ($8.3 \times 10^{-10} M$) and is saturable reaching a maximum at 50–60 ng/mL of $[^{125}I]$-NAPA-DP-insulin (32).

To study the cellular fate of insulin receptors photolabeled on the surface of isolated adipocytes, the experimental scheme summarized in Figure 5 has been used. Since endocytotic internalization is inhibited at 16°C (14), and since the insulin receptor is highly sensitive to tryptic degradation (33), these facts have been used to distinguish cell surface receptors from those that become translocated to the cell interior. Thus, at 16°C essentially all of the labeled receptors should be on the cell surface and accessible to tryptic degradation; hence trypsinization of the photolabeled cells at the end of the 16°C incubation period should result in the generation of tryptic fragments of the labeled cell surface receptors. In contrast, further incubation of the photolabeled cells at 37°C would allow endocytosis and internalization to occur. Therefore, trypsinization of the photolabeled adipocytes at the end of the 37°C incubation should degrade only the receptors that remain on the cell surface, while the

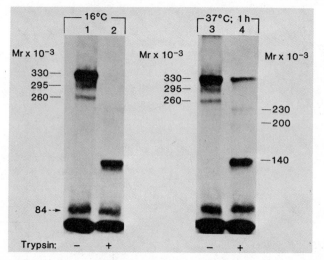

FIGURE 6. Generation of trypsin-insensitive (internalized) pool of photolabeled insulin receptor complexes at 37°C. Photolabeling of human adipocyte insulin receptors was carried out at 16°C as described in Figure 4, and the labeled cells were then further processed according to the protocol described in Figure 5. At the end of the 16°C photolabeling process, half of the labeled cells were immediately treated with trypsin as indicated, washed, and then solubilized. The rest of the labeled cells were incubated at 37°C for 1 hr and were then treated with trypsin as indicated, washed, and solubilized. In each instance trypsin (200 μg/mL) treatment was for 10 min at 37°C and the process was terminated by adding soybean trypsin inhibitor (400 μg/mL). Aliquots of the solubilized samples were analyzed on a 5 percent porous acrylamide gel under nonreducing conditions and autoradiogram of the dried gel is shown.

internalized pool of receptors should be inaccessible to trypsin in the incubation medium.

Using this experimental approach, we have photolabeled insulin receptors on intact human adipocytes at 16°C and then studied the cellular distribution of the labeled receptors both at the end of the labeling process at 16°C and after a 1 hr incubation of the labeled cells at 37°C. When adipocytes photolabeled at 16°C were trypsinized without further incubation at 37°C, all of the unreduced Mr 330,000, 295,00, and 260,000 insulin receptor species were completely converted into a major tryptic product of Mr 140,000 and a minor product of Mr 230,000 (Fig. 6), thus indicating that at 16°C, the labeled receptors were all on the cell surface. In contrast, when the cells photolabeled at 16°C were further incubated at 37°C for 1 hr and then trypsinized, a proportion of the Mr 330,000 receptor species became insensitive to tryptic degradation, indicating that this pool of receptors had been translocated to a trypsin-inaccessible (intracellular) compartment.

Figure 7 shows the time course of the intracellular accumulation of labeled intact insulin receptors (Mr 330,000) at 37°C. It can be seen that trypsin-insensitive (intracellular) receptors could be observed within 2 min of incubation of the photolabeled cells at 37°C, indicating that internalization of insulin receptor complexes in human adipocytes occurs very rapidly. The total intra-

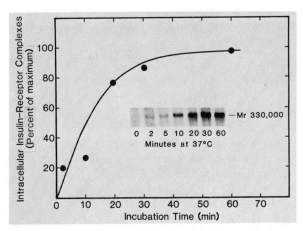

FIGURE 7. Time course of intracellular accumulation of insulin re tor complexes at 37°C. Isolated human adipocytes photolabeled at 16°C were further incubated at 37°C and at the times shown, the cells were trypsinized to remove labeled receptors still remaining on the cell surface. The cells were then solubilized and subjected to electrophoresis (under nonreducing condition) and autoradiography. The areas of the dried gel containing the trypsin-insensitive (intracellular) Mr 330,000 receptor forms were cut out and the radioactivity was measured in a γ counter. The results are expressed as percent of the maximal amount of intracellular-labeled insulin receptor complexes and the data shown represent the mean from three separate experiments. The inset shows a representative autoradiogram depicting a time-dependent increase in the intensity of the Mr 330,000 trypsin-insensitive receptor band.

cellular pool of labeled receptors reaches half-maximal amounts by 10 min and maximal amounts by about 30 min of incubation at 37°C; following this, the amount of intracellular receptor pool remains relatively constant for up to 60 min of incubation at 37°C. In other studies we have also found that in both rat (3) and human (32) adipocytes intracellular processing and degradation of the internalized receptors occurs and that this can be partially blocked by the lysosomotropic agent chloroquine, thus indicating possible lysosomal involvement in the degradation of internalized insulin receptor complexes in adipocytes. In contrast to the findings described here for adipocytes, photoaffinity labeling studies show that in cultured IM-9 human lymphocytes, a cell line in which demonstrable glucoregulatory effects of insulin are lacking, insulin receptor complexes are shed into the incubation media (34). These examples demonstrate the usefulness of photoaffinity labeling techniques in characterizing and studying the dynamics of insulin receptor complexes in different cell types.

REFERENCES

1. P. Gorden, J.-L. Carpentier, P. Freychet, and L. Orci, *Diabetologia* **18**, 263–274 (1980).

2. B. I. Posner, M. N. Khan, and J. J. M. Bergeron, *Endocrine Rev.* **3**, 280–298 (1982).

3. P. Berhanu, J. M. Olefsky, P. Tsai, P. Thamm, D. Saunders, and D. Brandenburg, *Proc. Natl. Acad. Sci. USA* **79**, 4069–4073 (1982).

4. J. M. Olefsky, S. Marshall, P. Berhanu, M. Saekow, K. Heidenreich, and A. Green, *Metabolism* **31**, 670–690 (1982).

5. M. Fehlmann, J.-L. Carpentier, A. Le Cam, P. Thamm, D. Saunders, D. Brandenburg, L. Orci, and P. Freychet, *J. Cell Biol.* **93**, 82–87 (1982).

6. S. Marshall, A. Green, and J. M. Olefsky, *J. Biol. Chem.* **256**, 11464–11470 (1981).

7. J. R. Gavin III, J. Roth, D. M. Neville, Jr., P. De Meyts, and D. N. Buell, *Proc. Natl. Acad. Sci. USA* **71**, 84–88 (1974).

8. I. D. Goldfine, *Biochim. Biophys. Acta* **650**, 53–67 (1981).

9. B. I. Posner, J. J. M. Bergeron, Z. Josefsberg, M. N. Khan, R. J. Khan, B. A. Patel, R. A. Sikstrom, and A. K. Verma, *Recent Prog. Hormone Res.* **37**, 539–582 (1981).

10. H. T. Haigler, F. R. Maxfield, M. C. Willingham, and I. Pastan, *J. Biol. Chem.* **255**, 1239–1241 (1980).

11. M. Rodbell, *J. Biol. Chem.* **239**, 375–380 (1964).

12. S. Marshall and J. M. Olefsky, *J. Clin. Invest.* **66**, 763–772 (1980).

13. O. G. Kolterman, J. Insel, M. Saekow, and J. M. Olefsky, *J. Clin. Invest.* **65**, 1273–1284 (1980).

14. S. C. Silverstein, R. M. Steinman, and Z. A. Cohn, *Ann. Rev. Biochem.* **46**, 669–722 (1977).

15. J. M. Olefsky and M. Kao, *J. Biol. Chem.* **257**, 8667–8673 (1982).

16. C. De Duve, T. De Barsy, B. Poole, A. Trouet, P. Tulkens, and F. van Hoof, *Biochem. Pharmacol.* **23**, 2495–2531 (1974).

17. S. O. Lei and B. Schofield, *Biochem. Pharmacol.* **22**, 3109–3114 (1973).

18. P. Cuatrecasas and M. D. Hollenberg, *Advan. Protein Chem.* **30**, 251–451 (1976).

19. S. Marshall and J. M. Olefsky, *J. Biol. Chem.* **254**, 10153–10160 (1979).

20. A. Green and J. M. Olefsky, *Proc. Natl. Acad. Sci. USA* **79**, 427–431 (1982).

21. R. A. Pullen, D. G. Lindsay, S. P. Wood, I. J. Tickle, T. Blundell, A. Wollmer, G. Krail, D. Brandenberg, H. Zahn, J. Gliemann, and S. Gammeltoft, *Nature* **259**, 369–373 (1976).

22. C. C. Yip, C. W. T. Yeung, and M. Moule, *Biochemistry* **19**, 70–76 (1980).

23. P. Thamm, D. Saunders, and D. Brandenburg, "Photoreactive Insulin Derivatives: Preparation and Characterization," in *Insulin: Chemistry, Structure and Function of Insulin and Related Hormones*, D. Brandenburg and A. Wollmer (eds.), Walter de Gruyter, Berlin, New York, 1980, pp. 309–316.

24. D. Saunders, P. Thamm, and D. Brandenburg, "Photoreactive Insulin Derivatives: Chemical and Physical Properties," in *Insulin: Chemistry, Structure and Function of Insulin and Related Hormones*, D. Brandenburg and A. Wollmer (eds.) Walter de Gruyter, Berlin, New York, 1980, pp. 317–325.

25. M. H. Wisher, M. D. Baron, R. H. Jones, P. H. Sönksen, D. J. Saunders, P. Thamm, and D. Brandenburg, *Biochem. Biophys. Res. Commun.* **92**, 492–498 (1980).

26. C.-C. Wang, J. A. Hedo, C. R. Kahn, D. J. Saunders, P. Thamm, and D. Brandenburg, *Diabetes* **31**, 1068–1076 (1982).

27. S. Jacobs, E. Hazum, Y. Shechter, and P. Cuatrecasas, *Proc. Natl. Acad. Sci. USA* **76**, 4918–4921 (1979).

28. D. Brandenburg, C. Diaconescu, D. Saunders, and P. Thamm, *Nature* **286**, 821–822 (1980).

29. L. Kuehn, H. Meyer, R. Rutschmann, and P. Thamm, *FEBS Lett.* **113**, 189–192 (1980).

30. P. Gorden, J.-L. Carpentier, M. L. Moule, C. C. Yip, and L. Orci, *Diabetes* **31**, 659–662 (1982).

31. U. K. Laemmli, *Nature (London)* **227**, 680–685 (1970).

32. P. Berhanu, O. G. Kolterman, A. Baron, P. Tsai, D. Brandenburg, and J. M. Olefsky, *J. Clin. Invest.* **72**, 1958–1970 (1983).

33. T. Kono and F. W. Barham, *J. Biol. Chem.* **246**, 6210–6216 (1971).

34. P. Berhanu and J. M. Olefsky, *Diabetes* **31**, 410–417 (1982).

C

INTRACELLULAR RECEPTORS AND HORMONE INTERNALIZATION IN RAT LIVER SUBCELLULAR FRACTIONS

BARRY I. POSNER, MASOOD N. KHAN, AND JOHN J. M. BERGERON*

Departments of Medicine and *Anatomy, McGill University and the Royal Victoria Hospital, Montreal, Quebec, Canada

1.   INTRODUCTION

It is now generally accepted that receptors for peptide hormones exist intracellularly. Our work has focused on isolating and characterizing the receptor-enriched intracellular entities (1, 2). We have restricted our analyses to rat liver, an organ for which subcellular fractionation methodology is well advanced. Our earlier work provided evidence for receptors in Golgi fractions (1). This was based upon the following observations:

1.   Golgi fractions bound hormones in a different pattern from purified plasma membrane, thus indicating that plasma membrane contamination did not account for the binding in Golgi fractions.

2.   Freeze-thawing enhanced binding to Golgi fractions but not plasma membranes, indicating that the receptors in the former were within vesicles.

3.   The receptors in Golgi fractions were more stable on extended incubation than those in plasma membranes.

4.   Electron microscope radioautography demonstrated [125I]-labeled hormone bound to lipoprotein-containing vesicles.

5.   The pattern of regulation of Golgi and plasma membrane receptors has been shown to differ for both insulin and prolactin receptors (3, 4).

More recently we have demonstrated that Golgi fractions are heterogeneous and contain lipoprotein-filled vesicles with and without enzymes of terminal glycosylation (5, 6).

It is the purpose of this chapter to summarize in detail the methodologies we employ for isolating receptor-rich vesicles from rat liver as well as the major methods for characterizing these structures. In all our studies Sherman or Sprague-Dawley rats (150–250 g each) have been used. The animals are fed *ad libitum* to the day before use and are fasted overnight before the experiment. They are sacrificed by decapitation and exsanguinated before the livers are removed. All sucrose solutions (w/w) are prepared with reagent grade material (Fisher Scientific Limited, Pittsburgh, PA). In earlier studies the rats received ethanol (0.6 g/100 g body wt) in a 50 percent (w/v) solution by stomach tube 90 min prior to sacrifice (3, 4). In more recent studies the use of ethanol has been discontinued (6, 7).

2. SUBCELLULAR FRACTIONS

2.1. The Preparation of Golgi Fractions by Differential Centrifugation

The procedure was developed in the early 1970s by Ehrenreich et al. (8) and represented the first method in which Golgi fractions were resolved on what was thought to be structural and functional grounds.

2.1.1. REAGENTS

Sucrose solutions: 0.25 M, 0.60 M, 0.86 M, 1.00 M, and 1.15 M.

2.1.2. PROCEDURE

Livers are collected individually or in batches in ice-cold 0.25 M sucrose (5 mL/g liver), weighed, minced with scissors, and drained. All subsequent procedures are carried out in a cold room at 4°C. The same volume of ice-cold 0.25 M sucrose is added to the minced tissue, which is transferred to a Potter–Elvejhem glass Teflon homogenizer where it is homogenized with six full strokes of the motor-driven Teflon pestle at 1000 rpm.

1. The homogenate is centrifuged at 4°C at $8800g_{max}$ (8000 rpm in a Beckman J2-21 using a JA-17 rotor) for 10 min.
2. The supernatant is decanted into 25 mL polycarbonate tubes on ice (the pellet was discarded) and then centrifuged at $200,000g_{av}$ (52,000 rpm in a Spinco L2-65 or L2-65B using a 60-Ti rotor) for 30 min.
3. A discontinuous sucrose gradient is prepared in polyallomer (SW-27 rotor) or cellulose nitrate (SW-40 rotor) tubes while the above centri-

fugation steps are proceeding. The sucrose solutions ($0.25\,M$, $0.60\,M$, $0.86\,M$, $1.00\,M$; prepared the day before and stored ice-cold) and centrifuge tubes are placed in crushed ice. Each succeeding layer of sucrose is placed beneath the others using a syringe with a long needle. The volume of each sucrose solution added is 7.0 mL for SW-27 rotor tubes and 4.0 mL for SW-40 rotor tubes.

4. The supernatant from step 2 is discarded and the pellet vortexed in $0.25\,M$ sucrose before decanting into a Dounce homogenizer with a loose-fitting pestle. The suspension is adjusted to a sucrose concentration of $1.15\,M$ (by adding appropriate volumes of $2.0\,M$ and $0.25\,M$ sucrose and distilled water) and gently homogenized to yield an even suspension.

5. The microsome suspension is slowly injected beneath the four sucrose layers (see step 3) using a syringe and long needle so as to fill the tube (volume used is 10.0 mL for SW-27 and 4.0 mL for SW-40 rotor tubes).

6. Centrifugation is at $100,000g_{av}$ for 190 min (25,000 rpm, SW-27) or $200,000g_{av}$ for 95 min (40,000 rpm, SW-40) to generate the following fractions: via flotation from the microsome suspension:
   (a) Golgi light (Gl) at $0.25/0.60\,M$ sucrose interface.
   (b) Golgi intermediate (Gi) at $0.60/0.86\,M$ sucrose interface.
   (c) Golgi heavy (Gh) at $0.86/1.00\,M$ sucrose interface.
   (d) Small vesicles (SV) at $1.00/1.15\,M$ sucrose interface.

7. Each fraction is removed from the gradient with a 90° angle needle and syringe, placed in a separate cellulose nitrate tube, and (if it is desirable to preserve isotonicity) diluted to $0.25\,M$ sucrose as follows:
   (a) Gl, fill with $0.25\,M$ sucrose.
   (b) Gi, add equal volume of distilled water and fill wtih $0.25\,M$ sucrose.
   (c) Gh, add 2 volumes of distilled water and fill with $0.25\,M$ sucrose.
   (d) SV, add 2.5 volumes of distilled water and fill with $0.25\,M$ sucrose.

8. Samples are then centrifuged at $200,000g_{av}$ for 30 minutes (53,00 rpm, 60-Ti rotor).

For binding studies all pellets are resuspended in 25 mM Tris/10 mM MgCl$_2$, pH 7.4.

2.1.3. COMMENT

The subfractions generated as described above have distinctive morphological features. Gl consists largely of vesicles containing lipoprotein particles. Gi is similar but somewhat more heterogeneous. The vesicles in this fraction show a wider range of size and there are some tubular and flattened saccular elements as well. The Gh fraction is quite heterogeneous with lipoprotein-containing vesicles being minority elements. There is an abundance of flattened saccules and tubular elements and a significant proportion of small vesicles. SV, formerly part of our Gh fraction prepared without a 1.0 M sucrose layer, consists largely of small vesicles. It is not clear to what extent these represent vesiculated plasmalemma or endocytotic vesicles.

The yield of each fraction (mg/g liver) is approximately: Gl, 0.10–0.15; Gi, 0.25–0.35; Gh, 0.40–0.55; and SV, 1.3–2.1. It is now appreciated that various endoplasmic-membrane marker enzymes are present in Golgi elements (9, 10). However, the enzymes enriched in the Golgi and characteristic of this organelle are the various terminal glycosyltransferases (11).

2.2. The Isolation of Nonlysosomal, Non-Golgi Vesicles by Percoll Gradient Fractionation

Recently it has become apparent that vesicles highly enriched in peptide hormone receptors and active in the internalization of hormone receptor complexes can be resolved from structures apparently enriched in glycosyltransferases (5, 6). These structures morphologically resemble the lipoprotein-containing elements that cosediment with glycosyltransferases but are heavier, devoid of glycosyltransferases, and contain modest levels of acid phosphatase and other lysosomal enzymes (about one-fourth to one-third the concentration in lysosomes). Because they share features of both Golgi vesicles and lysosomes, we have referred to them as intermediate, or "unique," vesicles to emphasize their distinctiveness (2, 6). The following method resolves intermediate, or "unique," vesicles from Golgi intermediate or heavy fractions on an isoosmotic, continuous, self-generating Percoll gradient. We are confident that in the near future, a more general quantitative scheme for preparing these receptor-rich intracellular structures will be available.

2.2.1. REAGENTS

1. 0.25 M sucrose solution (8.55 g sucrose/100 mL distilled water).
2. 62 percent sucrose solution (62 g sucrose/100 mL distilled water).
3. 2.5 M sucrose solution (85.5 g sucrose/100 mL distilled water).
4. 25 mM Tris-HCl, 10 mM MgCl$_2$, pH 7.4.
5. Percoll (Pharmacia Fine Chemicals, Sweden) 100 percent solution in H$_2$O.
6. Density marker beds (Pharmacia Fine Chemicals, Sweden).

2.2.2. PROCEDURE

1. The sucrose concentration of a freshly prepared Golgi intermediate (or heavy) fraction is determined by measuring its density (weigh 100-μL aliquots in triplicate) and computing the concentration from tabulated specific gravities of sucrose solutions (12).

2. The Golgi fraction (5–10 mL; 1 mg/mL protein) is diluted to 24 mL (the volume of the centrifuge tube) with 100 percent Percoll solution (4.13 mL) and water or 2.5 M sucrose as required to yield a final solution of 17.2 percent (v/v) Percoll, 0.25 M sucrose (final density = 1.05 g/mL).

3. Centrifuge at 60,000g_{av} for 30 min at 4°C (Spinco Ti 60) to generate a continuous gradient *in situ*.

4. Twelve 2 mL fractions are collected sequentially from the top of the centrifuge tube by pumping a 62 percent sucrose solution into the bottom of the tube.

5. The density of individual fractions is determined by weighing 100 μL aliquots in triplicate or by running an identical tube with density marker beads (13).

2.2.3. COMMENT

Most of the assays for marker enzymes, protein, and hormone binding can be done in off-the-gradient fractions. Where it is desirable to remove Percoll, the fraction is diluted 1:3 with 25 mM Tris-HCl, 10 mM MgCl$_2$ (pH 7.4), and centrifuged at 82,000g_{av} for 120 min at 4°C (SW-27 rotor). The supernatant is removed with a Pasteur pipette and the membranous material resting on the Percoll pellet is resuspended in a small volume (2 mL) of Tris-HCl, MgCl$_2$ buffer and either assayed immediately or frozen at −20°C.

The analysis of fractions from the Percoll gradients by the Lowry protein method is complicated because of the interference of Percoll. We have devised a modified Lowry procedure for protein estimation in which absorbance at 750 and 420 nm of unknowns, bovine serum albumin standards in 0.25 M sucrose, and Percoll solutions is determined (14). In this procedure Percoll-containing samples develop a thick white precipitate on the addition of 1.2 N NaOH which disappears after 20 min in a boiling water bath. Since the relation between the concentration of protein or Percoll and the absorbance values at the above two wavelengths is linear, one can devise a simple equation for computing protein concentrations. The method is suitable for samples containing as much as 30 percent Percoll (14).

3. ENZYME ASSAYS

3.1. Galactosyltransferase [EC 2.4.1.38]

This enzyme, involved in terminal glycosylation, is highly enriched in Golgi elements (15). The assay is by a modification of the method of Bretz and Staubli (16).

3.1.1. REAGENTS

1.	Sodium cacodylate buffer	0.35 M
	$MnCl_2$	0.32 M
	β-Mercaptoethanol (pH adjusted to 6.6)	0.31 M
2.	UDP-[^{3}H]galactose in H_2O	10 μCi/mL
3.	UDP-galactose	10 mM
	Adenosine triphosphate	50 mM
4.	Ovomucoid	175 mg/mL
5.	Triton X-100 in H_2O	2 percent (w/v)
6.	Phosphotungstic acid in 0.5 N HCl	1.0 percent (w/v)

3.1.2. PROCEDURE

1. The assay solution is prepared by mixing solutions 1, 2, 3, 4, and 5 in the ratio 5:1:4:4:4 (vols.).

2. Samples containing 2–50 μg protein in a volume up to 220 μL are mixed with 180 μL of assay solution and assayed in triplicate. Duplicate controls in which sample is added after terminating the reaction are prepared in parallel.

3. After incubation at 37°C for 30 min the reaction is stopped by adding 2 mL of ice-cold phosphotungstic acid–HCl and the mixture is vortexed before leaving the tubes on ice for 30 min.

4. The tubes are then centrifuged at 1600g_{av} for 10 min.

5. The pellet is washed two or three times with 2 mL aliquots of phosphotungstic acid and then once with 2 mL of ether–ethanol, 1:1 (v/v), and left to dry overnight at room temperature before dissolving in 0.5 mL Protosol (New England Nuclear) or 1 mL of 2 M NH$_4$OH.

6. The solution is neutralized with glacial acetic acid and counted in 12 mL of Aquasol-2 (New England Nuclear).

Enzyme activity is calculated as pmols of galactose incorporated into protein/ 30 min/mg protein.

3.2. Sialyltransferase [EC 2.4.99.1]

This enzyme is assayed by a modification of the method of Bretz et al. (11).

3.2.1. REAGENTS

1.	Sodium cacodylate buffer	0.4 M
	β-mercaptoethanol	0.16 M
2.	CMP-[^{3}H]-sialic acid in H_2O	10 μCi/mL

3. CMP-*N*-acetyl-neuraminic acid   10 m*M*
   (ammonium salt)

4. Asialofetuin [Fetuin (Sigma) is acid   175 mg/mL
   hydrolyzed in 0.05 *N* H_2SO_4 by the method
   of Spiro (17) and the lyophilized protein is
   dissolved in H_2O].

5. Triton X-100 in H_2O 2 percent (w/v)

6. Phosphotungstic acid in 0.5 *N* HCl   1 percent (w/v)

7. Trichloroacetic acid in H_2O (TCA)   10 percent (w/v)

All solutions are stored at $-20°C$ except for solutions 5–7, which can be stored at 4°C.

3.2.2. PROCEDURE

1. The assay solution is prepared by mixing solutions 1 to 5 in the ratios 25:10:10:10:10 (vols.).

2. Samples containing 1–8 µg protein in a volume up to 35 µL are mixed with 65 µL of the assay solution. Duplicate controls in which sample is added after terminating the reaction are prepared in parallel.

3. After incubating at 37°C for 30 min the reaction is stopped by adding 1 mL of phosphotungstic acid and the mixture is vortexed and left on ice for 30 min prior to centrifuging at $1600g_{av}$ for 10 min.

4. The pellet is washed two or three times with 2 mL ice-cold TCA and once with 1 mL ether–ethanol, 1:1 (v/v), and left overnight at room temperature to dry.

5. The dried pellet is dissolved in 0.5 mL Protosol or 1 mL 2 *M* NH_4OH before neutralizing with glacial acetic acid and counting in Aquasol-2.

Enzyme activity is calculated as nmols of CMP–neuraminic acid incorporated into protein/30 min/mg protein.

3.3. Acid Phosphatase [EC 3.1.3.2]

In distinguishing between various subcellular elements it is often important to measure this enzyme. With minor modifications, our procedure is based on that of Gianetto and deDuve (18).

3.3.1. REAGENTS

1. β-glycerophosphate, disodium salt   0.5 *M*
   sodium acetate buffer, pH 5.0   0.6 *M*

2. Triton X-100 in H_2O 1 percent (w/v)

3. Trichloroacetic acid (TCA)   16 percent (w/v)

3.3.2. PROCEDURE

1. The reaction mixture is prepared in phosphorus-free clean glass tubes by mixing 50 μL of solution 1 and 50 μL of solution 2 with sample containing 2–25 μg of protein.

2. The volume is adjusted to 500 μL with distilled water. Control tubes are those without added sample.

3. After 60 min at 30°C the reaction is stopped by adding 500 μL of 16 percent TCA.

4. The clear supernatant is collected after centrifugation at $2400g_{av}$ for 15 min and inorganic phosphorus is determined by the method of Chen et al. (19).

The results are corrected for readings of the control incubations. A unit of enzyme is micromoles of Pi released/hr/mg protein.

4. HORMONE BINDING

In order to maximize binding to the receptor-rich vesicles they must be frozen and thawed four times or incubated in the presence of 0.1 percent Triton X-100 to permeabilize the vesicles. This latency is explained as due to the presence of receptors on the inner aspect of the vesicles. Hormone binding is measured essentially as previously described (3, 4, 20).

4.1. Reagents

1. [^{125}I]-labeled hormone.

2. 125 mM Tris-HCl, 50 mM $MgCl_2$, 0.5 percent bovine serum albumin (BSA), pH 7.4.

3. Unlabeled hormone prepared in solution 2 (insulin, oPRL and bGH, 50 μg/mL; hGH, 20 μg/mL).

4.2. Materials

Glass fiber filters (2.4 cm, Reeve Angel or Whatman 934-AH) presoaked for 24 hr in 25 mM sodium acetate buffer, pH 5.0, containing 0.1 percent BSA.

4.3. Procedure

1. Solution 1 (200 μL) is incubated in triplicate with 800 μL of sample (20–100 μg protein) and 100 μL of solution 2 (final volume, 1.0 mL) for 24–30 hr at 4°C with constant shaking.

2. Duplicate control tubes for determining nonspecific binding are run under identical conditions except that 100 μL of solution 2 is replaced by 100 μL of solution 3.

3. The incubations are terminated by adding 3 mL of an ice-cold 1:5 dilution (with H_2O) of solution 2.

4. Bound and free radioactivity are separated by filtration on presoaked glass fiber filters using a Millipore manifold assembly.

5. After filtration the filters are washed with 20 mL of a 1:5 dilution of solution 1.

6. Radioactivity retained on the filters is counted in a γ-scintillation counter as described elsewhere (20).

Specific binding is the difference between radioactivity bound in the absence (total binding) and in the presence (nonspecific binding) of excess unlabeled hormone and is expressed as a percent of total radioactivity in the incubation. In circumstances where the sample is suspended in 25 mM Tris-HCl, 10 mM $MgCl_2$, 0.1 percent BSA, a 1:5 dilution of solution 2 is added to the incubation.

5. INTERNALIZATION OF INSULIN AND OTHER PEPTIDE HORMONES

5.1. Internalization into Subcellular Fractions

The uptake of [^{125}I]-labeled insulin and prolactin into rat liver subcellular elements has been studied in detail (21–24). The methodology involves the injection of [^{125}I] hormone (10–15 × 10^6 cpm) into the internal jugular or portal vein of the rat with subsequent sacrifice at specific times postinjection followed by rapid preparation of the subcellular fractions as described above. Radioactivity in the individual fractions is readily measured in a standard γ-scintillation spectrometer (21). Uptake into particular fractions is expressed as cpm/mg protein (specific activity) or as cpm/g liver (in which the specific activity is multiplied by the protein yield of that fraction per gram of liver).

Several points are noteworthy: (i) Injection of [^{125}I] hormone by the internal jugular vein is technically less tedious and more rapid than injection via the portal route. It is thus especially useful when a number of animals are to be processed within a short period of time. The extent of uptake following injection via the jugular vein is about 60 percent that following portal vein injection. (ii) The handling of the liver and the processing of all subcellular fractions must be done at 4°C to minimize both dissociation of $[^{125}I]$ hormone from receptors and degradation of $[^{125}I]$ hormone.

5.2. Methods for Quantitative Radioautography of Subcellular Fractions

Subcellular fractions are routinely processed for random sampling by the filtration protocol outlind by Baudhuin et al. (25) as modified by Wibo et al. (26). Briefly, after fixation in 2.5 percent glutaraldehyde in 0.05 M sodium cacodylate buffer, pH 7.4, Golgi fractions are recovered onto Millipore membranes (Type HA, 0.45-μm pore size) using the automated filtration apparatus of Baudhuin et al. (25) and then postfixed in 1 percent OsO_4 and block-stained in uranyl acetate. Membrane pellicles are then dehydrated, embedded in Epon 812, and thin sections are cut with block face orientated in order to assure a cross section through the depth of the filtered pellicle. These thin sections can then be viewed directly in the electron microscope following grid staining in uranyl acetate and lead citrate. This method, which has been standardized by Dr. B. Kopriwa (27), is as follows:

5.2.1. REAGENTS

1. Celloidin (Randolph Finishing Products, Carlstadt, NJ).
2. Isoamylacetate (Tousimis, New Jersey).
3. Ilford L-4 nuclear emulsion (Ilford Canada, Markham, Ontario).
4. Gold chloride (Canlab, Montreal, Canada).
5. Potassium thiocyanate (Fisher Scientific Limited, Canada).
6. Potassium bromide (Fisher Scientific Limited, Canada).
7. Elon (p-methylaminophenol sulfate) (Kodak, New Jersey).
8. Anhydrous sodium sulfite (Fisher Scientific Limited, Canada).
9. Sodium thiosulfate (Fixer) (Fisher Scientific Limited, Canada).

5.2.2. EQUIPMENT

Semiautomatic coating apparatus (Averlaid, Toronto).

5.2.3. PROCEDURES

1. Precleaned microcope slides are further cleaned by wiping with lens tissue.
2. The slides are dipped into a solution of 1 percent celloidin in iso-amylacetate and dried vertically in a dust-free cabinet overnight.
3. Thin tissue sections ($\sim$ 50 nm in thickness) are placed on the celloidin-covered glass slides where they are covered with 5 nm of carbon using

an Edwards carbon evaporator especially modified to assure a uniform application of carbon.

4. The slides are subsequently dipped in Ilford L-4 nuclear emulsion (diluted 1:2.5 in distilled water) at 40°C using the semiautomatic dipping device to ensure covering by a monolayer of emulsion.

5. The slides are dried vertically and then stored in lightproof boxes at 8°C with added Drierite in each box.

6. After suitable exposure ($\sim$ 60 days) the emulsion is developed for "fine-grain" development by the "solution-physical" procedure after prior treatment with gold in order to stabilize the exposed latent images. Thus, slides are dipped vertically into distilled water (1 min), followed by a freshly prepared gold thiocyanate solution (0.4 mg of gold chloride in 100 mL of 0.5 percent potassium thiocyanate, 0.6 percent potassium bromide) for 1 min followed by 7 min development in freshly prepared Agfa-Gevaert developer [0.75 g Elon, 0.5 g anhydrous sodium sulfite, and 0.2 g potassium thiocyanate in 100 mL distilled water (27)].

7. Slides are subsequently placed in distilled water for 30 sec followed by fixer (2 min in 24 percent sodium thiosulfate).

8. They are then washed in five changes of distilled water.

9. Sections are finally transferred to EM grids by flotation of the cut celloidin-emulsion couplet onto the surface of distilled water.

The key feature of the above technique involves the use of gold deposition about the exposed latent images. This treatment ensures the symmetrical deposition of silver about the exposed latent images by the Agfa-Gevaert developer. The final visualized micrograph is therefore one of exposed latent images and not, as for all other radioautographic methods (28), a micrograph showing developed silver crystals where the latent images have been randomly developed.

REFERENCES

1. B. I. Posner, J. J. M. Bergeron, Z. Josefsberg, M. N. Khan, R. J. Khan, B. A. Patel, R. A. Silkstrom, and A. K. Verma, *Rec. Prog. Horm. Res.* **37**, 539 (1981).

2. B. I. Posner, M. N. Khan, and J. J. M. Bergeron, *Endocr. Revs.* **3**, 280 (1982).

3. B. I. Posner, Z. Josefsberg, D. Raquidan, and J. J. M. Bergeron, *Proc. Natl. Acad. Sci. USA* **75**, 3302 (1978).

4. B. I. Posner, Z. Josefsberg, and J. J. M. Bergeron, *J. Biol. Chem.* **254**, 12394 (1979).

5. M. N. Khan, B. I. Posner, A. K. Verma, R. J. Khan, and J. J. M. Bergeron, *Proc. Natl. Acad. Sci. USA* **78**, 4980 (1981).

6. M. N. Khan, B. I. Posner, J. R. Khan, and J. J. M. Bergeron. *J. Biol. Chem.* **257**, 5969 (1982).

7. B. I. Posner, B. Patel, M. N. Khan, and J. J. M. Bergeron, *J. Biol. Chem.* **257**, 5789 (1982).

8. J. H. Ehrenreich, J. J. M. Bergeron, P. Siekevitz, and G. E. Palade, *J. Cell. Biol.* **59**, 45 (1973).

9. K. E. Howell, A. Ito, and G. E. Palade, *J. Cell. Biol.* **79**, 581 (1978).

10. M. G. Farquhar, J. J. M. Bergeron, and G. E. Palade, *J. Cell. Biol.* **60**, 8 (1974).

11. R. Bretz, H. Bretz, and G. E. Palade, *J. Cell. Biol.* **84**, 87 (1980).

12. Scientific Tables, in *Documenta Geigy*, K. Diem (ed.), Geigy Pharmaceuticals, Ardsley, NY, 1962. p. 320.

13. J. R. Mickelson, M. L. Breaser, and B. B. Marsh, *Anal. Biochem.* **109**, 225 (1980).

14. M. N. Khan, R. J. Khan, and B. I. Posner, *Anal. Biochem.* **117**, 108, (1981).

15. M. G. Farquhar and G. E. Palade, *J. Cell Biol.* **91**, 77 (1981).

16. R. Bretz and W. Staubli, *Eur. J. Biochem.* **77**, 181 (1977).

17. R. G. Spiro, *J. Biol. Chem.* **235**, 2860 (1960).

18. R. Gianetto and C. deDuve, *Biochem. J.* **59**, 432 (1955).

19. P. S. Chen, Jr., T. Y. Toribara, and H. Warner, *Anal. Chem.* **28**, 1756 (1956).

20. B. I. Posner, J. J. M. Bergeron, and Z. Josefsberg, *J. Biol. Chem.* **253**, 4067 (1978).

21. Z. Josefsberg, B. I. Posner, B. Patel, and J. J. M. Bergeron, *J. Biol. Chem.* **254**, 209 (1979).

22. B. I. Posner, B. Patel, A. K. Verma, and J. J. M. Bergeron, *J. Biol. Chem.* **255**, 735 (1980).

23. B. I. Posner, A. K. Verma, B. A. Patel, and J. J. M. Bergeron, *J. Cell Biol.* **93**, 560 (1982).

24. B. I. Posner, B. Patel, M. N. Khan, and J. J. M. Bergeron, *J. Biol. Chem.* **257**, 5789 (1982).

25. P. Baudhuin, P. Evrard, and J. Berthet, *J. Cell Biol.* **32**, 181 (1967).

26. M. Wibo, A. Amar-Costesec, J. Berthet, and H. Beaufay, *J. Cell Biol.* **51**, 52 (1971).

27. B. M. Kopriwa, *Histochemie* **37**, 1 (1973).

28. B. M. Kopriwa, *Histochemie* **44**, 210 (1975).

D

MEASUREMENT OF INSULIN-STIMULATED TYROSINE PROTEIN KINASE ACTIVITY IN PREPARATIONS DERIVED FROM CULTURED 3T3-L1 PREADIPOCYTES AND HUMAN PLACENTA

L. M. PETRUZZELLI, L. STADTMAUER, R. HERRERA, AND O. M. ROSEN
Department of Molecular Pharmacology, Albert Einstein College of Medicine, Bronx, New York

1. INTRODUCTION

Insulin stimulates the phosphorylation of its own receptor in intact cells and in cell-free extracts (1–4). In cell-free preparations the insulin receptor becomes phosphorylated principally on tyrosine residues in the β subunit (Mr = 95,000) of the receptor (2, 3), whereas in intact cells both serine and tyrosine residues in this subunit are phosphorylated (1). The tyrosine protein kinase activity responsible for the β subunit phosphorylation copurifies with the insulin receptor, suggesting that the receptor itself is a protein kinase (5–7). This is supported by the observation that phosphorylation of the receptor *in vitro* occurs by an intramolecular reaction (8). It is not known which subunit of the receptor contains the active site of the protein kinase, although it has been demonstrated that the β subunit contains an ATP binding site (9, 10). The insulin-stimulated protein kinase also phosphorylates tyrosine residues on exogenous substrates such as casein, histone, and angiotensin II (1, 11). In this chapter we outline methods for assaying the insulin-stimulated tyrosine protein kinase activity derived from either cultured 3T3-L1 adipocytes or human placental membranes.

2. PHOSPHORYLATION OF THE INSULIN RECEPTOR IN MEMBRANES

Insulin-stimulated phosphorylation of tyrosine residues in the β subunit of the insulin receptor is difficult to detect in plasma membranes. It becomes easier

Research of L. M. Petruzzelli was supported by NIH Training Grant T 32 GM 7288; reseach of L. Stadtmauer and R. Herrera supported by NIH Training Grant 5T 32 AM 07329; and research of O. M. Rosen supported by NIH Grant 5 RO1 AM 09038 and ACS Grant BC 12 N.

to assess as purification of the insulin receptor protein kinase proceeds (see below). Membranes from cultured 3T3-L1 adipocytes (12) are prepared by sonicating 10^7 cells in 1 mL of 10 mM Tris-HCl buffer (pH 7.5), 5 mM MgCl$_2$, 25 mM benzamidine, and 0.25 M sucrose for 15 sec at 75 V using a Brinkman polytron. The homogenate is centrifuged at 10,000g for 15 min, and membranes are collected from the resultant supernatant fluid by centrifugation at 130,000g for 1 hr. The pellet is resuspended in the same buffer at a protein concentration of 10–50 mg/mL. Human placental membranes are prepared as described in ref. 13 and resuspended in 50 mM Tris-HCl buffer, pH 7.4. The reaction mixture for insulin-stimulated protein phosphorylation contains 0.1–1 mg membrane protein plus 2 mM MnCl$_2$, 10 mM MgCl$_2$, 20 mM HEPES buffer (pH 7.4), 5–10 percent glycerol (optional), 30 mM NaCl (optional), and BSA* at a final concentration of 100 μg/mL. Sodium vanadate (50 μM) may be included to inhibit dephosphorylation. This mixture, in a final volume of 50 μL, is incubated in the presence or absence of insulin (0.1–1.0 μg/mL) for 10 min at 23°C. The reaction is initiated by the addition of 10 μL of ATP to give a final concentration of 100 μM (10 cpm/fmol) and is terminated after 5–10 min by the addition of 15 μL of a fivefold concentrate of SDS-PAGE buffer containing 0.3 M Tris-HCl buffer (pH 6.8), 50 percent glycerol, 10 percent SDS, 0.11 M dithiothreitol, and 1 M mercaptoethanol. Samples are heated to 100°C for 5 min and subjected to electrophoresis in a 7.5 percent SDS-PAGE (14). Skeletal muscle glycogen phosphorylase migrates at the approximate position of the β subunit of the insulin receptor and can be used as an electrophoretic marker. Following staining and destaining, the gel is incubated at 60°C in 1 M NaOH for 1 hr. This procedure selectively hydrolyzes seryl phosphate residues in proteins as described in ref. 15. The gel is next incubated for 5 min in 1 M HCl at room temperature, washed repeatedly with destaining solution (10 percent methanol, 10 percent acetic acid), dried and autoradiographed with Kodak XAR or XS film and a Dupont·Quanta III intensifying screen. The treatment with hot alkali is useful when phosphorylation of the insulin receptor is studied in impure fractions since it releases a substantial amount of the ^{32}P whose incorporation into proteins has been catalyzed by the more abundant serine protein kinases.

3. PHOSPHORYLATION OF THE INSULIN RECEPTOR IN DETERGENT EXTRACTS OF MEMBRANES

Chilled, freshly prepared 10 percent TX-100 (Triton X-100) is added to membranes at 4°C to achieve a final concentration of 2 percent. The 3T3-L1 membranes are vortexed intermittently for 1 hr and the placental membranes are stirred for 3 hr. The Triton extract, which generally contains from 2–5 fmol

---

* The following abbreviations are used: BSA, bovine serum albumin; PAGE, polacrylamide gel electrophoresis; TX-100, Triton X-100; SDS, sodium dodecyl sulfate; DTT, dithiothreitol; WGA, wheat germ agglutinin; NEM, N-ethylmaleimide.

of insulin-binding activity per microliter determined as described in (13, 16), is collected following centrifugation at 130,000g for 1 hr. The supernatant contains 50–95 percent of the insulin-binding activity detected in the membranes. Assays are performed as previously described with 10–250 μg of protein at either 4°C or at 23°C for 5–12 min (see above). The final concentration of TX-100 in the assay has little effect on the tyrosine protein kinase activity.

To help establish the identity of the [^{32}P]-labeled 95,000-dalton band as a subunit of the insulin receptor, disulfide reducing agents are omitted from the SDS–PAGE buffer. Under these conditions, the receptor migrates as a high molecular weight (Mr $\geq$ 300,000) oligomer, and there is no dissociation to yield a radioactive 95,000-dalton band. Both reduced and unreduced [^{32}P]-labeled receptors are immunoprecipitable by antibodies to the insulin receptor (6). For quantification, the β subunit can be excised from the dried gel and the ^{32}P content determined by liquid scintillation spectrometry.

4. PHOSPHORYLATION OF THE INSULIN RECEPTOR AFTER PURIFICATION BY CHROMATOGRAPHY ON WHEAT GERM AGGLUTININ–AGAROSE

The insulin receptor in the Triton X-100 extract can be purified further on an agarose-bound wheat germ agglutinin resin (Vector Laboratories, Burlingame, CA) (17). Batches of resin are pretested for recovery of insulin-stimulated protein kinase activity. Before applying the sample, each milliliter of resin is first washed with 5 mL of 50 mM HEPES buffer (pH 7.6), containing 0.01 percent SDS, 0.15 M NaCl, and 0.1 percent TX-100 (buffer A). It is then washed with 50 mL of 50 mM HEPES buffer (pH 7.6), containing 0.15 M NaCl, 0.1 percent TX-100 (buffer B), and finally with 50 mL of 50 mM HEPES buffer (pH 7.6), containing 0.15 M NaCl, 0.1 percent TX-100, and 10 mM MgSO$_4$ (buffer C). The TX-100 extract is applied and reapplied to the wheat germ resin a minimum of five times at room temperature. Approximately 300,000 fmol of insulin-binding activity may be applied to 20 mL (4 × 2.5 cm) of resin; however, this value varies with different lots of resin and must be determined for each batch purchased. After application of the sample at room temperature, the column is cooled to 4°C and washed with 25 mL of buffer C per mL of resin. A volume of buffer C (equal to the void volume) containing 5 mM EDTA and 0.3 M N-acetylglucosamine is applied, and the column is then turned off and incubated at 23°C for 30 min. The insulin receptor is eluted with this buffer at 23°C in 3–6 fractions each equal to one-half of a column volume. Most of the activity elutes in the first three fractions. The recovery from wheat germ agglutinin–agarose is about 50–75 percent of the applied insulin-binding activity from either 3T3-L1 cells or human placenta. The step yields a 10- to 20-fold purification of insulin-binding and insulin-activatable protein kinase activities. The resin can be reused after washing with buffer A, buffer B, and buffer C as described, and is best stored in 0.04

C. The properties of the protein kinase activity eluted from wheat germ agglutinin–agarose are described below.

5. PHOSPHORYLATION OF THE INSULIN RECEPTOR FOLLOWING PURIFICATION BY AFFINITY CHROMATOGRAPHY ON INSULIN-SEPHAROSE

The insulin-dependent tyrosine protein kinase activity can be further purified by affinity chromatography using insulin covalently bound to sepharose beads (8, 13). The wheat germ agglutinin–agarose eluate is applied to the resin (1 mg of protein/mL resin) and allowed to adsorb for 1 hr at 23°C. The column is then cooled to 4°C and washed with 50 mL/mL resin of 50 mM HEPES buffer (pH 7.4), containing 0.5 M NaCl, and 0.1 percent TX-100. One void volume of a solution of 0.15 M sodium acetate buffer (pH 5.5), containing 0.5 M NaCl, 0.1 percent TX-100, and 1 mM DTT is allowed to pass through the column at 23°C, following which the column is closed for 10 min. The insulin receptor is then eluted at 23°C using this buffer. Fractions (0.5 mL) are collected into tubes containing 30 μL of 1 M HEPES buffer (pH 9), 0.1 percent TX-100, 1 mM DTT, and 250 μg soybean trypsin inhibitor (Boehringer).

Phosphorylation of the insulin receptor, purified from insulin-Sepharose, is performed in a final volume of 60 μL containing 0.06 percent TX-100, 67 mM HEPES buffer (pH 7.4), 0.3 M NaCl, 12 mM MgCl$_2$, 2 mM MnCl$_2$, 0.1 M sodium acetate, 100 μg/mL BSA, and 170 μg/mL of soybean trypsin inhibitor. An equivalent amount of insulin-binding activity from a wheat germ agglutinin eluate elicited the same amount of protein phosphorylation under these conditions as under those described in the section on the wheat germ agglutinin purification. For assays in which the receptor is to be resolved by SDS-PAGE, 0.2–1.5 fmol of insulin-binding activity is incubated in reaction mixture containing 1 μg/mL insulin for 10 min at 23°C. ATP is then added to yield a final concentration of 25 μM (50 cpm/fmol) in a final assay volume of 60 μL and the reaction is allowed to proceed at 23°C for 5 min. The incorporation of ^{32}P into the receptor is proportional to time for 10 min. For phosphorylation of exogenous substrates approximately 2.5–5 fmol of insulin-binding activity are used in each assay. The receptor is preincubated in the presence of insulin for 10 min. ATP is added for 5–10 min followed by the addition of the substrate for 5–30 min (see below).

6. PHOSPHORYLATION OF EXOGENOUS SUBSTRATES BY THE INSULIN-ACTIVATED PROTEIN KINASE

6.1. Assay for Histone Phosphorylation

The insulin receptor kinase is able to catalyze the transfer of the γ-phosphate of ATP to specific tyrosine residues of several different proteins and peptides in an insulin-dependent manner. Stimulation by insulin varies between 3- and 10-fold as it does in the case of β subunit autophosphorylation and can be conveniently assayed using either the protein kinase present in the WGA eluate or the fully purified insulin receptor. Phosphorylation of a prototypical substrate, histone H2B, can be assayed in the following ways:

1.   The wheat germ eluate (3–15 fmol of insulin-binding activity) or purified receptor is preincubated with and without insulin (1 μg/mL) in the presence of 50–250 μg/mL of BSA for 10–15 min at room temperature under the conditions described above. [γ-^{32}P] ATP is added to yield a final concentration of 100 μM (10 cpm/fmol) in a 40–60-μL reaction mixture. After incubation at room temperature for 5–10 min a 5 μL aliquot of histone H2B is added (final concentration of 0.4 mg/mL). Phosphorylation of histone proceeds at a constant rate for 5–10 min at 23°C. If PAGE is to be used to quantitate incorporation of ^{32}P into the substrate, the reaction is stopped by the addition of SDS-PAGE sample buffer and subjected to electrophoresis in 10 percent SDS-PAGE as described above. An alternative method to quantitate [^{32}P] incorporation involves precipitation by trichloroacetic acid. At the end of the incubation, BSA is added to each tube (final concentration of 1 mg/mL) and the reaction is stopped by the addition of 0.5 mL of 10 percent trichloroacetic acid containing 10 mM sodium pyrophosphate. The mixture is then centrifuged at 5000 rpm in a Sorvall SM-24 rotor for 10 min and the supernatant fluid is discarded. The pellet is resuspended in 0.25 mL of 0.5 N NaOH and incubated at 55°C for 60 min. Following neutralization with 0.25 mL of 0.5 N HCl, the [^{32}P]-labeled protein is reprecipitated by the addition of 1 mL 10 percent trichloroacetic acid containing 10 mM sodium pyrophosphate, filtered on glass fiber filters (Enzo), washed with 10 volumes of 5 percent trichloroacetic acid and assayed by liquid scintillation spectrometry. This procedure measures primarily the incorporation of ^{32}P into tyrosine residues on histone since most of the phosphate on serine residues (catalyzed by contaminating histone kinases) has been hydrolyzed. Appropriate blanks include activity measured in the absence of insulin and in the absence of both insulin and histone. The results from the trichloroacetic acid assay are equivalent to those obtained with the PAGE assay if the gels have been treated with NaOH as described above (19).

2.   To measure the fully activated enzyme without the lag in substrate phosphorylation observed during the time required for autophosphorylation, the enzyme can be preactivated in the presence of insulin and ATP and recovered free of excess insulin and ATP following gel filtration (19). For small amounts of activated enzyme the following procedure is used. In a final volume of 60 μL, 40–150 fmol of insulin-binding activity are incubated in the standard reaction mixture with 0.3–1 μg of insulin per mL for 10–15 min at 23°C. ATP is then added (final concentration, 50–200 μM) for 10–20 min at 23°C. [γ-^{32}P] ATP can be used if it is of interest to also monitor phosphorylation of the insulin receptor. The mixture is acidified with 15 μL of 1 M MES buffer, pH 6.0, and after 3–6 min is applied to a 1-mL column of Sephadex G-75 (in a 1-mL pipette tip) previously equilibrated in 10 mM HEPES buffer, pH 6,

containing 0.1 percent TX-100. The column, placed in a 1 mL Eppendorf centrifuge tube, is centrifuged in an International clinical centrifuge for 30 sec. Six to seven fractions are collected sequentially by overlaying the column with a series of 70 μL aliquots of buffer, each of which is followed by centrifugation. The active enzyme is obtained in fractions 3 and 4, while discharged and unbound insulin and ATP are eluted after fraction 5. The fractions containing protein kinase activity are neutralized with 10 μL 1 M HEPES buffer, pH 7.4, and assayed as described above, except that the preincubation with insulin is omitted and the reaction is initiated by the addition of [γ-^{32}P] ATP. For larger volumes of receptor (up to 300 μL) a G-75 column (15 × 0.7 cm) can be used.

6.2. Assays for Peptide Phosphorylation

Tyrosine-containing peptides such as angiotensin II can serve as substrates for the insulin-dependent protein kinase (11). The 40 μL assay mixture containing 2 mM angiotensin II is as described above. The reaction is initiated by the addition of [γ-^{32}P] ATP (50 μM; 8–10 cpm/fmol) and the incubation is for 10–15 min at 23°C. Two methods are employed to quantitate phosphorylation of angiotensin and other peptides:

1. *Phosphocellulose Paper (20).* The reaction is stopped by addition of 50 μL of 5 percent trichloroacetic acid. Following centrifugation at 3000g for 10 min to remove precipitated proteins, two 40 μL aliquots of supernatant fluid are spotted on duplicate 2-cm^2 pieces of phosphocellulose paper. The papers are then washed in the following sequence: (i) 15 min in 30 percent acetic acid, (ii) three 10-min washes in 15 percent acetic acid, and (iii) 5 min in acetone. The papers are then dried and counted. The radioactivity bound to phosphocellulose in assays carried out without peptide is subtracted from assays performed in the presence of peptide.

2. *High-Voltage Paper Electrophoresis.* The reaction mixture described above is stopped with 3 μL of 0.2 M EDTA. Aliquots (10 μL) of reaction mixture are spotted in the center of a 34 × 10-in. piece of Whatman 3 MM paper, and electrophoresis is performed at pH 3.5 (pyridine–acetic acid–water 0.5:5.0:94.5 v/v/v) at 2000 V for 2 hr. The dried paper is subjected to autoradiography. To quantitate [^{32}P] incorporation, spots corresponding to the phosphorylated peptide, which can be visualized with ninhydrin as described in ref. 10, are cut out and counted. Phosphorylation of angiotensin II occurs at a constant rate for 60 min; however, incubation for 10–15 min under these conditions is sufficient to measure enzyme activity.

7. STABILITY OF THE INSULIN-ACTIVATED PROTEIN KINASE

The stability of the enzyme depends upon the state of purity. Following chromatography on wheat germ agglutinin, agarose activity is stable for 90 min

TABLE 1.   Effect of Heat on Protein Kinase and Insulin-Binding
Activities of the Insulin Receptor

Temperature (°C)	Protein Kinase Activity $T/2$ (min)	Insulin-Binding Activity (percent)
40	10	75
45	2.5	80
50	1.0	70

at 23°C, pH 7.4. At higher temperatures protein kinase activity is lost while insulin-binding activity is retained (Table 1).

The wheat germ agglutinin–agarose eluate was incubated at the indicated temperatures in the presence of 1 mg/mL bovine serum albumin. $T/2$ is defined as the time required for 50 percent loss of catalytic activity using histone as substrate.

Insulin binding was measured as described in ref. 13. The insulin-binding activity (percent or original) was measured when the protein kinase activity has been reduced 50 percent.

N-ethylmaleimide can be used to selectively inactivate the protein kinase. Thirty percent of the protein kinase activity remains following incubation with 1 mM NEM for 30 min at 23°C, and 100 percent loss of activity occurs with 2.5 mM NEM. Under these conditions insulin-binding activity remains unaffected.

The enzyme in the wheat germ agglutinin eluate can be stored at $-20°C$ for 1 month without loss of activity but should not be frozen and thawed more than once. After 3 months at $-20°C$ approximately one-third of both the protein kinase and insulin-binding activities remain.

The insulin-Sepharose-purified receptor (3 μg protein/mL) has a half-life of 60 min at 23°C. It can be stored at $-20°C$ in the presence of 250 μg/mL of soybean trypsin inhibitor but there is a 25 percent loss of activity after thawing once.

REFERENCES

1.   M. Kasuga, F. A. Karlsson, and C. R. Kahn, *Science* **215**, 185–187 (1982).
2.   M. Kasuga, Y. Zick, D. L. Blithe, F. A. Karlsson, H. U. Haring, and C. R. Kahn, *J. Biol. Chem.* **257**, 9891–9894 (1982).
3.   L. M. Petruzzelli, S. Ganguly, C. J. Smith, M. H. Cobb, C. S. Rubin, and O. M. Rosen, *Proc. Natl. Acad. Sci. USA* **79**, 6792–6796 (1982).
4.   J. Avruch, R. A. Nemenoff, P. J. Blackshear, M. W. Pierce, and R. Osathanondh, *J. Biol. Chem.* **257**, 15162–15166 (1982).
5.   E. van Obberghen and A. Kowalski, *FEBS Lett.* **143**, 179–182 (1982).

6. M. Kasuga, Y. Fujita-Yamaguchi, D. Blithe, and C. R. Kahn, *Proc. Natl. Acad. Sci. USA* **80**, 2317–2141 (1983).

7. L. M. Petruzzelli and O. M. Rosen, unpublished.

8. R. Herrera and O. M. Rosen, unpublished.

9. M. A. Shia and P. F. Pilch, *Biochemistry* **22**, 717–721 (1983).

10. E. van Obberghen, B. Ross, A. Kowalski, H. Gazzano, and G. Ponzio, *Proc. Natl. Acad. Sci. USA* **80**, 945–949 (1983).

11. L. Stadtmauer and O. M. Rosen, *J. Biol. Chem.* **258**, 6682–6685 (1983).

12. C. S. Rubin, A. Hirsch, C. Fung, and O. M. Rosen, *J. Biol. Chem.* **253**, 7570–7578 (1978).

13. T. Siegel, S. Ganguly, S. Jacob, O. M. Rosen, and C. S. Rubin, *J. Biol. Chem.* **256**, 9266–9273 (1981).

14. U. K. Laemmli, *Nature* **227**, 680–685 (1970).

15. J. A. Cooper and T. Hunter, *Mol. Cell Biol.* **1**, 165–178 (1981).

16. P. Cuatrecasas, *Proc. Natl. Acad. Sci. USA* **69**, 318–322 (1972).

17. J. A. Hedo, L. C. Harrison, and J. Roth, *Biochemistry* **20**, 3385–3393 (1981).

18. P. Cuatrecasas and I. Parikh, *Meth. Enzymol.* **34**, 670–688 (1974).

19. O. M. Rosen, R. Herrera, Y. Olowe, L. M. Petruzzelli, and M. H. Cobb, *Proc. Natl. Acad. Sci. USA* **80**, 3237–3240 (1983).

20. J. E. Casnellie, M. L. Harrison, L. J. Pike, K. E. Hellstrom, and E. G. Krebs, *Proc. Natl. Acad. Sci. USA* **79**, 282–286 (1982).

E

A HIGH-RESOLUTION ELECTRON MICROSCOPIC MARKER OF OCCUPIED INSULIN RECEPTORS

Monomeric Ferritin-Insulin

LEONARD JARETT AND ROBERT M. SMITH

Department of Pathology and Laboratory Medicine, University of Pennsylvania School of Medicine, Philadelphia, Pennsylvania

1. INTRODUCTION

A number of laboratories perform correlative ultrastructural and biochemical analyses of biological processes. These studies have been particularly prevalent in both endocrinology and pharmacology where effects of hormones, drugs, and other agents on cellular structure may be related to their biochemical functions. Our laboratory has used a correlative approach to study the interaction of insulin, a major anabolic hormone in mammalian organisms, with its target tissues. We were interested in determining the ultrastructural nature of the events involved in the binding, degradation, internalization, and processing of the hormone and its receptor. In addition, we wanted to determine the effects of various agents or disease states that modify these processes. Biochemical studies by several investigators (for review see ref. 1) have led to important speculations about the organization and the cellular processing of the hormone receptor complex. The development of reliable ultrastructural methodologies has complemented these studies and provided a more complete understanding of the biological processes involved.

Morphological analyses have used different techniques from the biochemical studies. These techniques have included light and electron microscopic autoradiography using [^{125}I]-labeled insulin (2–5), light microscopy using fluorescently labeled insulin (6), and high-resolution electron microscopy (7–16). High-resolution electron microscopic analyses of hormone receptor sites requires that a ligand, either the native hormone, an agonist, or a monovalent antibody to the receptor, be chemically modified to make it electron dense. This process can be accomplished either by conjugating to it an electron-dense molecule such as ferritin, hemocyanin, or gold, or by linking it to a product, such as peroxidase, which can be chemically treated to produce an electron-dense product. We elected to use ferritin as the electron-dense molecule because of its availability, size, and chemical characteristics. Several hormones, including epidermal growth factor (17), luteinizing hormone (18), luteinizing hormone-releasing factor (19), and melanocyte-stimulating hormone (20) have also been linked to ferritin and used to describe the distribution of occupied receptor sites on various target tissues.

In order for the conjugate to be a valid marker for the insulin receptor and allow certain analyses to be made, a set of strict criteria must be met. Monomeric ferritin-insulin (Fm-I) fulfills these criteria which include (i) the conjugate contains immunologically active insulin which is indistinguishable from native insulin; (ii) the biologically active insulin is equivalent in potency to the immunologic concentration of insulin and is indistinguishable from native insulin; (iii) the specificity and affinity of the conjugate for the insulin receptor is equal to native insulin; (iv) the conjugate is stable during storage and incubation with tissues; (v) the conjugate is monovalent and monomeric in terms of both insulin and ferritin; and (vi) the final conjugate contains no free, unconjugated insulin. This chapter describes a rapid, reproducible method for preparing a monomeric ferritin-insulin conjugate. The methodology has been previously described (13); much of the present data comes from a recent routine preparation chosen for illustrative purposes.

This monomeric ferritin-insulin conjugate has provided a method for studying the organization of the insulin receptor on cell surfaces, insulin uptake and recycling as well as documenting the effects of a variety of agents on the distribution of insulin receptors on cell surfaces, and on insulin uptake and distribution in intracellular structures (7–12, 14–16).

2. PREPARATION AND CHARACTERIZATION OF MONOMERIC FERRITIN-LABELED INSULIN

2.1. Materials

Porcine insulin (lot PJ5682; 23.1 U/mg) was a gift from Dr. R. Chance (Eli Lilly Co., Indianapolis, IN). Horse spleen ferritin (6X crystallized, cadmium free) was purchased from Miles Laboratories (Elkhart, IN.) and was used without prior purification. Glutaraldehyde (25 percent, EM grade, stored in glass ampules under inert gas) was purchased from Electron Microscopy Sciences (Fort Washington, PA). Bio-Gel A (1.5 M) was a product of Bio-Rad Laboratories (Richmond, CA). Bovine serum albumin and collagenase were purchased from Sigma Chemical (St. Louis, MO). and [^{125}I] was purchased from Amersham (Arlington Heights, IL). Other reagents and supplies were purchased from standard sources or as indicated in the text.

2.2. Preparation of Monomeric Ferritin-Labeled Insulin (Fm-I)

Figure 1 summarizes the standard protocol used to prepare Fm-I. Ferritin was superactivated with glutaraldehyde by using a modification of a previously

1. Superactivation of ferritin: 15 mg ferritin in 4 mL 0.05 M sodium phosphate buffer, pH 8.0, is mixed for 1 hr with 0.2 mL 2.5 percent glutaraldehyde. The activated ferritin is separated from the excess glutaraldehyde by Sephadex G-200 column chromatography.

2. Conjugation to insulin: The superactivated ferritin is mixed for 6 hr with 7 mg porcine insulin which was dissolved in 0.1 M HCl and diluted in phosphate buffer.

3. Neutralization of unreacted aldehyde groups: 2 mL of 2.25 M lysine-HCl is added and the reaction mixture is stirred for 16 hr at room temperature.

4. Concentration of ferritin and ferritin-insulin: The reaction mixture is ultracentrifuged at 40,000 rpm for 90 min. The supernatants are discarded and the pellets resuspended in less than 5 mL of phosphate buffer.

5. Purification of monomeric ferritin-insulin: The resuspended material from step 4 is applied to a Bio-Gel 1.5 M agarose column and eluted with phosphate buffer; the ferritin oligomer peak is discarded and the ferritin monomer peak is collected.

6. Further purification: Steps 4 and 5 are repeated.

7. Concentration, storage, and characterization of monomeric ferritin-insulin: The monomeric ferritin-insulin is centrifuged at 40,000 rpm for 90 min and the pellets resuspended in 1–2 mL phosphate buffered saline, pH 7.4. The conjugate is stored at 4°C. Characterization was performed by RIA, radioreceptor assay and bioassay as described in the text.

FIGURE 1. Summary of the preparation of monomeric ferritin-insulin.

described method (21). Fifteen milligrams of ferritin was diluted in 4 mL of 0.05 M sodium phosphate buffer, pH 8.0, (phosphate buffer). The ferritin concentration was determined by measuring the absorption at 440 nm and using the extinction coefficient of OD_{440} 1.000 = 0.65 mg ferritin (22). A freshly opened vial of glutaraldehyde was diluted to 2.5 percent with phosphate buffer and 0.20 mL of the cross-linker was added to the ferritin suspension with constant stirring. The final molar ratio in the suspension was >500:1 (glutaraldehyde to ferritin). The excess glutaraldehyde in the original reaction resulted in virtual saturation of the reactive amino groups in the ferritin by the bifunctional glutaraldehyde, providing more than 100 activated amino groups. The reaction modestly increased the amount of ferritin oligomers. The ferritin as purchased contained 5–7 percent oligomeric forms which was increased to 12–15 percent after the superactivation with glutaraldehyde.

The suspension was stirred for 1 hr at room temperature and was then applied to a 3 × 30-cm Sephadex G-200 column and eluted with phosphate buffer to separate the superactivated ferritin from the free glutaraldehyde. The void volume material containing the superactivated ferritin was diluted, if necessary, to about 20 mL with phosphate buffer. Porcine insulin was dissolved in 0.1 M HCl and diluted with phosphate buffer to a concentration of 7 mg/mL. One milliliter of the insulin solution was slowly added to the activated ferritin with constant vigorous initial mixing and then slowly stirred at room temperature for 6 hr. The molar ratio was about 35:1 (insulin to ferritin). At the end of this incubation unreacted aldehyde groups in the ferritin were blocked by adding 2 mL of 2.25 M lysine-HCl in phosphate buffer and stirring for another 16 hr at room temperature.

The molecular nature of the reaction between the activated ferritin and insulin is not known. The pH of the reaction (pH 8.0) would favor cross-linking occurring through the ε amino groups of B-29 lysine rather than the N-terminal amino groups. Insulin, because of its high concentration, probably exists as dimers or hexamers at pH 8.0 (23). If an insulin dimer or hexamer were linked to ferritin via a single amino group, upon dilution of the conjugate when dimers and hexamers dissociate into monomers, one should find high concentrations of free insulin. Since this was not found, it appears likely that cross-linking occurs between aldehyde groups and the small amount of monomeric insulin present. As the monomeric insulin couples to ferritin, the equilibrium between monomers, dimers, and hexamers would dissociate to monomers, assuring a constant concentration of reactive monomeric insulin. Blocking the unreacted aldehyde groups was essential to prevent nonspecific binding of the ferritin monomer insulin conjugate (Fm-I) to cell membranes and to prevent oligomer formation during subsequent centrifugations of the conjugate.

The mixture was centrifuged at 40,000 rpm (102,000g) for 90 min to concentrate the ferritin-insulin and free ferritin. (Since the Fm-I preparation contained both bound and unbound ferritin, as indicated below, all further reference to Fm-I will assume the presence of unbound ferritin.) Tubes were immediately removed from the centrifuge and supernatants, containing unconjugated insulin, removed as completely as possible. Pellets were resuspended in a minimal volume of phosphate buffer (<5 mL) and applied to a 3 × 45-cm Bio-Gel A 1.5 M agarose column and eluted with phosphate buffer. The ferritin migrated as two distinct bands; the first was present in the void volume and contained ferritin oligomers which were discarded. The second and only additional band was found at the molecular weight of monomeric ferritin 440,000 daltons and collected. The monomer fraction was concentrated by ultracentrifugation as described above, and the pellets were resuspended in phosphate buffer and rechromatographed on the Bio-Gel column. There was virtually no oligomer band associated with the rechromatographed ferritin. The monomer fraction was collected and the Fm-I concentrated by ultracentrifugation as before. The final pellets were resuspended in 1–2 mL of 0.9 percent NaCl in 0.05 M sodium phosphate, pH 7.4, and the conjugate was stored at 4°C. Under the conditions described, the final solution contained about 7 μg of insulin, or 0.1 percent of the initial insulin, and about 41 percent of the initial ferritin. The average ferritin-to-insulin ratio was 15:1.

2.3. Determination of Free, Unlabeled Insulin

Free insulin, that is, insulin not attached to ferritin, was determined by adding 2.25×10^8 cpm of [^{125}I]insulin to a preparation after blocking activated aldehyde groups on the ferritin. [^{125}I]insulin should serve as a tracer and be removed from the Fm-I in parallel with free insulin. The results of purification of Fm-I are shown in Table 1. Less than 0.0001 percent of added [^{125}I]insulin was recovered in the final Fm-I fraction, demonstrating that the centrifugation and

TABLE 1.   Separation of Unreacted [^{125}I]insulin from Monomeric Ferritin-Insulin during Purification of the Conjugate

Preparation Step	Percentage of Total [^{125}I]Insulin Recovered
1. Neutralization of unreacted aldehyde groups; [^{125}I]insulin added[a]	100.0
2. Ferritin pellets following first ultracentrifugation	8.5
3. Fm-I fraction from first Bio-Gel column	0.4
4. Fm-I pellets following second ultracentrifugation	0.04
5. Fm-I fraction from second Bio-Gel column	0.001
6. Purified Fm-I	0.0001

[a] Following the addition of lysine to block unreacted aldehyde groups on the activated ferritin, 2.25×10^8 cpm of [^{125}I]insulin was added to the reaction mixture.

chromatographic column steps effectively remove free insulin. In this preparation free insulin would be present to the extent of less than 0.1 percent of the total insulin present in purified Fm-I.

2.4.   Determination of Insulin Concentration and Activity

Insulin concentration in the purified Fm-I was determined using a routine radioimmunoassay, and the results of a typical radioimmunoassay are shown in Figure 2. Fm-I competed with [^{125}I]insulin for binding to the anti-insulin antibody in an identical dose-dependent manner to native porcine insulin standard. Molar ratios of ferritin to insulin in Fm-I were calculated assuming molecular weights of 450,000 and 6000 for ferritin and insulin, respectively.

Biological activity of Fm-I was determined by comparing the ability of Fm-I and native porcine insulin to stimulate glucose oxidation in adipocytes. Adipocytes were prepared from 120-g male Sprague–Dawley rats by previously published methods (7). Cells were incubated with 0.2–4 ng porcine insulin per milliliter or similar concentrations of Fm-I as determined by radioimmunoassay and the conversion of [^{14}C]glucose to $^{14}CO_2$ was determined by published methods (24). Figure 3 shows the results of a bioassay performed on the same Fm-I preparation studied in Figure 2. Fm-I stimulated the oxidation of glucose to CO_2 in a dose-dependent manner similar to native insulin, with biological activity essentially identical to the concentration of insulin determined by radioimmunoassay. This would suggest that immunologically active insulin was also accessible to the insulin receptor, and that any damage to or inactivation of insulin as a result of its linkage to ferritin was without effect on its biological activity. This finding is similar to previously published results with other selective modifications of insulin (25) at B-29 lysine.

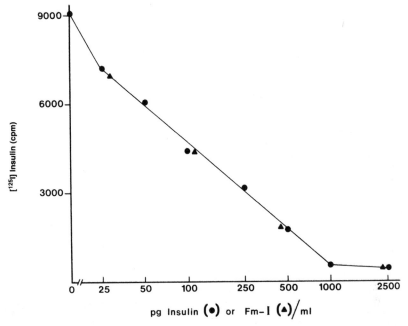

FIGURE 2. Determination of insulin concentration in monomeric ferritin-insulin by radioimmunoassay. The purified monomeric ferritin-insulin was serially diluted with RIA buffer. Aliquots of 200 μL were incubated in a final volume of 1 mL with 10^4 cpm [^{125}I]insulin in a standard insulin RIA. Porcine insulin was used as standards. The data showed that monomeric ferritin-insulin (▲) reacted in a dose-dependent manner identically to native porcine insulin (●). These data, when corrected for dilutions, showed that the insulin concentration in the monomeric ferritin-insulin was approximately 4.5 μg/mL.

The apparent molar ratio of ferritin to insulin (15:1) and the equivalent determination of immunological and biological activities of insulin suggest that few if any ferritin molecules contain more than one insulin molecule. The statistical probability of having more than one insulin linked to a ferritin is low when only 8 percent of the ferritin molecules contain insulin. Furthermore such conjugates would be difficult to detect by current assays. If multiple insulins were coupled to a single ferritin, the biological and immunological activities would not be expected to be equal. Thus the insulins would be readily accessible to the anti-insulin antibody, but only one insulin combined with the ferritin would bind to a receptor and cause a biological effect. The remaining insulin molecules on the ferritin would be unlikely to have access to a receptor due to steric inhibition by the ferritin molecule. This we have shown to be the case (13). Thus incubation of superactivated ferritin with insulin for 18 hr (instead of 6 hr) increased the amount of insulin coupled to ferritin with the result that the insulin determined immunologically was four times that determined biologically.

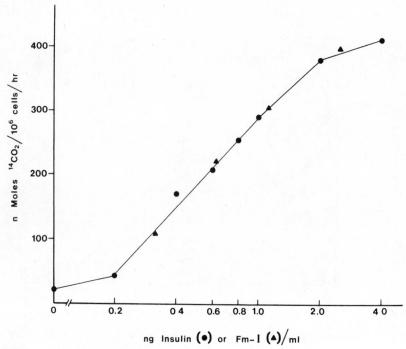

FIGURE 3.   Determination of the biological activity of monomeric ferritin-insulin in an adipocyte glucose oxidation assay. The monomeric ferritin-insulin preparation assayed in Figure 2 was diluted on the basis of the RIA results to appropriate concentrations and added to the reaction vessels. Porcine insulin standards were prepared and assayed simultaneously. The conversion of [^{14}C]glucose to $^{14}CO_2$ was determined by published methods (24). The results of this assay showed that monomeric feritin-insulin (▲) stimulated glucose oxidation in adipocytes in a dose-dependent manner identically to native porcine insulin (●) and that the biological activity of the conjugated hormone was identical to its immunological concentration.

2.5.   Specificity of Fm-I Binding to Insulin Receptors

The binding of Fm-I to the insulin receptor was directly assessed by comparing the competition of Fm-I or native insulin with [^{125}I]-labeled insulin for binding to receptors. Adipocytes, IM-9 lymphocytes, H4(IIEC3) cultured hepatoma cells, adipocyte plasma membranes, and liver plasma membranes were incurred with 0.4 ng/mL [^{125}I]-labeled insulin, prepared as described in ref. 26, in the presence of increasing concentrations of native insulin or Fm-I. Incubation conditions are given in detail in the legends to the figures. Receptor-bound insulin was determined by microfuge gradient centrifugation through 0.25 M sucrose in 0.05 M sodium phosphate buffer, pH 7.4, [IM-9s, H4(IIEC3)s, adipocytes, and liver plasma membranes] or by microfuge gradient centrifugation through dinonyl phthalate (adipocytes) as previously described (27). The results with cells are shown in Figures 4–6. As might have been expected from the biological activity assay, Fm-I competed with [^{125}I]insulin for binding to adipocyte insulin receptors in a dose-dependent manner identical to similar concentrations of native insulin. Similar data with isolated adipocyte plasma membranes have been published (13). The ultrastructural distribution pattern of insulin receptors was shown not to be significantly different on the various cell types (28). Thus, receptor sites on adipocytes are predominantly grouped, while receptors on liver membranes are present mostly as single sites. These differences might affect the binding of Fm-I to different tissues if ferritin interferes even slightly in the binding process. However, binding data thus far have indicated that Fm-I binding in all tissues studied was identical with native insulin.

2.6. Stability of the Conjugate and Reproducibility of the Method

To test the stability of the Fm-I, preparations were stored at 4°C for up to 6 months with no demonstrable loss of insulin activity or dissociation of the

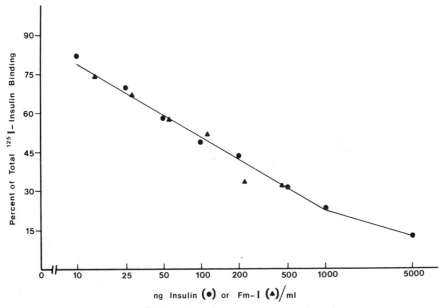

FIGURE 4. Comparison of monomeric ferritin-insulin and porcine insulin binding to IM-9 lymphocytes. IM-9 lymphocytes were incubated for 60 min at 15°C with 0.4 ng/mL [^{125}I]insulin and increasing concentrations of monomeric ferritin-insulin (▲) or porcine insulin (●). A 75-μl aliquot of the incubation mixture was layered over 300 μL 0.25 M sucrose in 10 mM sodium phosphate buffer and the cells pelleted in a microfuge. The pellets were counted to determine cell-associated [^{125}I]insulin. Nonspecific binding was determined in the presence of 25 μg/mL porcine insulin. The values reported represent specifically bound [^{125}I]insulin. These data show that monomeric ferritin-insulin competes with [^{125}I]insulin for binding to the IM-9 lymphocyte receptor almost identically to native porcine insulin.

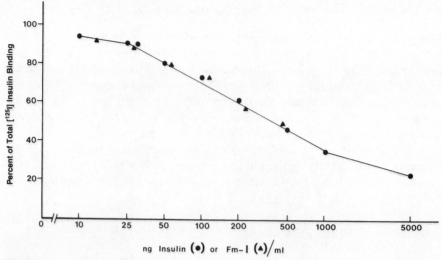

FIGURE 5. Comparison of monomeric ferritin-insulin and porcine insulin binding to H4(IIEC3) cultured hepatoma cells. HE(IIEC3) hepatoma cells were incubated for 60 min at 24°C with 0.4 ng/mL [125I]insulin and increasing concentrations of monomeric ferritin-insulin (▲) or porcine insulin (●). Total and specific binding of [125I]insulin was determined as described in Figure 4. The results indicate that monomeric ferritin-insulin is indistinguishable from porcine insulin in its ability to compete with [125I]insulin for binding to the IIEC3 hepatoma insulin receptor.

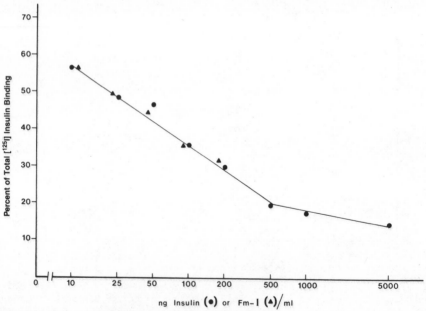

FIGURE 6. Comparison of monomeric ferritin-insulin and porcine insulin binding to rat adipocytes. Intact rat adipocytes were incubated for 30 min at 24°C with 0.4 ng/mL [125I]-insulin and increasing concentrations of monomeric ferritin-insulin (▲) or porcine insulin (●). A 300-μL aliquot of the incubation mixture was placed in a microfuge tube and then overlayered with 100 μL of dinonyl pthalate. The tubes were microfuged for 1 min and the cell layer cut from the microfuge tube for counting. Nonspecific binding in the presence of 25 μg/mL porcine insulin was subtracted from total binding. The results show that monomeric ferritin-insulin is indistinguishable from porcine insulin in its ability to compete with [125I]insulin for binding to rat adipocytes.

76

TABLE 2. Stability of Monomeric-Ferritin Insulin during Storage at 4°C

Elapsed Time from Preparation Date	Pellet	Supernatant
	(ng recovered)	
3 days	915.4 ± 26.6	4.2 ± 0.6
2 weeks	927.2 ± 17.0	2.7 ± 1.1
5 weeks	896.3 ± 16.5	3.2 ± 0.7
9 weeks	905.1 ± 12.2	4.6 ± 1.2
26 weeks	918.7 ± 18.8	2.9 ± 1.6

An aliquot of monomeric ferritin-insulin was ultracentrifuged at 40,000 rpm for 90 min after being stored for the indicated time period at 4°C. The supernatant was removed and the pellet resuspended to its original volume. Insulin concentrations of both the pellet and supernatant were determined by RIA, and the results expressed in terms of the total insulin recovered. The small amount of insulin activity found in the supernatants was probably due to incomplete sedimentation of the ferritin.

conjugate (Table 2). Aliquots were ultracentrifuged (as above) to sediment Fm-I, the supernatants were removed and saved, and pellets resuspended back to original volume. Insulin concentrations of both were determined by radioimmunoassay. The small amount of insulin present in the supernatants did not increase but remained virtually constant over 6 months, and was therefore attributed to a small amount of ferritin present which failed to sediment. Similar protocols were performed after incubating cells or membrane fractions with Fm-I, and the data (not shown) indicate that under incubation conditions insulin did not dissociate from the conjugate.

During the past 2 years at least 25 preparations of Fm-I have been made in our laboratory by a number of individuals. The results, provided the prescribed protocol was followed, have been very consistent as demonstrated in Table 3. Modifications, such as increasing the time of incubation of insulin with activated ferritin, have resulted in predictable differences (see above) (13).

TABLE 3. Reproducibility of the Preparation of Monomeric Ferritin-Insulin

Analysis	Mean	Range
Ferritin:Insulin (molar ratios)	15.2:1	10.2–17.1:1
Immunologic:Biologic (concentrations)	1:1	0.9–1.1:1
Recovery of insulin	0.10	0.094–0.112
Total insulin recovered (μg)	7.0	6.6–7.8

The above analyses have been made on 25 separate preparations of monomeric ferritin-insulin during the past 3 years. The results indicate that the current method has been highly reproducible.

3. ELECTRON MICROSCOPIC STUDIES

3.1. Estimation of Oligomer Contamination of Fm-I

In order to assess the relative purity of the Fm-I and the amount of contamination with oligomeric forms, Fm-I was diluted in deionized water with 0.1 percent bacitracin (added as a wetting agent) and applied to a carbon-coated formvar-coated 300-mesh copper grid. The samples were negatively stained with 2.5 percent ammonium molybdate in 2.0 percent ammonium acetate. The specimen was observed in a JEOL 100C × electron microscope and random areas of the specimen were photographed. The total number of ferritin particles and the number of closely aligned and probably oligomeric ferritin molecules were counted. These results were compared to those found for a similar dilution of cationic ferritin (Miles Laboratories Inc., Elkhart, IN) which is known to be entirely monomeric. Electron micrographs of Fm-I in Figure 7 and cationic ferritin (not shown) demonstrated that Fm-I was essentially identical in appearance to cationic ferritin. Quantitation of Fm-I demonstrated that the concentration of oligomeric ferritin was less than 3 percent of the total (data not shown).

3.2. Use of Fm-I to Localize Occupied Insulin Receptors

Incubation of various tissues with ferritin insulin has been described in detail elsewhere (7–12, 14–16, 18) and is outlined in the legends to subsequent figures. After incubation cells were washed by centrifugation through buffer

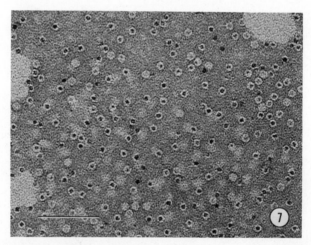

FIGURE 7. Electron micrograph of negatively stained monomeric ferritin-insulin. The lack of closely approximated ferritin particles, which would be observed with ferritin oligomers, indicates that the conjugate is virtually pure monomeric ferritin. Bar = 0.1 μm, magnification = 200,000.

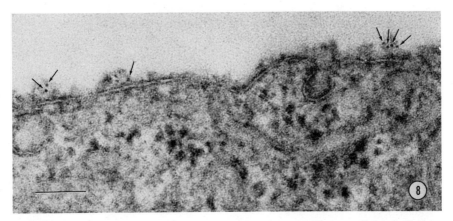

FIGURE 8. Electron micrograph of Fm-I receptor sites on intact rat adipocytes. Isolated adipocytes were prepared and incubated with 40 ng/mL Fm-I for 30 minutes at 37°C in Krebs–Ringer phosphate buffer, pH 7.4. The cells were washed and prepared for electron microscopy by previously published methods (8). The arrows indicate Fm-I molecules bound to the insulin receptor in the glycocalyx of the adipocyte plasma membrane. Insulin receptors were found predominantly in small groups on the rat adipocyte and these groups did not aggregate during prolonged incubation (9). Bar = 0.1 μm, magnification = 175,000.

and fixed with 2 percent glutaraldehyde in 0.1 *M* sodium cacodylate (membrane preparations) or in Krebs–Ringer phosphate buffer (intact cell preparations). The tissues were routinely postfixed in 2 percent OsO_4 in 0.1 *M* sodium cacodylate buffer, stained in block with uranyl acetate, and embedded in Spurr resin. Thin sections were stained with saturated alcohol-uranyl acetate and examined in the electron microscope. Fm-I receptor quantitation has been described in detail elsewhere (11).

Monomeric ferritin-insulin has been used to qualitatively and quantitatively determine the original distribution, microaggregation, and endocytosis of insulin receptors on a variety of cell types. A comprehensive review of those studies has been prepared (28). Our analyses have shown that there are significant differences in the native distribution of insulin receptors, both in terms of the location of the receptor sites relative to specialized structures such as microvilli and in terms of the organization of the receptor sites into groups of multiple receptors. Two cell types which demonstrate some of these differences are shown in Figures 8, and 9a,b. A number of studies have proven that insulin receptors on the rat adipocyte are normally grouped together and the groups are randomly distributed over the entire cell surface (9, 11, 12). The receptor sites do not aggegegate and are randomly endocytosed in smooth pinocytotic invaginations (15). Figure 8 demonstrates Fm-I binding to rat adipocytes.

In contrast to the rat adipocyte, the insulin receptors on the 3T3-L1 adipocyte are initially located on the microvillous projections of the cell and are found primarily as single or paired receptor sites (Fig. 9a). During incubation the insulin receptors appear to microaggregate and move to the cell surface where

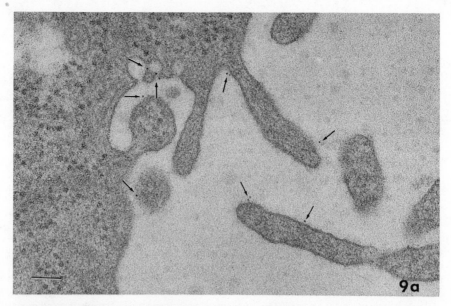

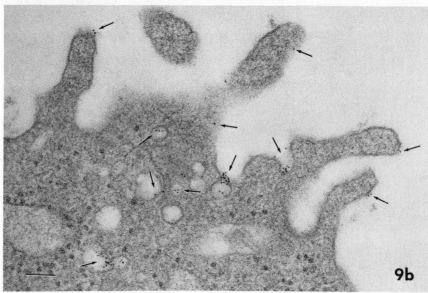

FIGURE 9. Electron micrograph of Fm-I receptor sites on 3T3-L1 adipocytes. One aliquot of 3T3-L1 adipocytes was prefixed with 0.1 percent glutaraldehyde for 15 min at 4°C, diluted with 10 volumes of Krebs–Ringer buffer with 50 m*M* Tris-HCl (to inactivate the excess glutaraldehyde) pelleted and resuspended. Both prefixed and normal cultured 3T3-L1 adipocytes were suspended Krebs–Ringer phosphate buffer, pH 7.4, and incubated with 40 ng/mL Fm-I for 30 min at 37°C. Cells were washed and prepared for electron microscopy by routine methods. The arrows indicate Fm-I molecules bound to insulin receptors on the microvilli and pinocytotic vesicles. Quantitative analysis of the receptor distribution on the prefixed cells indicated that most of the receptors are initially located on the microvilli as single or paired receptor sites as shown in Figure 9*a*. On the normal or unfixed cells shown in Figure 9*b*, the receptors microaggregate into small clusters and move to the intervillous cell surface and are endocytosed in pinocytotic invaginations (28). Bar = 0.1 μm, magnification = 100,000.

they concentrate in smooth pinocytotic invaginations and coated pits, as shown in Figure 9*b*. The observation of these differences in the ultrastructure of the insulin receptor is only part of a growing body of evidence that the insulin receptor may not be identical on all cell types. Monomeric ferritin-insulin, as well as other similar conjugates, provides a technique which should facilitate detailed investigation of insulin receptor dynamics on a variety of insulin responsive and resistant cell types.

REFERENCES

1. J. M. Olefsky, S. Marshall, P. Berhanu, M. Saekow, K. Heidenreich, and A. Green, *Metabolism* **31**, 670 (1982).

2. J. J. M. Bergeron, G. Levine, R. Sikstrom, D. O'Shaughnessy, B. Kopriwa, N. J. Nadler, and B. I. Posner, *Proc. Natl. Acad. Sci. USA* **74**, 5051 (1977).

3. J.-L. Carpentier, P. Gorden, M. Amherdt, E. van Obherghen, C. R. Kahn, and L. Orci, *J. Clin. Invest.* **61**, 1051 (1978).

4. M. Fehlmann, J.-L. Carpentier, A. LeCam, P. Thamm, D. Saunders, D. Brandenburg, L. Orci, and P. Freychet, *J. Cell Biol.* **93**, 82 (1982).

5. I. D. Goldfine, A. L. Jones, G. T. Hradek, K. Y. Wong, and J. S. Mooney, *Science* **202**, 760 (1978).

6. J. Schlessinger, Y. Schechter, M. C. Willingham, and I. Pastan, *Proc. Natl. Acad. Sci. USA* **75**, 2659 (1978).

7. L. Jarett and R. M. Smith, *J. Biol. Chem.* **249**, 7024 (1974).

8. L. Jarett and R. M. Smith, *Proc. Natl. Acad. Sci. USA* **72**, 3526 (1975).

9. L. Jarett and R. M. Smith, *J. Supramol. Struct.* **6**, 45 (1977).

10. D. M. Nelson, R. M. Smith, and L. Jarett, *Diabetes* **27**, 530 (1978).

11. L. Jarett and R. M. Smith, *J. Clin. Invest.* **63**, 571 (1979).

12. L. Jarett, J. B. Schweitzer, and R. M. Smith, *Science* **210**, 1127 (1980).

13. R. M. Smith and L. Jarett, *J. Histochem. Cytochem.* **30**, 650 (1982).

14. R. M. Smith and L. Jarett, *Proc. Natl. Acad. Sci. USA* **79**, 7302 (1982).

15. R. M. Smith and L. Jarett, *J. Cell. Physiol.* **115**, 199 (1983).

16. L. Jarett and R. M. Smith, *Proc. Natl. Acad. Sci. USA* **80**, 1023 (1983).

17. J. A. McKanna, H. T. Haigler, and S. Cohen, *Proc. Natl. Acad. Sci. USA* **76**, 5689 (1979).

18. J. L. Lubarsky and H. R. Behrman, *Mol. Cell. Endocrinol.* **15**, 61 (1979).

19. C. R. Hopkins and H. Gregory, *J. Cell Biol.* **75**, 528 (1977).

20. A. DiPasquale, J. M. Varga, G. Moellmann, and J. McGuire, *Anal. Biochem.* **84**, 37 (1978).

21. Y. Kishida, B. R. Olsen, R. A. Berg, and D. J. Prockop, *J. Cell Biol.* **64**, 3331 (1975).

22. A. F. Schick and S. J. Singer, *J. Biol. Chem.* **236**, 2477 (1961).

23. B. H. Frank, A. H. Pekar, and A. J. Veros, *Diabetes* **21** (suppl. 2), 486 (1972).

24. J. Gliemann, *Diabetologia* **3**, 382 (1967).

25. M. J. Ellis, S. C. Darby, R. H. Jones, and P. H. Sonksen, *Diabetologia* **15**, 403 (1978).

26. J. B. Schweitzer, R. M. Smith, and L. Jarett, *Proc. Natl. Acad. Sci. USA* **77**, 4692 (1980).

27. G. T. Hammons, R. M. Smith, and L. Jarett, *J. Biol. Chem.* **257**, 11563 (1982).

28. R. M. Smith and L. Jarett, in *Insulin, Its Receptor and Diabetes*, M. D. Hollenberg (ed.), Marcel Dekker, New York, in press.

F

INSULIN-SENSITIVE cAMP PHOSPHODIESTERASE

TETSURO KONO

Department of Physiology, School of Medicine, Vanderbilt University, Nashville, Tennessee

1. INTRODUCTION

Insulin stimulates low K_m cAMP phosphodiesterase in rat liver and adipocytes (1–5) by increasing the V_{max} without changing the K_m (2–4), which is approximately 0.3–0.5 μM (1, 2). The increase in the V_{max} of the adipocyte enzyme is approximately 2.5–3.0-fold when the enzyme activity is determined in a crude microsomal fraction (P-2) (5). General characteristics of this enzyme have been reviewed (6), and a possible mechanism of insulin action on this enzyme has been discussed (7). The following methods are based on the original work of Manganiello and Vaughan (2) and include subsequent modifications (8, 9). In this chapter the word *water* refers to either distilled or deionized water.

2. TREATMENT OF FAT CELLS AND PREPARATION OF FRACTION P-2

2.1. Principle

Freshly prepared rat epididymal adipocytes are exposed to insulin; the cells are washed and homogenized in 0.25 M sucrose at pH 7.0; a crude microsomal fraction (P-2) is prepared by differential centrifugation; and fraction P-2 is suspended in 0.25 M sucrose at pH 7.5.

2.2. Materials

1. Buffer A—Krebs-Henseleit. 4-(2-hydroxyl)-1-piperazineethanesulfonic acid (HEPES) buffer (pH 7.4) (10) supplemented with 20 mg/mL fraction V bovine serum albumin and 2 mM sodium pyruvate or D-glucose.

2. Isolated rat epididymal adipocytes. Prepare fresh cells by the collagenase method (11), and suspend them in buffer A at an approximate concentration of 50 mg/mL. One Sprague-Dawley rat weighing 180–230 g should supply enough cells for eight tests.

3. 100 nM zinc insulin. Dilute 100 μL of 1 μM stock insulin (in 3 mM HCl containing 0.154 M NaCl) with 400 μL of buffer A shortly before use.

4. Buffer B—0.25 M sucrose in 10 mM N-tris(hydroxymethyl)methyl-2-amino-ethanesulfonic acid (TES) buffer, pH 7.0. Keep this buffer refrigerated, and take out the amount needed approximately 10 min before use.

5. Buffer C—0.25 M sucrose in 10 mM TES buffer, pH 7.5. Keep refrigerated.

The methods described in this chapter have been tested and improved over a period of several years in collaboration with F. W. Robinson, J. A. Sarver, Dr. R. H. Pointer, Dr. P. M. de Buschiazzo, Dr. H. Makino, J. E. Jordan, T. Pate, and Dr. M. Ueda. This and most of our original manuscripts were typed by Ms. Patsy Barrett. Our original work cited above was supported by USPHS Grant 5RO1 AM 06725 from NIH.

2.3. Procedures

Place 2 mL portions of a pooled adipocyte suspension, approximately 50 mg/mL, in 25 mL polyethylene vials and incubate at 37°C with gentle shaking (approximately 10–20 strokes/min). At 5 min add 20 μL of 200 nM insulin to the "plus insulin" vials leaving the "basal" vials as controls. At 15 min decant each cell suspension into a 12 mL plastic conical centrifuge tube, rinse each vial with 1 mL of buffer B at approximately 13–15°C, and add the rinse to the main cell suspension. Then wash the cells twice by centrifugation (see below) using 4 mL portions of buffer B at approximately 13–15°C. The washing is carried out by brief centrifugation of the cell suspension (in an International Clinical Centrifuge for 30 sec at half-maximum acceleration; approximately 260g for 30 sec) followed by aspiration of the aqueous phase and resuspension of the cells in fresh buffer. Next suspend the washed cells in 5 mL of buffer B at approximately 13–15°C and homogenize them in a 7 mL Dounce tissue grinder with eight strokes of a type B pestle (the tighter one). Transfer each homogenate into a 15 mL Corex centrifuge tube, place the latter in a Beckman JA-20 rotor (or a similar one), and immediately start the centrifugation at 2°C for 15 min at an 11,000-rpm setting (approximately 14,500g_{max}). The time for centrifugation includes the acceleration period, but not the deceleration time. Decant the supernatant (with some solidifed fat) into a cold 15 mL Corex centrifuge tube and run the centrifuge for 30 min at 20,000 rpm (approximately 48,000g_{max}) at 2°C. Remove the supernatant by decantation and wipe off the remaining solution with 6-in.-long Q-tips. Add 1 mL of ice-cold buffer C to the pellet, scrape it off the glass wall with a plastic spatula, and homogenize the suspension by pumping it forcefully in and out of an Oxford pipette. Keep the final preparation (fraction P-2) in ice, or freeze it at −20°C, until ready for assay.

2.4. Comments

The insulin-dependent stimulation of phosphodiesterase can be observed in the cell homogenate, but the enzyme activity, both in the basal and plus insulin states, is more stable in fraction P-2 than in the cell homogenate. We routinely run the first centrifugation for 2 min in a Beckman J-21 centrifuge set at 20,000 rpm. However, results obtained by this method may vary depending on the acceleration rate. The dose-response curve of insulin action on phosphodiesterase is biphasic with the maximum at approximately 1–3 nM (5). The stimulation is completed within 10 min at 37°C (5). The action of insulin is ATP dependent (8), but the external energy source (pyruvate or glucose) may be omitted under normal conditions. The basal enzyme activity is significantly low when cells are homogenized in TES buffer at pH 7.0, instead of in Tris buffer at pH 7.4 or 7.5 (9); the plus insulin activity is unaffected (9). The plus insulin activity is considerably reduced when cells are homogenized in the presence of 1 mM EDTA or dithiothreitol (5). When cells are homogenized at 10°C or less, fat from adipocytes may partially solidify and stick to the container wall, thereby trapping a large fraction of membranes including the plasma membrane and endoplasmic reticulum (5). Our strategy is to wash and homogenize fat cells at 13–15°C and separate the membranes from the fat before the latter solidifies in the refrigerated centrifuge. Alternatively, a "fat-free" homogenate may be obtained by centrifuging the cell homogenate for 2 min at room temperature at approximately 650g. The enzyme in fraction P-2 is highly stable at 0°C in buffer C (pH 7.5). However, the catalytic domain of the enzyme is easily split off by proteolysis, e.g., when the intrinsic protease is activated with dithiothreitol (12). We found a batch of "enzyme grade" sucrose that contained enough proteolytic activity to split the enzyme during an overnight refrigeration (Kono, unpublished). The liver enzyme is readily split by the intrinsic proteinase when the enzyme preparation is washed with a hypotonic solution (13).

3. PHOSPHODIESTERASE ASSAY

3.1. Principle

First, a fraction of [^{3}H]cAMP is decomposed to [^{3}H]AMP by phosphodiesterase from adipocytes. Second, after the enzyme is denatured by heat, [^{3}H]AMP is totally converted into [^{3}H]adenosine by 5-nucleotidase in snake venom. Finally, [^{3}H]adenosine is separated from unreacted [^{3}H]cAMP by column chromatography on AG 1-X2 (Bio-Rad). This method was first successfully applied to the fat cell enzyme by Manganiello and Vaughan (2).

3.2. Materials

1.   Buffer D = 50 mM sodium-acetate buffer, pH 4.0, with 1 mg/mL fraction V bovine serum albumin. Divide the solution into 20 mL portions, and keep frozen at 20°C.

2.   Buffer E = 50 mM Tris-HCl buffer, pH 7.5, with 1 mg/mL fraction V bovine serum albumin. Divide the solution into 20 mL portions, and keep frozen.

3.   20 mM cAMP. Dissolve 66 mg cAMP into 10 mL buffer D (pH 4.0). The solution may be refrigerated for several weeks or kept frozen for a longer period.

4.   20 mM AMP. Dissolve 93 mg AMP (Na$_2$ · 4 H$_2$O; M = 463) into 10 mL buffer E (pH 7.5). The solution may be refrigerated for several weeks.

5.   10 μM cAMP. Dilute 0.5 mL of fresh or frozen 20 mM solution with 9.5 mL of buffer D (keep frozen).

6.   20 μCi/mL [^{3}H]cAMP in buffer D (pH 4.0). Dilute 0.1 mL of 1 mCi/mL [^{3}H] cAMP (ammonium salt, [2,8-^{3}H], 30–50 Ci/mmol in 1:1 ethanol) with 4.9 mL buffer D (keep frozen).

7.   Substrate mixture. Mix 1.8 mL water, 2.0 mL 0.1 M TES buffer (pH 7.5), 50 μL 10 μM cAMP in buffer D, 50 μL 20 μCi/mL [^{3}H] cAMP in buffer

D, and 100 μL 200 mM MgSO$_4$ in water. The solution should be prepared shortly before use and kept in ice. The total volume is 4.0 mL, which is enough for 19 tests (including blanks) and for preparation of a standard sample.

8. "Balanced" 0.1 N HCl and 0.1 N NaOH. Titrate approximately 0.1 N HCl and NaOH against each other, and dilute the more concentrated solution with a calculated amount of water.

9. 5 mM cAMP plus 5 mM AMP. Mix 1 mL 20 mM cAMP in buffer D, 1 mL 20 mM AMP in buffer E, and 2 mL water. The solution may be refrigerated for several weeks.

10. Snake venom. Dissolve 10 mg *Crotalus atrox* venom (from Sigma) in 10 mL 0.1 M Tris-HCl, pH 8.0. Divide the solution into 2 mL portions, and keep frozen.

11. 5 mM adenosine in 200 mM EDTA, pH 7.0–8.0. Suspend 5.8 g EDTA (free acid) in approximately 75 mL water; titrate the suspension with 5 and 1 N NaOH to pH 7–8; dissolve 134 mg adenosine; and fill up the solution to 100 mL. Keep the solution refrigerated.

12. AG 1-X2 columns (0.7 × 21 mm). We prepare the columns under the following standardized conditions. First, draw a line at 21 mm above the glass filter of Econo-Columns (0.7 × 4 cm; from Bio-Rad) (see Figure 1). Then

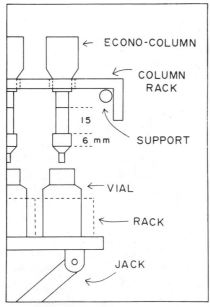

FIGURE 1. Column assembly for separation of [³H]adenosine from unreacted [³H]cAMP. Econo-Columns packed with AG 1-X2 in chloride form are inserted into the holes in a column rack; which is held at a proper height by two metal bars (although the cross section of only one bar is shown). Scintillation vials are inserted into a vial rack and placed on a Jiffy Jack, which is conveniently used to adjust the height of the vials.

insert the columns into the holes in a column rack; the one we use is Model CR-S (from Iso-lab), which has a total of 20 holes in two rows (the diameter of the holes are enlarged to accommodate Econo-Columns). Place an empty tray under the columns where vials are present in Figure 1. Fill the columns with water, tap them to eliminate air bubbles trapped in the glass filter, and close the bottom of the columns with caps. Add a slurry of AG 1-X2 (200– 400 mesh, chloride form from Bio-Rad) to the columns, and wait for 5 min. When the resin is mostly sedimented, remove the caps at the bottom and let the water drain. While the water is running, take out most of the resin plus water above the line marked on the column (see above) using an injection syringe fitted with a long needle. Add fresh water up to the rim of the columns, and scrape off the resin attached to the glass wall. Finally, when the sedimentation of the resin is completed, remove all the resin particles that are above the mark on the column.

3.3. Procedures

3.3.1. PHOSPHODIESTERASE ASSAY

Place 200 μL portions of the substrate mixture at the bottom of disposable test tubes (e.g., 16.8 × 95-mm polystyrene test tube from Sarstedt, No. 55-468), and put the latter in a water bath at 30°C. After approximately 2 min, add 50 μL of a phosphodiesterase preparation (fraction P-2; see Section 2) to the first test tube and start a stopwatch. Swirl the test tube and immediately put it back into a 30°C water bath. Add the rest of the enzyme preparations to the substrate mixture at 10-sec intervals. After exactly 5 min of incubation, stop the reaction by adding 100 μL of 0.1 N HCl and supplement the reaction mixture with 50 μL of 5 mM cAMP plus 5 mM AMP. Place a glass marble (which serves as a weight and a loose stopper) at the top of each test tube, and place all the test tubes at once in a water bath at 70–73°C for heat denaturation of phosphodiesterase. After 4 min move the test tubes to a room temperature water bath and keep them in there for 2 min. Neutralize the reaction mixture with 100 μL of 0.1 N NaOH and then add 50 μL of the snake venom solution. Place tight stoppers on the test tubes and incubate the latter for 20 min at 37°C. Terminate the reaction by adding 50 μL of the adenosine-EDTA solution and bring the test tubes to room temperature. Take out 500 μL of the final reaction mixture (which is now 600 μL) and apply it to the AG 1-X2 column (Fig. 1). After the solution is drained, rinse the inside of the column above the resin by adding 200, 200, and 300 μL portions of water in succession, letting the water completely drain after each addition. Now replace the water tray below the columns with scintillation vials as shown in Figure 1; elevate the jack until the bottom ends of the Econo-Columns are in the vials; and add 3 mL of water to each column for elution of [^{3}H]adenosine. When the 3 mL water is drained into the vial, fill the vial with 11 mL of ACS scintillation cocktail (from Amersham) or approximately 10 mL of any other cocktail miscible with water. Shake the mixture for 30 min (or manually shake vigorously and then leave 30 min without shaking) before the determination of radioactivity by the liquid scintillation counting method. For each set assayed, include two blank samples (50 μL buffer C). Prepare one or two standard preparations by adding 100 μL of the substrate mixture (12.5 pmol cAMP) and 3.9 mL water directly into a vial and mixing them with the scintillation cocktail.

3.3.2. PROTEIN ASSAY [by the Bradford Method (14)]

Place 100 μL of fraction P-2 (see Section 2) in a small disposable test tube (e.g., 12 × 55 mm, Sarstedt, No. 55-484). Add 1 mL of the "diluted" Bradford reagent (see below) to the test tubes, mix the solution with a vortex mixer, and measure the optical density of the mixture at 595 nm in 5–30 min. For the blank, use 100 μL of buffer C in place of the protein solution; and for the standard, use 10 μL of 1.2 mg/mL crystalline bovine serum albumin plus 90 μL of buffer C. Prepare the diluted Bradford solution by diluting the concentrated stock solution (from Bio-Rad) fourfold with water; filter the diluted solution and keep it at toom temperature. The glass cuvettes (or cells) stained with the Bradford solution should be rinsed twice with 0.5 mL methanol after each use.

3.3.3. COLUMN WASH

AG 1-X2 adheres strongly to glass walls. Therefore, we wash used Econo-columns by the following specific procedures. Hold the column upside down, and shoot out the resin into a bottle (see below) by applying compressed air at the bottom end of the column. Fill the column with tap water, and shoot out the water plus resin particles into the "radioactive" sink using compressed air as above. The columns should be almost free of the resin particles at this stage; repeat the above process if necessary. Then soak the columns with detergent (e.g., Micro) and make foams by scrubbing with a brush. Now inject tap water from the bottom end of the column; the last trace of resin particles will be carried away with the foam. Finally, wash the columns with deionized water. The used resin collected in a bottle (see above) may be regenerated by the standard method.

3.3.4. CALCULATION

Calculate the phosphodiesterase activity by Equation (1):

pmol cAMP decomposed/min/mL =

$$\frac{(\text{cpm of sample } - \text{ cpm of blank}) \times 60}{\text{cpm of standard}} \quad (1)$$

Estimate the protein concentration by Equation (2):

$$\mu g \text{ protein/mL} = \frac{(\text{OD of sample} - \text{OD of blank}) \times 120}{\text{OD of standard} - \text{OD of blank}} \tag{2}$$

Compute the specific activity (pmol/min/mg) from the values obtained by the above calculations.

3.4. Comments

All the reagents used in this assay are reasonably stable. However, [³H]cAMP slowly decomposes in the substrate mixture in the presence of Mg^{2+}. Nevertheless, the incubation time of the enzyme with the substrate mixture at 30°C may be increased from 5 min to 10 or 15 min, if necessary. Many samples can be analyzed in one assay set; however, we routinely handle eight enzyme preparations plus one blank in duplicates (18 samples in total). The decomposition of AMP by snake venom goes to completion; therefore, the reaction can be continued for more than 20 min (e.g., for 40 min) without any trouble. Although snake venom contains phosphodiesterase, it equally increases the radioactivity in the enzyme and blank samples. The water to be used for rinsing of resin-filled Econo-Columns should be kept in a specifically assigned container; the water would rapidly be contaminated with the resin particles that are inevitably brought in by the pipettes. Also, use specifically assigned pipettes for the handling of AG 1-X2 and for the addition of water to resin-filled columns. It is impossible to clean glass pipettes that are contaminated with AG 1-X2. Used glass scintillation vials can be conveniently washed with a "water fountain" and recycled, as described elsewhere (15).

REFERENCES

1. E. G. Loten and J. G. T. Sneyd, *Biochem. J.* **120**, 187–193 (1970).
2. V. Manganiello and M. Vaughan, *J. Biol. Chem.* **248**, 7164–7170 (1973).
3. B. Zinman and C. H. Hollenberg, *J. Biol. Chem.* **249**, 2182–2187 (1974).
4. E. G. Loten, F. D. Assimacopoulos-Jeannet, J. H. Exton, and C. R. Park, *J. Biol. Chem.* **253**, 746–757 (1978).
5. T. Kono, F. W. Robinson, and J. A. Sarver, *J. Biol. Chem.* **250**, 7826–7835 (1975).
6. S. H. Francis and T. Kono, *Mol. Cell. Biochem.* **42**, 109–116 (1982).
7. T. Kono, *Rec. Prog. Hormone Res.* **39**, 519–557 (1983).
8. T. Kono, F. W. Robinson, J. A. Sarver, F. V. Vega, and R. H. Pointer, *J. Biol. Chem.* **252**, 2226–2233 (1977).
9. F. V. Vega, R. J. Key, J. E. Jordan, and T. Kono, *Arch. Biochem. Biophys.* **203**, 167–173 (1980).
10. T. Kono and F. W. Barham, *J. Biol. Chem.* **246**, 6210–6216 (1971).

11. M. Rodbell, *J. Biol. Chem.* **239**, 375–380 (1964).

12. H. Makino, P. M. de Buschiazzo, R. H. Pointer, J. E. Jordan, and T. Kono, *J. Biol. Chem.* **255**, 7845–7849 (1980).

13. E. G. Loten, S. H. Francis, and J. D. Corbin, *J. Biol. Chem.* **255**, 7838–7844 (1980).

14. M. M. Bradford, *Anal. Biochem.* **72**, 248–254 (1976).

15. T. Kono and F. W. Robinson, *Anal. Biochem.* **63**, 592–594 (1975).

II

MEDIATORS AND METABOLIC METHODS

A

PHOTOAFFINITY LABELING OF ADIPOCYTE HEXOSE TRANSPORTERS

YOSHITOMO OKA AND MICHAEL P. CZECH

Department of Biochemistry, University of Massachusetts Medical Center, Worcester, Massachusetts

1. INTRODUCTION

Studies on hexose transport and its regulation in mammalian cells have classically relied on measurements of substrate flux across biological membranes of interest. Such flux measurements allow complex evaluations of apparent kinetic constants characteristic of the system under study. These experimentally obtained flux measurements and kinetic values have been extremely useful in providing insight into the molecular capabilities of hexose transport systems and about their regulation by insulin and other agents. Unfortunately, such kinetic parameters are not able to provide insight into the molecular structure of transport proteins, nor about their cellular locations and turnover rates. Because of these limitations, it has been necessary to develop more powerful technology designed to allow identification and characterization of membrane transporter structures. These considerations were the impetus for development of a hexose transporter photolabeling technique in our laboratory. The technique results in the covalent tagging of transporters with [3H]cytochalasin B, making identification of the transporter protein on dodecyl sulfate gels readily accomplished. This labeling procedure can be applied to hexose transporters in intact cells or isolated membrane fractions. We have succeeded in applying this photolabeling technique to hexose transporter identification in membranes from erythrocytes (1), adipocytes, and fibroblasts (2). The method is therefore effective in most, if not all, cell types. In this chapter we describe the technique as applied to the insulin-sensitive adipocyte.

2. PHOTOAFFINITY LABELING OF HEXOSE TRANSPORTERS IN ISOLATED MEMBRANE FRACTIONS FROM RAT ADIPOCYTES

The simplest system for photoaffinity labeling of hexose transporters involves the use of one or more isolated membrane fractions as starting material. The use of a broken cell system eliminates the problem of cell viability during the photolabeling reaction. The discoveries that insulin action in intact adipocytes leads to an apparent redistribution of hexose transporters from a low-density membrane fraction to a plasma membrane fraction (3, 4) necessitates that care be given to the particular membrane fraction being utilized. By carefully fractionating cells and applying the affinity labeling technique to the various membrane fractions, one can readily observe the apparent movement of labeled hexose transporters from a low-density microsome fraction to a plasma membrane fraction upon insulin treatment of the intact cells. The following procedures have been successfully utilized to achieve this goal.

2.1. Preparation of Isolated Membrane Fractions from Isolated Adipocytes

Fat cells are isolated from the epididymal fat pads of 140–170 g male rats (SD strain, Taconic Farms) by the method described by Rodbell (5). The fat pads are digested for 1 hr at 37°C in Krebs–Ringer phosphate buffer, pH 7.4, containing 3 percent bovine serum albumin (fraction V, Reheis Chemical Co.) and 1 mg/mL collagenase (Type I, Worthington Biochemical Co.). Isolated fat cells are then filtered through nylon chiffon and washed twice with the above buffer, and cells are incubated for 15 min at 37°C in the presence or absence of 2 mU/mL of insulin (porcine, Eli Lilly Co., Indianapolis, IN). The fat cells are rinsed twice with 10 mM Tris-HCl, 1 mM EDTA, 250 mM sucrose, pH 7.4 buffer, at room temperature and homogenized in the same buffer in a Potter–Elvejhem glass tissue homogenizer (capacity 55 mL) with Teflon pestle by 10 strokes using a Fisher Dyna-Mix stirrer at a setting of 7. All subsequent steps in the fractionation procedure are carried out at 4°C using this buffer unless otherwise noted.

Membrane fractions denoted as plasma membranes, high-density microsomes and low-density microsomes, are prepared by a differential centrifugation method described by McKeel and Jarett (6) and Cushman and Wardzala (3) with some modifications. Each homogenate is centrifuged at 12,000g for 15 min. The fat cakes are discarded and the supernatants saved for preparation of microsomal membranes. The pellets (plasma membranes, mitochondria, and nuclei) are resuspended, homogenized in a glass homogenizer by 10 strokes using a Fisher Dyna-Mix stirrer at a setting of 4, and centrifuged at 2500g for 10 min. The pellets containing primarily mitochondria and nuclei are discarded, while the resulting supernatants are recentrifuged at 28,000g for 30 min. These pellets containing the plasma membranes are resuspended in 2 mL of buffer (crude plasma membranes) and layered onto a discontinuous sucrose step gradient consisting of 10 mL each 55, 32, and 20 percent sucrose–water (w/w). The gradients are centrifuged at 104,000g (Beckman SW-28 rotor, 28,000 rpm) for 90 min and the 20–32 percent sucrose interphase is removed, diluted with 5 mM NaH$_2$PO$_4$, 1 mM EDTA, 250 mM sucrose, pH 7.4, and centrifuged at 146,000g for 1 hr before final resuspension of the plasma membranes in this buffer at approximately 2 mg protein/mL.

The 12,000g supernatant of cell homogenates previously obtained is centrifuged at 28,000g for 15 min to sediment the high-density microsomal membranes. The low-density microsome fraction is obtained by centrifuging the 28,000g supernatant at 146,000g for 1 hr, then resuspending in 5 mM NaH$_2$PO$_4$, 1 mM EDTA, 250 mM sucrose, pH 7.4, at a final concentration of 4–5 mg protein/mL. We use a 1 mL tuberculin syringe with 18g, 22g, and 27g needles in this order for final resuspension of the membrane fraction and obtain fine suspensions.

2.2. Photoaffinity Labeling of Transporters in Isolated Membranes

The methods of photoaffinity labeling of adipocyte hexose transporters are similar to those we have reported for labeling of hexose transporters in isolated membranes from human erythrocytes (1) or chicken fibroblasts (2). [^{3}H]cytochalasin B (10–15 Ci/mmol, New England Nuclear) in 100 percent ethanol is dried under nitrogen and resuspended in 5 mM NaH$_2$PO$_4$, 1 mM

EDTA, 250 mM sucrose, pH 7.4, at a concentration of 10 μM. The stock cytochalasin B solution is prepared daily just prior to use. The stock sugar solutions (D-glucose, 3-O-methylglucose, or D-sorbitol) are 2.7 M or 1.8 M. Membrane protein (500 μg), 500 mM D-glucose or D-sorbitol, and 0.5 μM [^{3}H]cytochalasin B are mixed well in a total volume of 500 μL in 1 cm pathlength quartz curvettes. Quartz curvettes are required instead of glass or plastic curvettes because the latter absorb UV light. After 30 min incubation at 4°C for equilibration of [^{3}H]cytochalasin B binding to membranes, samples are irradiated at 4°C twice for 5 sec each with a 1000-W Porta-Cure lamp (American Ultraviolet Co., PC-1421) at a distance of 18 cm. To attain the full intensity of the UV light, a 4 min warm-up period is required according to the literature of the company, but we actually warm the bulb for at least 20 min. The samples are mixed well between each irradiation and the reaction is stopped by shutting off the UV light with a metal shield. The samples are diluted with 2.5 mL of ice-cold 5 mM NaH$_2$PO$_4$, 1 mM EDTA, 250 mM sucrose, pH 7.4, and centrifuged at 115,000g (Beckman 40.3 rotor, 40,000 rpm) for 90 min, yielding pellets.

2.3. Sodium Dodecyl Sulfate Polyacrylamide Gel Electrophoresis of Photolabeled Samples

Pellets are resuspended with 150 μL of distilled water by using the ultrasonicator and then boiled for 2 min in the presence of 1 percent sodium dodecyl sulfate and 0.5 percent dithiothreitol in a total volume of 350 μL. They are electrophoresed on a 3 mm thick 10 percent polyacrylamide slab gel as described by Laemmli (7). The gel lanes are sliced into 1 mm wide strips with a Bio-Rad gel slicer and 0.5 mL of Protosol (New England Nuclear) is added to the gel slices, which are then shaken for several hours. The radioactivity in the gel slices is then monitored by adding 4 mL ACS or Econofluor (New England Nuclear) in a liquid scintillation spectrometer. Econofluor yields a better efficiency than ACS in this sytem.

The results of a typical experiment are shown in Figure 1. There are several labeled protein components, especially a large one near the dye front. With the exception of the labeled protein component of apparent Mr 46,000, none are inhibited by the presence of 500 mM D-glucose. Only this labeled protein component is increased in the plasma membrane fraction and decreased in the low-density microsomes in insulin-treated cells compared to controls (data not shown). The amount of the labeling in the Mr 46,000 protein component is approximately 0.3 pmol/mg low-density microsomes. When we compare this number with that reported as D-glucose-inhibitable cytochalasin B binding sites from Scatchard analysis of [^{3}H]cytochalasin B binding (3), we estimate that the efficiency of the photoaffinity labeling of transporters in isolated membranes is approximately 1 percent.

In order to obtain better efficiency of the labeling reaction, we have tried to irradiate the sample for much longer periods than a total of 10 sec. However, these maneuvers did not help because the radioactivity of the background also

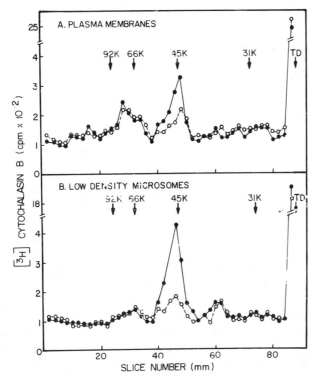

FIGURE 1. Photoaffinity labeling of isolated membrane fractions from control rat adipocytes. Plasma membranes and low-density microsomes were prepared from control rat adipocytes and photoaffinity labeled with 0.5 μM [³H]cytochalasin B in the presence of 500 mM D-sorbitol (●) or 500 mM D-glucose (○). Samples were then electrophoresed on a 10 percent sodium dodecyl sulfate polyacrylamide gel and incorporated [³H]cytochalasin B into protein was analyzed. See details in Section 2.1 to 2.3. Arrows depict the location of molecular weight markers. TD, tracking dye front.

increases under these conditions. When the concentration of [³H]cytochalasin B is increased (e.g., 1 or 2 μM), the absolute amount of the labeling increases; however, the percentage of inhibition of the labeling by 500 mM D-glucose decreases, probably because the binding of cytochalasin B to transporters is saturated. A method to improve the efficiency of labeling involves applying the membrane samples onto small plastic culture dishes (diameter, 32 mm) and irradiating from above, analogous to photoaffinity labeling of transporters in intact cells (see Section 3). This technique improves the efficiency of hexose transporter labeling approximately two- to threefold.

The chemical nature of the photoaffinity labeling of [³H]cytochalasin B to hexose transporters is not yet known. One possibility is that [³H]cytochalasin B itself is photoactivated by UV light and covalently inserts into the transporter. Using several kinds of glass filters (data not shown), we found that UV light with wavelengths of 260–320 nm is sufficient for affinity labeling of hexose transporters. Tryptophan and tyrosine are known to absorb UV light near 280 nm. Therefore, it is possible that tryptophan and/or tyrosine residues of the transporter near or on the cytochalasin B binding site is photoactivated and covalently bound to [^{3}H]cytochalasin B. This issue requires further investigation for clarification.

3. PHOTOAFFINITY LABELING OF HEXOSE TRANSPORTERS IN INTACT FAT CELLS

The method for labeling hexose transporters in intact cells is similar to that described for photoaffinity labeling in isolated membranes (Section 2.2), but there are several important modifications. [^{3}H]cytochalasin B (10–15 Ci/mmol; New England Nuclear) in 100 percent ethanol is dried under nitrogen and resuspended in Krebs–Ringer phosphate buffer, pH 7.4. 1.8 mL of fat cell suspension (3–3.5 × 10^6 cells/mL) is placed onto a plastic dish (diameter, 50 mm) and incubated at the indicated temperature with 0.5 μM [^{3}H]cytochalasin B and 10 μM unlabeled cytochalasin D, which has much less affinity for hexose transporters, in the presence or absence of 3-O-methylglucose for the indicated period. The samples (final volume, 2 mL) are then irradiated three times for 10 sec each with a 1000-W Porta-cure lamp (American Ultraviolet Co.) through a glass color filter (Farrand Optical Co., no. 7-54) which transmits only UV light from 260 to 400 nm at a distance of 26 cm. Cells are mixed well between each irradiation period. Irradiated cells are put in a prechilled glass homogenizer containing 25 mL of 10 mM Tris-HCl, 1 mM EDTA, 250 mM sucrose, pH 7.4 buffer, and homogenized as described in Section 2.1.

Irradiation through the glass color filter is necessary to maintain cell viability due to the harmful effects of other wavelengths of light emitted by the mercury lamp. The presence of 10 μM unlabeled cytochalasin D is required to prevent [^{3}H]cytochalasin B incorporation into actin (apparent Mr, 43,000) and other nontransport proteins (data not shown). The presence of 10 μM cytochalasin D does not affect the incorporation of 0.5 μM [^{3}H]cytochalasin B into transporters (data not shown).

Homogenates are centrifuged at 12,000g for 15 min, yielding a pellet which is used as a crude plasma membrane fraction without further purification. The reason for omitting further purification steps is that such steps lead to a significant loss of labeled transporters, making it difficult to compare quantitatively the transporters among different membrane fractions. The supernatant is centrifuged at 146,000g for 60 min, yielding a pellet of microsomes. In order to separate microsomes into low- and high-density microsomes, the 12,000g supernatant is centrifuged at 28,000g for 15 min, yielding a pellet of high-density microsomes. The resulting supernatant is recentrifuged at 146,000g for 1 hr, yielding a pellet of low-density microsomes. Analysis by SDS-PAGE and counting the incorporated radioactivity are performed as described in Section 2.3.

The results from an experiment where cells were preincubated with or without

100 mM 3-O-methylglucose for 30 min at 37°C and then irradiated with 0.5 μM [^{3}H]cytochalasin B and 10 μM unlabeled cytochalasin D are shown in Figure 2. Only the labeling of the apparent Mr 46,000 protein component is inhibited both in the plasma membranes and microsomes by the presence of 100 mM 3-O-methylglucose. When insulin-treated cells are irradiated, the labeling of the Mr 46,000 protein is increased approximately twofold in the plasma membranes and decreased by nearly 50 percent in microsomes (data not shown). The magnitude of these effects of insulin are consistent with previous reports showing membrane redistribution of hexose transport activity (4) or [^{3}H]cytochalasin B binding activity (3) in response to insulin. No significant change in cell number or passive diffusion of 3-O-methylglucose was found after irradiation, indicating that cell integrity is maintained under these experimental conditions. Furthermore, when control intact adipocytes are irradiated first, and then treated with insulin, the labeled protein component of apparent Mr 46,000 increases in the plasma membranes and decreases in the microsomes, demonstrating that the affinity-labeled transporters remain responsive to insulin (data not shown).

3.1. Determination of Cellular Disposition of Hexose Transporters

An important contemporary hypothesis on the regulation of hexose transport activity by insulin involves the concept that sequestered or intracellular hexose transporters are mobilized or exposed on the cell surface by the regulatory agent. Thus, it is of great interest to have an experimental tool that will differentiate hexose transporters that are exposed to the extracellular medium on

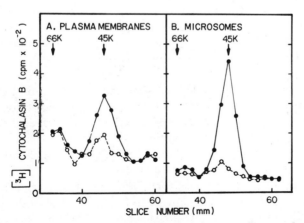

FIGURE 2.   Photoaffinity labeling of hexose transporters in intact rat adipocytes. Isolated adipocytes in Krebs–Ringer phosphate buffer containing 3 percent bovine serum albumin were incubated for 30 min at 37°C with 0.5 μM [^{3}H]cytochalasin B and 10 μM cytochalasin D in the presence (○) or absence (●) of 100 mM 3-O-methylglucose. Cells were then irradiated and homogenized and incorporated [^{3}H]cytochalasin B into protein was analyzed as described in Section 3.

the cell surface versus those that are sequestered and unexposed to the extracellular fluid. We have recently developed methodology using the photoaffinity labeling technique that allows the investigator to distinguish between exposed and unexposed hexose transporters. The strategy we employ involves the use of the D-glucose analogue ethylidene glucose which penetrates cells very poorly. Ethylidene glucose has the important properties of (i) inhibiting D-glucose transport activity, (ii) inhibiting [³H]cytochalasin B binding to hexose transporters, and (iii) having little or no capacity to be transported by the hexose transporters that it inhibits such that it penetrates cells extremely poorly. Thus, following incubation of cells with this glucose analogue for an appropriately brief period of time, cells would be exposed to medium concentrations of the hexose at their cell surface and little or no hexose in the intracellular compartment. If the intracellular concentration of this hexose were low enough to be incapable of affecting inhibition of the photolabeling reaction, hexose transporters in this cellular compartment would be labeled without interference from the competing hexose. In contrast, hexose transporters on the cell surface that are exposed to the medium concentration of ethylidene glucose would be inhibited in their photolabeling by [³H]cytochalasin B.

We have been able to develop methodology that fulfills the criteria of the experimental strategy described above. Intact adipocytes incubated with 50 mM ethylidene glucose for 1 min at 15°C results in the accumulation of 2 mM ethylidene glucose intracellularly. This concentration of hexose (2 mM) has no effect on the photoaffinity labeling reaction using 0.5 μM [³H]cytochalasin B, either in isolated membranes or in intact adipocytes (data not shown). Association of 0.5 μM [³H]cytochalasin B to transporters in intact fat cells was completed within 1 min at 15°C, and inhibition by the ethylidene glucose of [³H]cytochalasin B binding to transporters in isolated low-density microsomes was also rapid and completed within 1 min at 15°C (data not shown). Thus, in order to distinguish between hexose transporters that are exposed to the extracellular medium and those that are in an unexposed disposition, experimental conditions of the photolabeling reaction are utilized as described in Section 3 except that the combination of ethylidene glucose (50 mM) and 0.5 μM [³H]cytochalasin B are added together and incubated for 1 min at 15°C prior to irradiation. Such cells are compared to the condition where the [³H]cytochalasin B and 50 mM D-sorbitol are added. Unlabeled 10 μM cytochalasin D is present in both conditions. The plasma membrane and low-density microsome membranes are then prepared from the photolabeled cells according to the methods described previously.

Validation of the technique described for distinguishing sequestered versus exposed hexose transporters is depicted in Figure 3. Most of the transporters in control cells reside in the low-density microsome fraction, as previously reported (3, 4). The hexose transporters in this fraction are photolabeled without interference by the ethylidene glucose added to the medium (Fig. 3B). These data are consistent with the observation that the low-density microsome fraction is associated with enzyme markers that appear to be Golgi in origin (4, 8). In

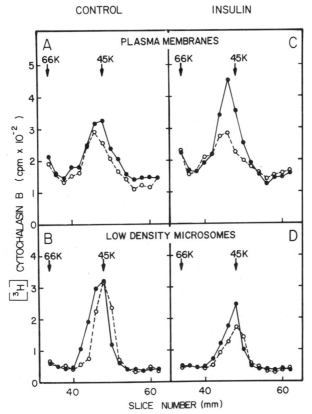

FIGURE 3. Effect of 1 min incubation with 50 mM ethylidene glucose on the photoaffinity labeling in control (left) and insulin-treated cells (right). Isolated adipocytes were incubated in Krebs–Ringer phosphate buffer containing 3 percent bovine serum albumin with (right-side panel) or without (left-side panel) 2 mU/mL insulin for 15 min at 37°C, then 10 μM cytochalasin D was added. Cells were then incubated with 0.5 μM [³H]cytochalasin B and 50 mM sorbitol (●) or 50 mM ethylidene glucose (○) for 1 min at 15°C and irradiated. After irradiation, cells were homogenized and the labeled protein analyzed in membrane fractions as described in Section 3.

contrast, insulin action in these cells results in the redistribution of transporters to the plasma membrane fraction where they are clearly inhibited in their photolabeling by the ethylidene glucose (Fig. 3C). The apparent exposure of hexose transporters in the plasma membrane fraction to the medium ethylidene glucose is consistent with the observation that the plasma membrane fraction is associated with 5′-nucleotidase activity (3, 4, 8). Thus, the data generated using this strategy are consistent with the hypothesis that insulin action is associated with the transition of hexose transporters from a sequestered to an exposed cellular location. It should be noted that our experience indicates that this method is not reliable for assessing the low amounts of transporters in the plasma membrane fraction of control cells or the low-density microsomes of insulin-treated cells. This problem is probably related to the fact that significant contamination of one membrane fraction by membranes of the other fraction leads to equivocal results when low numbers of transporters are present.

4. CONCLUSIONS

The methodology and validating data presented in this chapter demonstrate the utility of photolabeling techniques as applied to hexose transporters in insulin-sensitive adipocytes. Three distinct objectives can be attained using this methodology. First, identification of the [^{3}H]cytochalasin B binding component of the adipocyte hexose transporter can be readily achieved by photolabeling isolated membrane fractions from these cells. The apparent molecular weight of 46,000 that is obtained for the hexose transporter by this method agrees well with that obtained using antibodies against the red cell hexose transporter that cross-react with the adipocyte transport protein (9). Second, the adipocyte hexose transporter can be affinity labeled in intact, viable adipocytes. Subsequent to affinity labeling, the transporter retains its ability to respond to insulin by redistributing from the low-density microsomes to the plasma membrane fraction. Last, under certain conditions it is possible to distinguish between those transporters that reside in exposed positions on the cell surface and those that are sequestered or exist in the intracellular space. This latter technology may prove useful in further characterizing the membrane transformations that occur in response to the regulatory actions of insulin.

REFERENCES

1. C. Carter-Su, J. E. Pessin, R. Mora, W. Gitomer, and M. P. Czech, *J. Biol. Chem.* **257**, 5419 (1982).
2. J. E. Pessin, L. G. Tillotson, K. Yamada, W. Gitomer, C. Carter-Su, R. Mora, K. J. Isselbacher, and M. P. Czech, *Proc. Natl. Acad. Sci. USA* **79**, 2286 (1982).
3. S. W. Cushman and L. J. Wardzala, *J. Biol. Chem.* **255**, 4758 (1980).
4. K. Suzuki and T. Kono, *Proc. Natl. Acad. Sci. USA* **77**, 2542–2545 (1980).
5. M. Rodbell, *J. Biol. Chem.* **239**, 375 (1964).
6. D. W. McKeel and L. Jarett, *J. Cell Biol.* **44**, 417 (1970).
7. U. K. Laemmli, *Nature (London)* **227**, 680 (1970).
8. C. L. Oppenheimer, J. E. Pessin, J. Massague, W. Gitomer, and M. P. Czech, *J. Biol. Chem.* **258**, 4824 (1983).
9. T. J. Wheeler, I. A. Simpson, D. C. Sogin, P. C. Hinkle, and S. W. Cushman, *Biochem. Biophys. Res. Commun.* **105**, 89 (1982).

B

GLUCOSE TRANSPORT
AND METABOLISM
IN THE ADIPOCYTE

JØRGEN GLIEMANN
Institute of Physiology, University of Aarhus, Aarhus, Denmark

1. INTRODUCTION

Rodbell (1) was the first to prepare isolated rat adipocytes. He showed that the cells metabolize glucose and that this process is markedly enhanced by insulin. The present chapter will describe procedures for cell preparation and for measuring hexose transport and metabolism. The methods are designed for rat adipocytes but may, with minor modifications, be applied to adipocytes from other mammals. For preparation and handling of human adipocytes see refs. (2, 3).

The transport system of the adipocyte can exist in two extreme states: a "basal" and a maximally stimulated state. The latter is brought about by insulin at a maximally stimulating concentration and is well defined in the sense that the permeability of the cell membrane to a given hexose only varies little from cell batch to cell batch. Under these conditions most of the hexose transporters of the adipocyte are operational in the plasma membrane (4, 5). The basal state prevails when the cells are suspended in a buffered salt solution in the absence of stimulatory or inhibitory agents. Under these conditions most of the hexose transporters appear to reside in another cellular compartment other than the plasma membrane (4, 5). This state is less well defined since a number of nonhormonal treatments, and even mechanical trauma, may activate the hexose transport system (6, 7). For this reason it is essential to prepare the adipocytes as gently as possible. A good cell preparation should give about a 10-fold stimulation (or more) using insulin at a maximally stimulating concentration.

Insulin causes a dose-dependent increase in glucose uptake of each single adipocyte (8), and this seems largely explained by a dose-dependent translocation of transporters (4, 5). Several hormones (e.g., catecholamines, growth hormone) and numerous pharmacological agents also cause dose-dependent enhancements of glucose transport and metabolism. Such effects are difficult to study if basal transport is already elevated. This again stresses the importance of a good cell preparation.

2. PREPARATION OF ADIPOCYTES

2.1. Materials

1. Male rats weighing 140–200 g and fed *ad libitum*.

2. Thirty-mL plastic beakers, approximately 60×27 mm with a smooth and even bottom (e.g., NUNC, Kamstrup, Denmark, Catalog No. 536455; "bump" in the bottom may have to be removed).

3. Smooth 5×15-mm Teflon stir bar.

4. Nylon mesh with approximately 300-μm mesh size (e.g., Polyman, PES 300, Schweizerische Seidengazefabrik; AG, Zürich).

5. Round-bottom plastic tubes, approximately 17×100 mm (14 mL) (e.g., Greiner Laborteknik, Switzerland, Catalog No. 187301).

6. Collagenase [e.g., Worthington type I (CLS)].

7. Albumin (e.g., Sigma, bovine serum albumin, fraction V; Catalog No. A4503).

8. HEPES [4-(2-hydroxyethyl)-piperazinethanesulfonic acid] and salts, analytical grade.

9. A 37°C water bath and magnetic stirrer. It is convenient to use a magnetic stirrer with several magnets driven by the same motor. We use the following combination: Water bath 01 T 443 and magnetic stirrer MA 6 VS (both from Heto, Birkerød, Denmark). Six beakers, each with two "standard" fat pads, can be stirred simultaneously at 37°C.

2.2. Buffers

The composition (in mM) of the incubation buffer is as follows: Na^+, 134; K^+, 4.7; Ca^{2+}, 2.5; Mg^{2+}, 1.25; Cl^-, 141; $HPO_4^{2-}/H_2PO_4^-$, 2.5; SO_4^{2-}, 1.25; HEPES, 10, and albumin as required, usually 0.5–5 percent (w/v).

The buffer is conveniently prepared from the following stock solutions:

2.2.1. ALBUMIN

To prepare a 10 percent (w/v) albumin solution, dissolve 100 g bovine serum albumin in 500 mL of distilled water. Let stand overnight at 4°C. Pour the solution into dialysis tubing (e.g., Visking, width 27/32 in.) which has been soaked in distilled water. Dialyze against 5 L of distilled water for about 12 hr at 4°C, with two changes of distilled water. Empty the dialysis tubing and adjust the volume to 1 L. Filter first through paper (e.g., Whatman No. 41) and then through a 0.8-μm Millipore filter. Keep the solution cold during these procedures. Adjust pH. Store at $-20°C$ in convenient aliquots. Can be stored for 1 year or more.

2.2.2.   "Mixed Salts" ($10\times$ concentrated)

Weigh out 76.74 g NaCl, 3.51 g KCl, 3.06 g MgSO$_4$, 7H$_2$O, 3.63 g CaCl$_2$2H$_2$O, and dissolve in 1 L distilled water, free of pyrogens and bacterial contaminations. May be stored for 2 weeks at 4°C.

2.2.3.   "Buffer" ($10\times$ concentrated)

Weigh out 23.8 g HEPES and 3.42 g NaH$_2$PO$_4$·H$_2$O and dissolve in 1 L of water. Adjust to pH 7.4 at 37°C (equals 7.6 at 20°C). May be stored for 2 weeks at 4°C.

The buffer is prepared by mixing the albumin solution (plus water to give the required final albumin concentration) and "mixed salts" followed by "buffer."

2.3.   Comments to Materials and Buffers

Male rats are usually chosen because the epididymal fat pad is a suitable source of tissue. Parametrial fat from female rats may also be used and retroperitoneal fat from both sexes. Younger rats may also be used, but the yield of fat cells is small. The fat cells become more fragile when the rats get older and more obese (weight > 200 g).

HEPES has been found to be a suitable buffer. The pK is 7.4 at 37°C (9) and 10 mM is enough, at least around this pH. It should also be noted that albumin provides a considerable buffer capacity. Krebs–Ringer bicarbonate buffer (25 mM HCO$_3$) is also suitable, but one has to make sure that the buffer is always equilibrated with the correct gas phase (5 percent CO$_2$ for pH 7.4 at 37°C).

For preparation of fat cells (collagenase buffer) use Krebs–Ringer HEPES buffer containing 3.5 percent w/v bovine serum albumin, 0.5 mM glucose, and 0.5 mg/mL collagenase, pH 7.40, at 37°C. The collagenase buffer may be stored at $-20°C$ in the plastic beakers for 4 weeks.

For wash and incubation, use the same buffer (without collagenase) but adjust the albumin concentration and pH according to the particular requirements of the experiment.

2.4.   Procedure

1.   Decapitate the rat, remove the skin using one pair of scissors (dirty), and open the abdominal cavity with another. Displace testis to the abdominal cavity. Hold epididymis with a pair of tweezers and remove the epididymal fat pad by cutting (small scissors) in the angle between the vessel and the pad. Remove the fat pad gently and without crushing the tissue.

2.   Place the two pads in one 30-mL flat-bottom beaker containing 3 mL collagenase buffer and a stir bar. Make sure that the buffer is at least 25°C. The tissue may be minced using scissors, but the mincing should be quite coarse (1–2 mm-cubes).

3.   Place the beaker with the stir bar in the water bath at 37°C and start stirring. "Correct" stirring is essential but it is difficult to quantitate the speed since this is dependent on the geometry of beaker and stir bar. Make sure that the stir bar is well centered and does not hit the side of the beaker. Use the minimum speed, which disintegrates the tissue in 60 min. Incubate for about 45 min, that is, until the tissue is about 90 percent disintegrated. Keep an eye on the suspension. The timing may vary slightly from one batch of collagenase to another. Shaking may be used instead of stirring. In that case it is usually necessary to use about 100 cpm. Again, use the minimum mechanical treatment that disintegrates the tissue in about 60 min using 0.5 mg/mL crude collagenase.

4.   Shape the nylon mesh as a funnel (clip) and place it over the 14 mL round-bottom tube. Remove the stir bar from the beaker, shake the contents by hand, and pour the cells through the filter followed by a few milliliters of wash buffer. About 2 g of cells can be accommodated in one tube.

5.   Allow the cells (from up to four rats) to float for about 1 min and remove the infranatant, including sedimented debris, using a 14-gauge 12-cm needle. Add 10 mL of buffer, turn the tube *gently*, and remove the infranatant. Repeat this procedure three times.

6.   The packed-cell volume in this concentrated cell suspension is now measured. (It should be 40–45 percent.) Shake the suspension by hand; quickly fill a capillary tube (use suction) and seal and centrifuge for 1 min in a hematocrit centrifuge. The trapped extracellular buffer will be about 4 percent of the volume of packed cells.

7.   Dilute the cells with incubation buffer to the required cell concentration in terms of packed-cell volume.

2.5.   Testing the Cell Preparation

2.5.1.   THE PHYSICAL APPEARANCE

Watch the cells when they have been filtered through the nylon mesh and during the subsequent washings. They should float easily and should not adhere to the sides of the tube. There should be no large oil droplets on the surface of the suspension. After centrifugation in the hematocrit tube, the packed cells should be uniformly opaque and with only a thin film of oil on the top.

2.5.2.   MICROSCOPY

According to our experience, one cannot infer much more about the cell function from microscopy than from the gross physical appearance of the preparation. The nuclei should be easily stainable with methylene blue. The number of lipid droplets should, of course, be minimal, but some are always present. Dye exclusion using trypan blue seems of little value. Counting and sizing the cells is essential for the conversion from packed cell volume to cell number. This may be done on fresh preparations (6, 10, 11) or on osmium fixed cells (12, 13). The latter procedure is perhaps the most convenient because it can be carried out when the experiment is finished. As a rule of thumb the average cell volume is 100 pL, but this number is markedly dependent on the size and the nutritional condition of the animal.

3. MEASUREMENT OF HEXOSE TRANSPORT

The method was originally described by Whitesell and Gliemann (14). For bibliography and kinetic data see ref. 15.

3.1. Materials

1. 17 × 100-mm round-bottom plastic tubes (see step 5 in Section 2.1).

2. 11 × 50-mm round-bottom plastic tubes (e.g., minivials, Hansac, Hasselager, DK 8361).

3. Automatic pipettes (must not leak).

4. Albumin free buffer containing the transported hexose, for instance, 3-O-[^{14}C-methyl]-D-glucose.

5. 0.3 mM phloretin in 0.9 percent NaCl. This stopping solution is prepared by dissolving 137 mg phloretin in 500 μL DMSO, 1160 μL ethanol followed by dilution 1:1000 in 20°C 0.9 percent NaCl. It is important to add the phloretin stock solution dropwise to a vigorously stirring NaCl solution.

6. Silicone oil, density 0.99, viscosity 100 centistokes.

7. 550 μL polypropylene microfuge tubes (e.g., Milian, Switzerland, PAT-22).

8. Scalpel blade mounted onto a wrench (e.g., Bacho 222, 0–20 mm).

9. Metronome set at 120 beats/min.

3.2. Procedure

Experiments at physiological temperature are best carried out in a 37°C room if a rapidly transported sugar such as 3-O-methylglucose is used and the transport system is maximally stimulated. The reason is that incubations under these conditions should be carried out for 1–2 sec for measurements approximating the initial velocity of influx. However, a water bath can be used if one works rapidly.

For measurement of transport of 3-O-[^{14}C-methyl]glucose at a tracer concentration, proceed as follows:

1.   Place a 12 μL drop of albumin-free buffer containing 10^5 cpm of the tracer in a small tube. The 12 μL should be centered in the bottom of the tube.

2.   Add 1.0 mL 40.0 percent (v/v) cell suspension to a large tube.

3.   Shake the cell suspension by hand, quickly remove 40 μL and shoot it onto the 12 μL isotope buffer on "beat one." The other hand holds an automatic pipette with 3 mL stopping solution.

4.   Place the tip containing the stopping solution about 1 cm from the cell droplet on the side of the tube. Release on "beat 3" for 1 sec. The trick is to get the "front" of the stopping solution onto the cell suspension at the right time. The rest of the 3 mL serves as a large dilution volume.

5.   Add quickly (but do not splatter) 0.5 mL silicone oil on top of the phloretin solution and centrifuge for 40 sec at about 2000g in a rapidly accelerating centrifuge provided with a brake. Handle only two to four tubes at a time.

6.   Remove the cell pellet from the top of the silicone oil, for instance, using a bent piece of a pipe cleaner. The cells should coalesce in one pellet. Cells from a partially damaged preparation scatter around the rim of the tube. This procedure should be carried out within about 30 min after the centrifugation.

7.   Assay for radioactivity in a scintillation fluid miscible with water. It is convenient to use minivials.

Alternatively, proceed through step 4 above but stop by using 400 μL phloretin solution. Then:

8.   Suck 400 μL back from the 452 μL cell suspension and add this to a 550 μL polypropylene microfuge tube filled with 100 μL silicone oil.

9.   Centrifuge for 30 sec in a microfuge at about 10,000g, cut the tube through the oil layer using the scalpel blade mounted on the wrench, and assay the cell pellet for radioactivity.

3.3. Comments on Measurement of Hexose Transport

Measure zero-time uptake (extracellularly trapped buffer) by adding first a drop of phloretin solution, then isotope, and finally the rest of the phloretin solution. Measure infinite-time uptake (equilibrium distribution space for 3-O-methylglucose) by incubation for 10 min. The calculated space should be nearly the same (about 2 μL/100 μL packed cells) after incubation for 10, 20, and 30 min. If this is not the case, the cells may metabolize a trace contaminant of the hexose analogue and this should be purified, for instance, by paper chromatography.

The uptake of 3-O-methylglucose at a tracer concentration is approximately exponential with a half-time of 2–4 sec in maximally stimulated cells. The initial velocity of uptake (i.e., net influx) may therefore be calculated using early time points. For details, see ref. 15. Uptake-zero for 2 sec underestimates the initial velocity by about 30 percent in maximally stimulated cells.

The hexose transport system will become progressively saturated at higher 3-O-methylglucose concentrations and the K_m is about 4 mM. Equilibrium exchange of this hexose analogue is measured by adding unlabeled sugar at the same concentration to the isotope-containing solution and to the cell suspension. The cells should equilibrate for 30–60 min—the longer, the higher the methylglucose concentration. The uptake curve is exponential at any 3-O-methylglucose concentration under equilibrium exchange conditions.

The net uptake from the extracellular to the intracellular compartment (zero-trans entry) is measured by adding the sugar analogue to the isotope solution only (note that its concentration will decrease to one-third when mixed with the cell suspension). The uptake (or progress) curve is nonexponential ("flat") under zero-trans entry conditions (14, 15). The transport system appears to be kinetically symmetrical (15, 16).

Alternative methods have been described for measuring hexose transport (17–20). The latter reference describes a flow tube which allows measurement of 3-O-methylglucose uptake using incubation times of less than 1 sec.

4. MEASUREMENT OF 2-DEOXYGLUCOSE TRANSPORT AND PHOSPHORYLATION

2-deoxy-D-glucose is transported through the adipocyte membrane by the same mechanism as 3-O-methyl-D-glucose and D-glucose. Its affinity for the transporter is of the same magnitude as that of methylglucose and slightly higher than that of glucose. The transmembrane transport (1–2 sec incubations) is enhanced by ongoing glucose metabolism in contrast to the transport of methylglucose (21). A model has been proposed to explain this unexpected phenomenon (21, 22).

Once transported, 2-deoxyglucose is phosphorylated by hexokinase and trapped inside the cell. Uptake of 2-deoxyglucose is often taken as a measure of 2-deoxyglucose transport using 3 min incubations. However, it should be realized that the rate of phosphorylation is measured, and that this is only equivalent to the rate of transport when two conditions are fulfilled. The rate of phosphorylation must not be rate limiting for the uptake, and no dephosphorylation must occur. The first condition appears to be fulfilled using cells from normal fed rats and 2-deoxyglucose at a very low concentration, but not in the presence of 2-deoxyglucose (or glucose) at concentrations higher than about 50 μM (23). The second condition is not fulfilled in a strict sense since a dephosphorylation occurs (24). However, this is so slow in cells from fed rats that the error is negligible using 3 min incubations. This may not be the case when cells are prepared from animals in other nutritional conditions, and it is therefore not always easy to interpret the meaning of 2-deoxyglucose uptake measurements.

4.1. Materials

1. Use standard incubation vials (see step 5 in Section 2.1) and buffer containing 1 percent albumin. For 3 min incubations it is convenient to use 20 percent packed cell volume. At this time maximally stimulated cells will have taken up about 10 percent of the medium tracer at 37°C.

2. Microfuge tubes (see step 7 in Section 3.1).

3. Silicone oil (see step 6 in Section 3.1).

4.2. Procedure

Transfer 400 μL of cell suspension to microfuge tubes containing 100 μL silicone oil. Terminate the incubation by starting the microfuge, centrifuge for 30 sec, cut the tube through the oil layer, whirlmix the cell pellet in 2 mL scintillation fluid (minivial), and assay for radioactivity. With this relatively long incubation time the standard method can be employed (25), and it is not necessary to use a stopping solution.

5. MEASUREMENT OF THE RATE OF CONVERSION OF D-GLUCOSE TO PRODUCTS

D-glucose is transported across the membrane and subsequently metabolized to various products. In "standard" adipocytes from fed rats transport is probably the rate-limiting step at very low sugar concentrations, that is, about 200 μM or less. Thus, the rate of formation of the total metabolic products from labeled glucose will approximate the rate of glucose influx, and the backflux of glucose from the cell to the medium will be negligible. The highest responses to insulin in terms of "percent increase above basal" are obtained using low total glucose concentrations. The following section will deal with the metabolism of [^{14}C]- and [^{3}H] labeled glucose under these conditions.

5.1. Materials

The incubations may be carried out using 20-mL β-scintillation vials. Other materials as in Section 4.1.

5.2. Procedure

1. *Incubation.* Use 1 percent (v/v) cell suspension (approximately 10^5 cells/mL) for 1 hr incubation. About 10 percent of the tracer will be metabolized by maximally stimulated cells.

2. *Labeled Products Associated with the Cell Pellet.* Employ procedure in Section 4.2 and assay radioactivity using a scintillation fluid miscible with

water. Radioactivity will be present both in neutral lipids and in hydrophilic metabolites (26).

3. *Labeled Lipids.* (i) To 1 mL cell suspension add 10 mL toluene- or xylene-based scintillation fluid not miscible with water. The sample may be assayed directly in a β-counter if [^{3}H] labeled glucose is used (27). Transfer of (part of) the organic phase to another vial is necessary to avoid high background counts if [^{14}C] labeled glucose is used or if the cell suspension contains [^{125}I] labeled insulin. Alternatively, (ii) To 1 mL cell suspension add 5 mL 2-propanol-heptane 4:1 (forms a one-phase system) followed by 3 mL of heptane and 2 mL of water to split the phases. Count an aliquot of the upper phase (largely heptane).

4. *Labeled Glyceride Fatty Acids.* Evaporate the heptane off the upper phase [3 (ii)], add 0.5 mL 0.5 N KOH in 75 percent ethanol and incubate for 2 hr at 60°C, reacidify by the addition of 0.5 mL 1 N H$_2$SO$_4$ and redistribute in the isopropanol–heptane–water system. The fatty acids will be in the upper and the glycerol in the lower phase.

5. *CO$_2$.* Place a rectangular piece of filter paper in a β scintillation vial as that used for incubation. Moisten the paper with about 400 μL phenethylamine and press a piece of soft tubing (about 4 cm) into the opening of the vial. Place vial and tube horizontally (use a support) and add about 400 μL 8 N H$_2$SO$_4$ to the open end of the tube which is cut obliquely (6, 11). Terminate the incubation by carefully removing the stopper (must be well fitting, no screw caps), join the tubes and shake for 1 hr. The acid will liberate CO$_2$, which is subsequently bound to the amine. Some CO$_2$ is in the gas phase by the time the incubation vial is open. Nevertheless, the procedure can be carried out with almost 100 percent efficiency because CO$_2$ is heavier than air.

6. CHOICE OF PARAMETER FOR MEASURING INSULIN EFFECTS

6.1. Isotope: [U-^{14}C]Glucose

1. *Cell-Associated Radioactivity.* The highest incorporation into the cell pellet of insulin-stimulated cells is obtained at the extremely low glucose concentrations 100 nM (i.e., tracer alone) to 10 μM. At higher glucose concentrations more is converted to ^{14}CO$_2$ (maximum at 100–200 μM glucose) and less to cell-associated products. The reason for this apparent paradox (and others stated below) is probably that increasing glucose saturates labeled precursor pools (26). Using 100 nM [U-^{14}C]glucose, about 85 percent of the radioactive products are in the cell pellet and about 15 percent in CO$_2$. Release of radioactive metabolites, including lactate, into the medium is negligible.

2. *Lipids.* Use 10 μM glucose which gives the highest incorporation. This accounts almost for the total radioactivity in the cell pellet. Using tracer

alone, about one-third of the radioactivity associated with the cell pellet is in hydrophilic intermediates (26).

3. CO_2.   The highest conversion rate of the tracer is obtained using 100 μM. This accounts for 30–40 percent of the total conversion rate. This glucose concentration should also be used if [1-^{14}C]glucose is employed. The rate of conversion of that tracer to CO_2 is about twice that of [U-^{14}C]glucose.

6.2. Isotope: [3-^{3}H]Glucose

This tracer is frequently used mainly because its conversion to [^{3}H]lipids can be measured simply by the addition of scintillation fluid to the incubation vial (see step 3 in Section 5.2). About half is metabolized to [^{3}H]O$_2$ using glucose in the concentration range 15 nM (i.e., tracer alone) to 200 μM.

1. *Cell-Associated Radioactivity*.   The highest incorporation into the cell pellet of insulin-stimulated cells is obtained using 4–100 μM glucose. When even lower glucose concentrations are employed (e.g., 15 nM, tracer alone) the radioactivity in the cell pellet declines slightly due to a slow loss of hydrophilic metabolites to the medium.

2. *Lipids*.   Use about 50 μM unlabeled glucose, which gives the highest incorporation of the tracer. This accounts for almost all radioactivity in the cell pellet. Using tracer alone about two-thirds of the radioactivity associated with the cell pellet is in hydrophilic metabolites (26).

The variations in the recovery of labeled metabolites described above are much less in cells not stimulated by insulin. Therefore, the highest percent response to insulin is obtained when the incorporation into a given metabolite is maximal using insulin-treated cells.

7.   TROUBLE SHOOTING

What could be wrong if insulin stimulates hexose transport and glucose metabolism less than about 10-fold?

7.1. Mechanics

It is very important to use plastic acceptable for the cell surface. We do not know what the plastic surface characteristics should be ideally, but the charge distribution may be important. Some types of plastic as well as unsiliconized glass cause cell lysis, and this is easy to see when one has a well-working preparation to start with.

Even using suitable plastics, the mechanical treatment may easily become too harsh. Always use the minimum force in all steps and be careful that cells are not exposed to cold temperatures. Make sure that the bore in, for instance, disposable pipette tips is wide enough. If necessary, cut the tip. It should also be noted that a slight cell lysis is unavoidable, particularly when one is working with concentrated cell suspensions (e.g., 40 percent v/v). This makes the pipetting inaccurate because the suspension tends to creep more and more along the sides of the tip. It may be necessary to change the tip after each pipetting.

Vega and Kono (7) have noted that the basal rate of glucose transport and metabolism (but not the insulin-stimulated rate) decreases when the cells are preincubated in the presence of glucose for 30–60 min before they are used in an experiment. We have noted such recovery after the preparation "trauma" because our cells were already maximally insulin responsive shortly after their preparation. However, this apparent discrepancy may be caused by minor differences in the cell preparation procedure and a testing of such "recovery" is highly recommended in laboratories which start working with isolated fat cells.

7.2. Collagenase

The disintegration of the tissue is caused by the combined action of collagenase, an acid protease (28), and the mechanical treatment. Collagenase itself does not disintegrate the tissue, and we have to use the crude preparations since the active protease(s) has not been isolated. We have experience with preparations obtained from Worthington and Sigma, and there seems to be no systematic difference. We have for many years not seen collagenases producing cell lysis. However, some batches disintegrate the tissue so slowly that one is tempted to increase the mechanical force, which in turn may cause lysis. Cells made from several batches of collagenase have exhibited increased basal rates of glucose metabolism and therefore low responses to insulin. This is irrespective of whether the collagenase preparation has been designated "for preparation of fat cells." The rate of glucose transport and metabolism in the presence of insulin and ED_{50} for insulin varies only little between cells prepared from different batches of collagenase. All laboratories working routinely with fat cells buy a new batch of collagenase only after careful comparison with a batch known to produce cells with an adequate insulin response. It is therefore a great advantage for a person who starts working with fat cells to get a small amount of collagenase which is known to work. When the fat cell preparation gives satisfactory results, several new batches should be tested before a large amount is bought.

7.3. Albumin

We have not had "troubles" in our laboratory for many years using the Sigma bovine serum albumin prepared as described. "Trouble" usually means high basal glucose transport and metabolism rates. We have had this problem with the kind of albumin preparation (from Miles) which may be added directly to the buffer, and we therefore went back to the—admittedly—cumbersome dialysis and filtration procedure. The "insulinlike" effect of albumin is probably most often due to proteases, for instance, from the ubiquitous *B. subtilis*. Jordan and Kono (29) have reported that such activity can be reduced by treatment of the albumin preparation with trypsin.

We have also noted that some albumin preparations can reduce the insulin-stimulated rate of glucose metabolism dramatically without affecting the basal rate. This has been the case with preparations from Boehringer (fraction V), which are cheaper than those from Sigma. We were unable to remove this inhibitory activity.

REFERENCES

1. M. Rodbell, *J. Biol. Chem.* **239**, 375 (1964).

2. O. Pedersen and J. Gliemann, *Diabetologia* **20**, 630 (1981).

3. O. Pedersen, E. Hjøllund, H. Beck-Nielsen, H. O. Lindskov, O. Sonne, and J. Gliemann, *Diabetologia* **20**, 636 (1981).

4. E. Karnieli, M. J. Zarnowski, P. J. Hissin, I. A. Simpson, L. B. Salans, and S. W. Cushman, *J. Biol. Chem.* **256**, 4772 (1981).

5. T. Kono, K. Suzuki, L. Dansey, F. W. Robinson, and T. L. Blevins, *J. Biol. Chem.* **256**, 6400 (1981).

6. J. Gliemann, *Diabetologia* **3**, 382 (1967).

7. F. V. Vega and T. Kono, *Archiv. Biochem. Biophys.* **192**, 120 (1979).

8. J. Gliemann and J. Vinten, *J. Physiol. (London)* **236**, 499 (1974).

9. N. E. Good, G. D. Winget, W. Winter, N. Connolly, S. Izawa, and R. M. M. Singh, *Biochemistry* **253**, 7857 (1978).

10. M. Di Girolamo, S. Mendlinger, and J. W. Fertig, *Am. J. Physiol.* **221**, 850 (1971).

11. J. Gliemann, *Diabetes* **14**, 643 (1965).

12. J. E. Foley, A. L. Laursen, O. Sonne, and J. Gliemann, *Diabetologia*, **19**, 234 (1980).

13. F. M. Hansen, J. H. Nielsen, and J. Gliemann, *Europ. J. Clin. Invest.* **4**, 411 (1974).

14. R. R. Whitesell and J. Gliemann, *J. Biol. Chem.* **254**, 5276 (1979).

15. J. Gliemann and W. D. Rees, in *Current Topics in Membranes and Transport*, Vol. 18, R. Martin and A. Kleinzeller (eds.), Academic Press, New York, 1983, p. 339.

16. L. P. Taylor and G. D. Holman, *Biochim. Biophys. Acta* **642**, 325 (1981).

17. J. Vinten, J. Gliemann, and K. Østerlind, *J. Biol. Chem.* **251**, 794 (1976).

18. E. Schoenle, J. Zapf, and E. R. Froesch, *Am. J. Physiol.* **237**, E325 (1979).

19. M. P. Czech, *J. Biol. Chem.* **251**, 1164 (1976).

20. J. Vinten and H. Galbo, *Am. J. Physiol.* **244**, E129 (1983).

21. J. E. Foley, R. Foley, and J. Gliemann, *J. Biol. Chem.* **255**, 9674 (1980).

22. J. E. Foley and J. Gliemann, *Int. J. Obesity* **5**, 679 (1981).

23. J. E. Foley, R. Foley, and J. Gliemann, *Biochim. Biophys. Acta* **599**, 689 (1980).

24. J. E. Foley and J. Gliemann, *Biochim, Biophys. Acta,* **648**, 100 (1981).

25. J. Gliemann, K. Østerlind, J. Vinten, and S. Gammeltoft, *Biochim. Biophys. Acta* **286**, 1 (1972).

26. J. Gliemann, W. D. Rees, and J. E. Foley, unpublished.

27. A. J. Moody, M. A. Stan, M. Stan, and J. Gliemann, *Horm. Metab. Res.* **6**, 12 (1974).

28. T. Kono, *J. Biol. Chem.* **244**, 1772 (1969).

29. J. E. Jordan and T. Kono, *Anal. Biochem.* **104**, 192 (1980).

III

IMMUNOLOGICAL AND IMMUNOCHEMICAL INVESTIGATIONS

A

CYTOTOXIC MECHANISMS IN INSULIN-DEPENDENT DIABETES MELLITUS

**MOHAMMAD ALI GHALAMBOR,
HARRY G. RITTENHOUSE, STANLEY A. SCHWARTZ,
SUMER BELBEZ PEK, DIANE AR,
AND DALE L. OXENDER**

*The University of Michigan, Departments of Biological Chemistry,
Internal Medicine, Pediatrics, and Epidemiology, Ann Arbor, Michigan
and Abbott Laboratories, Chicago, Illinois*

1. INTRODUCTION

The notion that humoral (1–4) and cellular (5–9) immunoregulatory mechanisms may be impaired, at least in part, in some phases of the pathogenesis of insulin-dependent diabetes mellitus (IDDM) is suggested from preliminary studies on drug-induced diabetes in experimental animals and studies of other autoimmune diseases. Investigations conducted by Jensen et al. (10) on a cyclophosphamide-derivative-induced diabetes mellitus and of Buschard and Rygaard's (8) passive transfer of streptomycin-induced diabetes mellitus from mouse to mouse indicate a possible importance of reduced suppressor cell activity. In addition, results obtained from studies of other autoimmune diseases indicate that the activity of suppressor cells may be diminished (11–13).

Evidence for a cell-mediated immune mechanism resulting in β cell destruction is obtained from studies on the activity of T lymphocyte subsets; the activity of these cells on specific or nonspecific target cells is used to assess cell-mediated immunity in IDDM (14). The majority of patients with IDDM have augmented K cell activity immediately following the onset of the disease which gradually returns to normal within 1 year (9). Furthermore, it has been demonstrated that high K cell activity occurs simultaneously with high antibody-dependent cellular cytotoxicity (ADCC) and elevated levels of islet cell antibodies (ICA), which suggests that both humoral and cell-mediated immune mechanisms might play a role in the destruction of β cells.

A number of phenomena indicate that IDDM results from the effect of toxic substances on β cells, the most important of which are (i) binding of anti-human immunoglobulin-fluorescein-conjugated antibodies (Ab) to islets, pancreatic sections and islet cells pretreated with serum, or plasma from IDDM patients (1, 15, 16), (ii) inflammation and lymphocytic infiltration in islets of patients with recently diagnosed onset (17, 18), (iii) inhibition of leukocytic migration following exposure to pancreatic extracts or islet cells (19, 20), (iv) correlation between the incidence of viral infections and subsequent appearance of cases of IDDM (21–23), and (v) increased number of low-affinity erythrocyte-rosetting human K cells (9, 24). Furthermore, the major histocompatibility complex containing genes that specifically code for cell surface proteins is known to be involved in a variety of immunological phenomena including initiation of Ab synthesis and certain interactions between the cells and subcellular components of islet cells (25, 26).

Cytotoxicity mediated by humoral and/or cellular mechanisms has been reported to be active against allogeneic human insulinoma cell lines (27). In addition, augmented complement-dependent antibody-mediated cellular cytotoxicity has been observed in association with IDDM (28–33). Using BB Wistar rats with spontaneous diabetes as an experimental model, Dyrberg et al. (34) have obtained evidence for cell-mediated immune mechanisms that include (i) presence of lymphocyte antibodies in sera of diabetic animals, (ii) modification, or elimination, of the syndrome by treatment with antilymphocyte antibodies (35), (iii) possible passive transfer of diabetes by lymphocytes from diabetic rats to mice (36) and (iv) the presence of lymphopenia before and after the onset of diabetes (37, 39).

Concerning the humoral immune mechanisms, islet-cell-specific Ab (ICA) in sera of patients with IDDM can be determined by various assay systems. These ICA are of different types depending on their immunological specificity—that is, islet cell cytoplasmic Ab, islet cell surface Ab (ICA-S), complement-dependent cytotoxic Ab, and antibody-dependent cellular cytotoxic (ADCC) Ab. Reports from several laboratories have documented that ICA are present in sera of more than 70 percent of patients with IDDM (1–3, 40–43). These circulating antibodies are uncommon in patients with non-insulin-dependent diabetes mellitus (Type II) and their presence in these patients indicates prognosis of insulin-dependent diabetes (3, 41, 44). The ICA directed against cytoplasmic antigen(s) are not specific for β cells since they are recognized by all four types of endocrine cells of the islets of Langerhans (45). Membrane-reactive ICA, or ICA-S, have been determined quantitatively (45) and their prevalence seems to parallel that of the anticytoplasmic Ab. Such antibodies may cause islet cell lysis either by complement-dependent cytotoxicity (29, 32, 33) or by ADCC involving K-cell-mediated mechanisms (9, 31, 46–49).

Presently little is known about the islet cell antigens to which ICA are directed. Since the ICA present in the sera from IDDM patients are not species specific, these sera can be conveniently used with animal pancreatic islets as substrate (29, 34, 50, 51). Thus, single islet preparations from rats or hamsters could serve as a diagnostic tool for detection of ICA in sera of patients with IDDM.

This chapter describes the procedure for detection of ICA in patients with IDDM using islets as substrate. The ICA activity demonstrated by sera from patients with insulin-dependent diabetes mellitus is attributed to the serum immunoglobulin fraction and confirmed by radioisotopic techniques as well as by fluorescence microscopy.

2. PREPARATION OF ISLETS

2.1. Materials

Male Syrian golden hamsters (80–120 days old).

Hanks' balanced salt solution (HBSS), pH 7.4 [Grand Island Biological Co., Grand Island, NY (GIBCO)].

Collagenase, Worthington Type IV.

Ficoll, 30 percent (Sigma Chemical Co., St. Louis, MO) dialyzed against distilled water and lyophilized. The powder is then dissolved in HBSS, pH 7.4, to give a final concentration of 25 percent.

Solutions of 23, 20.5, and 11 percent (w/v) of Ficoll are prepared by dilution of the stock 25 percent solution with HBSS.

Dimethyl dichlorosilane (Sigma) 1:100 w/v in water, is used to siliconized 16×25-mm culture tubes, 20-mL beakers, Pasteur pipettes, glass Petri dishes, and capillary pipettes.

2.2. Procedure

Islets of Langerhans are isolated by a modification of the method of Ballinger and Lacy (52) as follows: male Syrian golden hamster, 80–120 days of age, are sacrificed by cervical dislocation and their pancreata are immediately removed. The pancreata are freed of fat and lymph nodes, placed in 20 mL siliconized beakers containing 8 mL of HBSS, pH 7.4, at 4°C and thoroughly minced with three pairs of dissecting scissors to obtain pieces approximately 1–1.5 mm^3 in size. The homogenate is transferred to a screw-capped 16×125 mm culture tube and diluted with cold HBSS to give about 3 mL/pancreas. The suspension is allowed to sediment at $1g$ at 4°C for 1 min after which the supernatant solution containing the remaining fat is discarded. The sediment is taken up in HBSS again, the centrifugation step is repeated, and the supernatant solution is removed by Pasteur pipette and discarded. The remaining pellet usually contains approximately 1.0 mL of homogenate and residual HBSS/pancreas. The homogenate is partially digested with collagenase (Worthington Type IV), 1000 U, in 1 mL buffer per pancreas at 37°C for 10 min with vigorous shaking. The digestion mixture is diluted with cold HBSS to 10 mL and shaken vigorously to stop the enzymatic reaction. The digestion tubes are centrifuged at $300g$ at 4°C for 1 min in a swinging bucket rotor and the supernatant fluids are withdrawn with a Pasteur pipette and discarded. The pellets are suspended in 3 mL of HBSS per pancreas, mixed, and the centrifugation step is repeated. The washed tissue homogenate is suspended in 4 mL of 25 percent Ficoll, 400-DL (Sigma), and the suspension is transferred to a siliconized culture tube. Then 2-mL portions of 23, 20.5, and 11 percent Ficoll in HBSS, pH 7.4, are carefully layered on top of the suspension by allowing the Ficoll solution to run slowly from a pipette against the tilted side of the culture tube above the suspension. The tubes are centrifuged in a swinging bucket rotor at $250g$ at 4°C for 12 min with no braking. Intact free islets are located at 11 and 20.5 percent Ficoll interface and are carefully removed with a Pasteur pipette. The islet portions are suspended in 5 mL of HBSS at 4°C, mixed, and centrifuged at $200g$ at 4°C for 5 min. The washing step is repeated once and the washed islets are suspended in 10 mL of cold HBSS. Individual intact islets are selected under a dissecting microscope from a plastic Petri dish using a bent-tip Pasteur pipette. Islets are found to be of uniform shape and size and the yield is approximately 200 usable islets per hamster pancreas.

3. CYTOTOXICITY ASSAY METHODS

3.1. Trypan Blue Dye Method (Sigma)

Serum samples are taken from patients with insulin-dependent diabetes mellitus (Type I diabetes) and non-insulin-dependent diabetes mellitus (Type II diabetes) ranging in age from 5 months to 55 years, with the duration of disease from 1 month to 5 years. Sera obtained from nondiabetic hospitalized patients and healthy adult donors are used as controls. All samples are stored at -20°C until used.

3.1.1. MATERIALS

Serum samples.
Rabbit anti-hamster islets antiserum (prepared by authors).
Bovine insulin (Sigma), 400 μg/mL.
Ham's medium containing 13 percent heat-inactivated fetal calf serum (FCS) (GIBCO).

Fetal calf serum (GIBCO).

Hamster islet preparation (prepared by authors).

Trypan blue dye, 2 percent in water (Sigma).

Guinea pig complement preparation (authors).

3.1.2. Procedure

Serum samples are heat inactivated at 56°C for 30 min and incubated with 4 μg of bovine insulin/100 μL to saturate all binding sites on the endogenous insulin antibodies (Ab). Since the concentration of bound Ab on the surface of islet cells may be a critical variable in complement-mediated cytotoxicity, a small number of hamster islets per assay is routinely employed. Ten to 12 intact islets are suspended in 25 μL of Ham's medium in 6 mm diameter microtiter plate wells (Cook Engineering Co.) and incubated at 4°C for 2 days. To a microtiter plate well containing 10–12 hamster pancreatic islets, 50 μL of human serum to be tested are added and the mixture is incubated at 37°C for 1 hr. Then 20 μL aliquots of fresh guinea pig complement are added at hourly intervals for 5 hr and the mixture is incubated for 17 hr at 37°C. An additional 20 μL aliquot of guinea pig complement is added and the mixture is incubated at 37°C for 2 hr. Fifty microliters of 2 percent trypan blue are added, mixed, and incubated at 23°C for 5 min and a wet mount of the mixture is examined with a phase-contrast microscope within 2 min. The extent of cytotoxicity is determined by (i) assessment of cellular uptake of the vital dye and (ii) morphological determination of the extent of disruption of the islet surface by phase-contrast microscopy.

Positive cytotoxicity is defined as the uptake of trypan blue by more than 90 percent of the outer islet cells (extending from the surface of the islet to one-third of the islet radius toward the center) plus morphologic disruption of the normally compact and dense islet structure.

The assay is performed using duplicate serum samples. Each experiment contains at least one known noncytotoxic human serum sample and one positive cytotoxic sample (serum sample from a rabbit immunized against a hamster islet cell tumor homogenate).

Under the experimental conditions described, the following criteria should be satisfied.

1. Hamster islets incubated with negative-control serum samples from normal healthy donors in the presence of complement remain morphologically identical to the freshly prepared hamster islets.

2. Hamster islets incubated in Ham's medium containing guinea pig complement, without serum, retain their normal morphological characteristics and appear identical to the untreated hamster islets when examined microscopically (Fig. 1A).

3. Hamster islets incubated with serum samples from Type II diabetic

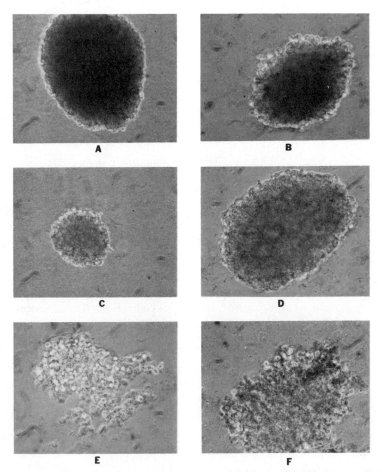

FIGURE 1. Trypan blue cytotoxicity assay using hamster islets. The experiments were carried out as described in Section 2.1. All microtiter wells contained 100 µL of culture medium, 10–12 hamster islet and one of the following: (A) fresh guinea pig C, no serum; (B) fresh guinea pig C and serum from a Type II diabetic patient; (C) serum from a Type I diabetic patient and heat-inactivated guinea pig C; (D) Type I diabetic serum; (E and F) serum from Type I diabetic patient and fresh guinea pig complement.

patients and fresh guinea pig complement appear normal with no detectable damage to the outer cells. The trypan blue-stained cells in these samples as well as other negative samples are less than 5 percent of the total cell population (Fig. 1B).

4. Hamster islets incubated with sera from Type I diabetic patients in Ham's medium without complement show no cytotoxic effects or damage to the islets (Fig. 1C,D).

5. When sera from the patients with Type I diabetes (see criterion 4) are incubated with hamster islets in the presence of guinea pig complement,

islet cell morphology is dramatically affected. In addition, trypan blue uptake by islet cells exceeds 90 percent (Fig. 1E,F).

3.1.3. COMMENTS

The cytotoxicity assay applied to 20 samples from Type I diabetic patients, 11 samples from Type II diabetics, 4 nondiabetic controls, and 28 samples from healthy adult subjects revealed the following:

1. Complement-dependent cytotoxicity against hamster islets was found in 37 percent of the Type I diabetic patients. None of the serum samples from Type II diabetics, however, caused any detectable damage to hamster islets. This finding indicates that these sera are incapable of inducing complement-dependent cellular cytotoxicity in hamster islets in the presence, or absence, of exogenously added guinea pig complement.

2. Not all of the normal healthy control serum samples were negative. One of 28 samples induced lysis of hamster islet cells in the presence, or absence, of complement. In addition, a heat-inactivated serum sample from 1 out of 11 Type I diabetic patients was cytotoxic against hamster islets in the absence of exogenous complement.

3.2. Immunofluorescence Techniques

3.2.1. MATERIALS

Pancreas samples (Dept. of Pathology, U. of Michigan Med. Center).
Diabetic and control serum samples.
Fresh guinea pig complement preparation.
Anti-C_1q-fluorescein isothiocyanate (FITC) conjugate.
Sheep anti-human complement conjugated with FITC (Miles, Elkhart, IN).
Hanks' balanced salt solution (HBSS).

The reaction of common antigens found in the cytoplasm of all the endocrine cells in the islets of Langerhans with ICA present in the sera of IDDM patients results in the formation of Ag-Ab complexes, which in the presence of complement react with anti-C fluorescein isothiocyanate conjugated immunoglobulins to form immunofluorescent (IF) staining.

3.2.2. PROCEDURE

The pancreas section is incubated with 100 μL of undiluted patient's serum, followed by addition of 100 μL of 1:2 dilution of fresh guinea pig serum (HBSS) as a source of complement. After 60 min the tissues are washed in

HBSS and treated with 100 μL of 1:10 dilution of sheep anti-human C_3, or anti-C_1q fluorescein isothiocyanate (FITC) conjugate for 60 min at room temperature, followed by 3 hr at 4°C. Then the tissue sections are washed thoroughly in 2-mL portions of HBSS three times, wet mounted, and examined under an epi-fluorescent microscope. The follwing controls are included:

1. *Serum control*, in which normal healthy donor serum is used instead of the patient's serum.
2. *Complement control*—Heat-inactivated guinea pig serum is substituted for the fresh guinea pig serum.
3. *Positive control*—A serum known to give a positive test in this procedure is run concomitantly.

3.2.3. COMMENTS

1. Unfixed 5 mm cryostat sections from blood group O donors should be used throughout.
2. The diabetic sera are first assayed for ICA before use.
3. Positive complement-fixing islet cell antibodies(CF-ICA) often give brighter fluorescence than the corresponding IgG anti-human IgG system and the cytoplasm staining is confluent.
4. In the samples with negative results, the islets are darker than the exocrine portion of pancreas which shows some fluorescence at the apices of zymogen-bearing cells, since these cells have a tendency to concentrate C.
5. There is no difference in the results when sheep anti-C_3-FITC, anti-C_1q-FITC, or anti-C_4-FITC conjugates are employed (53).
6. The sera that consistently show positive immunofluorescence with the whole islets also routinely stain the dispersed islet cells in complement-fixation tests (CFT) (30, 40) which appears to be more selective during follow-up. This suggests that CF-ICA are separate species of Ab that can be activated independently of other types of ICA (53).

3.3. Complement-Mediated Cytotoxicity Assay Using ^{51}Cr Release

3.3.1. MATERIALS

Na_2 $^{51}CrO_4$, 50 Ci/mmol, New England Nuclear.
Diabetic and normal control sera.
Hanks' balanced salt solution (HBSS).
L-Glutamine, 30 mg/mL HBSS (Calbiochem, Los Angeles, CA).
Gentamicin, 8 mg/mL HBSS (Schering Corp., Kenilworth, NJ).
Fetal calf serum.

RPMI 1640 culture medium (GIBCO).

Complete medium, RPMI 1640 culture medium (93 mL) are mixed with 1 mL of gentamicin solution, 5 mL of heat-inactivated fetal calf serum, and 1 mL of glutamine solution.

Fresh and heat-inactivated guinea pig complement.

Triton X-100, 0.20 percent in distilled water (Sigma).

Rabbit anti-rat islet serum (author's).

Rat islet cells.

3.3.2. PROCEDURE

Islet cells are labeled with ^{51}Cr in 1.0 mL of complete medium supplemented with 1.0–2.0 μmol (50–100 μCi) of Na$_2$ ^{51}CrO$_4$ for 60 min at 37°C. Cells are harvested by centrifugation at 100g for 5 min, washed with two 10 mL portions of HBSS, and, centrifuged (30, 54, 55). The pellet is resuspended in 5 mL of complete medium and incubated at 37°C for 2 hr. Then 1 × 10^4 islet cells containing 0.5–1.0 μCi of ^{51}Cr in 100 μL of medium are dispensed in microculture plates. The test serum, 50 μL of a 1:10 dilution, is added to each well, mixed, and the cell suspensions are incubated at 37°C for 30 min. The cultures are centrifuged at 100g for 5 min and the serum present in the supernatant fluid is withdrawn and discarded. The cell pellets are washed twice with 200 μL of RPMI 1640 culture medium and resuspended in 100 μL of the same. A 100 μL aliquot of a 1:10 dilution of fresh guinea pig complement is added to each well and incubated at 37°C for 30 min. After centrifugation at 100g for 5 min, a 100 μL aliquot of the supernatant fluid from each well is removed and assayed for ^{51}Cr in a γ counter.

The following controls are included in each set of experiments (Table 1):

1. *Total release.* Triplicate wells containing 100 μL of islet cells are lysed by the addition of 50 μL of 0.20 percent Triton X-100 solution and 50 μL of culture medium.

2. *Positive controls.* Consist of three wells receiving 50 μL of 1:2 dilutions of a hyperimmune serum prepared in rabbits against rat islet cells, 100 μL of islet cell suspension, and 50 μL of guinea pig complement.

3. *Spontaneous isotope release.* Rabbit hyperimmune serum is incubated with islet cells in the absence of complement.

4. *ICA-negative controls.* Sera from healthy normal human donors are incubated with complement and target cells side by side with the test sera.

5. *HBSS.* Fresh complement and target cells are incubated in the absence of antiserum, instead of which an equal volume of HBSS is included.

6. *Complement controls.* Test sera are incubated with islet cells and heat-inactivated complement.

TABLE 1.   Assay of Complement-Dependent Cytotoxicity[a]

Test No.	Serum Source	Complement[b]	[51]Cr Release[c] (percent)
1	None (PBS)	Fresh	8–11
2	Negative	Fresh	9–15
3	Positive	None	8–12
4	Positive A-inactivated	Fresh	8–14
5	Positive	A-inactivated	8–14
6	Positive	Fresh	48–58
7	Total release	—	85–95

[a] Assays were carried out as described in Section 2.2. To microtiter plate wells 100 μL of islet cell suspensions and 50 μL of the following were added as indicated: 1, PBS; 2, Negative serum; 3, positive serum; 4, serum heated at 56°C for 30 min; 5, 6, positive serum and allowed to adsorb.
[b] Cells are washed and resuspended in 100 μL of culture medium and treated with 100 μL of the following: 1, 2, fresh complement; 3, PBS; 4, 6, fresh complement, 5, heat-inactivated complement.
[c] After centrifugation at 100g for 5 min at 24°C, 100 μL aliquots of the supernatant fluids were used for determination of radioactivity. Percent ^{51}Cr release is calculated as described.

3.3.3.   CALCULATIONS

Percent cytotoxicity is calculated from the arithmetic mean values of ^{51}Cr of triplicate determinations as follows:

$$\text{Percent }^{51}\text{Cr release} = \frac{(\text{super. cpm} \times 2) - \text{spontaneous release}}{(\text{super. cpm} \times 2 + \text{pellet cpm}) - \text{spontaneous release}}$$

4.   ANTIBODY-DEPENDENT CELLULAR CYTOTOXICITY

4.1.   Materials

Peripheral blood.
Ca$^+$ Mg$^+$-free Hanks' balanced salt solution (HBSS, GIBCO, Grand Island, NY).
RPMI 1640 culture medium.
HEPES buffer, 0.025 M, pH 7.3 (Sigma).
Fetal calf serum (FCS; GIBCO).
Gentamicin, 8 mg/mL (Schering Corp., Kenilworth, NJ).
L-Glutamine, 30 mg/mL.
Sephadex G-10 (Pharmacia Fine Chemicals, Piscataway, NJ).
HBSS.
Sheep red blood cells (SRBC).

Neuraminidase, 100 μL/mL (Worthington).

Ficoll-Hypaque (Pharmacia).

Minimal essential medium (MEM; GIBCO).

Percoll (Pharmacia), 36.5, 40, 42.5, 45, 47.5, and 50 percent solution in distilled water.

Sodium chromate ($Na_2 {}^{51}CrO_4$, New England Nuclear, Boston, MA).

Islet cell suspension, 10^6 cells/mL of HBSS.

Normal total immunoglobulins solution, 30 mg/mL (prepared from heat-inactivated pool sera) by diluting the Ig in PBS, pH 7.3.

Diabetic total immunoglobulins solutions, 30 mg/mL (prepared from heat-inactivated pool sera) by appropriate dilution in PBS, pH 7.3.

Complete medium. RPMI 1640 culture medium (93 mL) are mixed with 1 mL of 8 mg/mL gentimicin, 5 mL of heat-inactivated fetal calf serum, and 1 mL of 30 mg/mL of L-glutamine solution.

4.2. Procedure

Diabetic patients of both sexes with various duration of disease (3–19 years) are evaluated. Normal age-matched subjects are used as controls.

4.2.1. PREPARATION OF MONONUCLEAR CELLS

Peripheral blood is withdrawn into heparinized (20 μL/mL, preservative-free; Fellows Laboratories, Oak Park, IL) syringes (56) and diluted with an equal volume of HBSS and centrifuged at 400g for 20 min at 24°C. The cell band is harvested, suspended in complete medium, and washed three times with same.

4.2.2. PURIFICATION OF LYMPHOCYTES

Lymphocytes (PBL) are separated from adherent cells by chromatography on a Sephadex G-10 column according to the method of Ly and Mishell (57) as modified by Berlinger et al. (58) as follows: peripheral blood mononuclear cells (PBMC) are suspended in RPMI 1640 culture medium supplemented with 10 percent calf serum and are applied to a 25 × 1-cm column of Sephadex G-10 which has been equilibrated with the same medium. After a 45 min incubation at 24°C, the column is eluted with one bed volume (20 mL) of warm (37°C) medium to remove the nonadherent cells. The PBMC are resuspended in complete medium.

4.2.3. PREPARATION OF T LYMPHOCYTES

T lymphocytes are prepared by the method of Gupta et al. (59) as follows: 4 × 10^6 PBL depleted of adherent cells are mixed with 250 μL of heat-inactivated FCS preadsorbed with sheep red blood cells (SRBS) and 1 mL of 1 percent packed volume of neuraminidase desialated SRBC (25 units/mL in 5 percent SRBC suspension). The cell suspension is incubated at 37°C for 5 min, centrifuged at 300g for 3 min at 24°C, and incubated at 4°C for 1 hr. The suspension is centrifuged at 100g for 1 min and E rosettes containing SRBC and T lymphocytes are separated from non-T lymphocytes by density gradient centrifugation on 20 percent Ficoll-Hypaque at 450g for 20 min at 24°C. SRBC present in T-lymphocyte-containing rosettes are lysed by treatment with 1 mL of distilled water, followed by 1 mL of double strength MEM. T cells are then suspended in RPMI 1640 culture medium and washed in same three times. The T cells are resuspended in complete medium and incubated at 37°C for 24 hr prior to use.

4.2.4. ENRICHMENT OF ADCC EFFECTOR CELLS

ADCC effector cells are enriched using a discontinuous gradient of Percoll (Pharmacia) according to the method of Timonen and Saksela (60). Percoll solution is mixed with varying volumes of RPM 1640 culture medium and 2-mL aliquots of 50–37.5 percent in 2.5 percent increments are gently layered into a 15 × 130-mm plastic tube. Lymphocytes depleted of adherent cells are carefully layered on top of the gradient, and the tubes are centrifuged at 300g for 45 min at 24°C. Each cell fraction is withdrawn with a Pasteur pipette and washed separately in RPM 1640 culture medium. Under the conditions described, the least dense band at the interface of 37.5 percent Percoll layer consistently contains the highest NK-enriched cells.

4.2.5. TARGET CELL PREPARATION

Rat islet cells are prepared by dispersion of islets of Langerhans of rat pancreas as described in this series. Isolated, single intact islet cells are used in cytotoxicity assays not more than 4 hr after preparation. To 0.8 mL aliquots of complete medium containing 1×10^6 islet cells, 100 μCi sodium chromate (Na$_2$ ^{51}CrO$_4$) are added. The islet cell suspension is incubated at 37°C for 1 hr in a humidified 5 percent CO_2, 95 percent air atmosphere with intermittent shaking. The cells are harvested by centrifugation at 400g for 2 min at 24°C. The pellets are resuspended in 2 mL of complete medium and washed three times. The final pellet is resuspended in 2 mL of the complete medium and diluted with same to a final concentration of 2×10^5 cells/mL.

4.2.6. ASSAY FOR ADCC

The ADCC activity is assayed according to the method of Perlmann and Perlmann (61) as modified by Handwerger and Koren (62) as follows: 50 μL of increasing concentrations of effector cells are added to 50 μL of complete medium containing 1×10^4 ^{51}Cr-labeled islet target cells and 100 μL of 1:10, 1:100, and

1:1000 dilutions of total immunoglobulins from normal and diabetic patients corresponding to 3000, 300, and 30 μg of immunoglobulin protein, respectively. Microculture plates are incubated in a humidified incubator at 37°C for 4 hr and centrifuged at 300g for 10 min at 24°C. A 100 μL aliquot from the supernatant fluid of each well is assayed for ^{51}Cr in a γ counter. The percent cytotoxicity and percent ADCC activity is calculated using the arithmetic mean value of triplicate determination of counts per incubation as follows:

4.2.7. NOTES

1. All experiments are carried out in triplicate tubes.
2. In each experiment the following controls are included in triplicate.

   (a)   normal pooled total Ig with rat islet cells,
   (b)   spontaneous release tubes containing [^{51}Cr]-labeled target cells, but no added effector cells, and
   (c)   a known positive ADCC control.

5.   DEMONSTRATION OF ICA IN DIABETIC SERA

5.1.   Indirect Immunofluorescence Technique

Serum samples tested in cytotoxicity assays are also analyzed for the presence of ICA using cryostat and/or frozen sections of fresh human blood group type O cadaveric pancreas. Serum-treated pancreas sections are stained with FITC-conjugated goat anti-human IgG and examined by fluorescence microscopy. The serum samples from Type I diabetics with positive complement-dependent cytotoxicity contain cytoplasmic islet cell antibodies as observed by fluorescence microscopy, whereas sera from Type II diabetic patients, nondiabetic control patients, and healthy adult subjects do not display any detectable ICA activity by the same technique.

5.2.   ICA Activity of Immunoglobulins

5.2.1.   MATERIALS

Hanks' balanced salt solution (HBSS).
Serum samples from normal controls and diabetic patients.
Saturated ammonium sulfate solution, 70 percent. To 100 mL of distilled water in a flask, add 70 g of crystalline ammonium sulfate (Enzyme Grade, Sigma) slowly, allowing to dissolve by stirring the mixture on a stirrer, cool and dilute to 200 mL total volume with distilled water.

5.2.2. PROCEDURE

An aliquot (2.5 mL) of 70 percent ammonium sulfate solution is added dropwise to 1 mL of serum sample from a Type I diabetic patient (with known positive complement-mediated cytotoxicity toward hamster islets) with constant stirring. The turbid suspension obtained is incubated at 4°C for 4 hr and centrifuged at 10,000g for 15 min at 4°C. The pellet is dissolved in 0.5 mL of HBSS. Both the ammonium sulfate (A.S.) soluble fraction and the precipitable fractions are dialyzed against 1 L of HBSS at 4°C for 48 hr with three changes of buffer at 12 hr intervals. After dialysis the retentates from both fractions are centrifuged at 10,000g at 4°C for 15 min and the supernatant fluids saved. The A.S. precipitable fraction is adjusted to 1.0 mL and the soluble fraction to 4 mL with HBSS. Aliquots (50 μL) from the precipitable fraction (total immunoglobulin) and 200 μL of the A.S. soluble fraction containing the serum albumin are tested with hamster islets for complement-dependent cytotoxicity using the assay procedure described. In our experience the total immunoglobulin (Ig) fraction induced complement-dependent cytotoxicity to an extent similar to that of an identical quantity of the same unfractionated serum when tested side by side. The soluble fraction containing primarily serum albumin did not cause any detectable complement-dependent lysis of hamster islets. The 50 percent saturated ammonium sulfate precipitate obtained from normal healthy control sera and the known noncytotoxic serum samples obtained from sera of patients with Type I diabetes mellitus did not display any detectable complement-dependent lysis of hamster islet cells when tested in the same experiment.

6. DETECTION OF INSULIN ANTIBODIES

6.1. Materials

Serum samples.
Polyethylene glycol (PEG, 7000 D, 6000 M.W.) (Siegfried Zotingen, Switzerland); 30 percent in distilled water [^{125}I]labeled insulin (porcine, monoiodinated, S.A. = 100 μCi/μg, New England Nuclear).
Hanks' balanced salt solution (HBSS).

6.2. Procedure

To 1.0 mL of each of 30 serum samples from juvenile patients with Type I diabetes mellitus, 1.0 μCi (10 μL) of [^{125}I]iodinated insulin is added, mixed, and the mixture is incubated at 4°C for 3 days. Then the total Ig fraction is precipitated by the addition of 2.0 mL of 30 percent PEG, followed by 16 hr incubation at 4°C. The precipitates are harvested by centrifugation at 10,000g

for 10 min at 4°C. The pellets are resuspended in 2 mL of 20 percent PEG solution, mixed, and centrifuged at 10,000g for 10 min. The pellets are washed in 2 mL of 20 percent cold PEG solution and assayed for ^{125}I content after solubilization in 2 N NaOH. The amount of radioactivity recovered in PEG-ppt obtained from sera from Type I diabetic patients was invariably greater than those of the normal control sera obtained from healthy individuals. No correlation was found, however, between the presence of insulin antibodies and IDDM serum cytotoxic factor(s).

REFERENCES

1. G. F. Bottazzo, A. Florin-Christensen, and D. Doniach, *Lancet* **2**, 1279 (1974).

2. N. K. MacLaren, S. W. Huang, and J. Fogh, *Lancet* **1**, 997. (1975).

3. A. Lernmark, Z. R. Freedman, C. Hofmann, A. H. Rubenstein, D. F. Steiner, R. L. Jackson, R. J. Winter, and H. S. Traisman, *N. Engl. J. Med.* **299**, 375 (1978).

4. R. Lendrum, G. Walker, A. G. Cudworth, C. Theophanides, D. A. Pyke, A. Bloom, and D. R. Gamble, *Lancet* **2**, 1273 (1976).

5. A. C. MacCuish, J. Jordan, C. J. Campbell, L. J. P. Duncan, and W. J. Irvine, *Diabetes* **23**, 693 (1974).

6. J. Nerup, O. O. Anderson, G. Bendixen, J. Egberg, R. Gunnarsson, H. Kromann, and J. Poulsen, *Proc. R. Soc. Med.* **67**, 506 (1974).

7. A. C. MacCuish, J. Jordon, C. J. Campbell, L. J. P. Duncan, and W. J. Irvine, *Diabetes* **24**, 36 (1975).

8. K. Buschard and J. Rygaard, *Acta Pathol. Microbiol. Scand. (c)* **86**, 277 (1978).

9. P. Pozzilli, M. Sensi, A. Gursuch, G. F. Bottazzo, and A. G. Cudworth, *Lancet* **2**, 173 (1979).

10. F. K. Jensen, H. Muntefering, and W. A. K. Schmidt, *Diabetologia* **13**, 545 (1977).

11. S. Horowitz, W. Borcherdring, A. Vishnu Moorthy, R. Gheney, H. Schulte-Wissermann, R. Hong, and A. Goldstein, *Science* **197**, 999 (1977).

12. A. D. Steinberg, N. L. Gerber, M. E. Gershwin, R. Morton, D. Goodman, T. M. Chused, J. A. Hardin, and D. R. Barthold, in *Suppressor Cell in Immunity*, S. K. Singhal and N. R. St. C. Sinclair (eds.), The University of Western Ontario, Canada, 1975, p. 174.

13. A. J. Strelkauskas, R. T. Gallery, J. McDowell, Y. Borel, and S. F. Schlossman, *Proc. Natl. Acad. Sci. USA* **75**, 5150 (1978).

14. J. L. Salam, J. Clot, M. Andary, and J. Miroutze, *Diabetologia* **16**, 35 (1979).

15. R. Lendrum, D. G. Nelson, D. A. Pyke, G. Walker, and D. R. Gamble, *Brit. Med. J.* **1**, 553 (1976).

16. M. Christy, J. Nerup, G. F. Bottazzo, D. Doniach, R. Platz, A. Suejgaard, L. P. Ryder, and L. P. Thomsen, *Lancet* **2**, 142 (1976).

17. W. Gepts, *Diabetes* **14**, 619 (1965).

18. J. Egberg, K. Junker, H. Kromann, and J. Nerup, in "Immunological Aspects of Diabetes Mellitus," O. O. Anderson, T. Deckert, and J. Nerup (eds.), *Acta Endocrinol 175*, Copenhagen, Denmark, 1975, p. 129.

19. J. Nerup, O. O. Anderson, G. Bendixen, J. Egberg, and J. E. Poulsen, *Diabetes* **20**, 424 (1971).

20. A. C. MacCuish and W. J. Irvine, *Clinics in Endocrinol. and Metabol.* **4**, 435 (1975).

21. D. R. Gamble, K. W. Taylor, and H. Cumming, *Brit. Med. J.* **4**, 260 (1973).

22. A. G. Cudworth, in *Advanced Medicine*, Vol. 16, A. J. Bellingham (ed.), Pitman Medical, Bath, England, 1980, p. 123.

23. A. B. Jensen, H. S. Rosenberg, and A. L. Notkins, *Lancet* **2**, 345 (1980).

24. W. H. West, R. B. Boozer, and R. B. Heberman, *J. Immunol.* **120**, 90 (1978).

25. H. O. McDevitt, *N. Engl. J. Med.* **303**, 1514 (1980).

26. D. Götze, in *The Major Histocompatibility System in Man and Animals*, D. Götze (ed.), Springer-Verlag, New York, 1977, pp. 1–7.

27. S. W. Huang and N. K. MacLaren, *Science* **191**, 64 (1976).

28. A. Charles, B. Sharma, N. Waldeck, E. Dodson, and S. Nobel, *Diabetes* **28**, 397 (1979).

29. H. G. Rittenhouse, D. L. Oxender, S. B. Pek, and D. Ar, *Diabetes* **29**, 317 (1980).

30. M. J. Doberson, J. E. Schartt, F. Ginsberg-Fellner, and A. L. Notkins, *N. Engl. J. Med.* **303**, 1493 (1980).

31. G. S. Eisenbarth, M. A. Morris, and R. M. Scearce, *J. Clin. Invest.* **64**, 403 (1981).

32. L. A. Idahl, J. Sehlin, I. B. Taijedal, and L. E. Thornell, *Diabetes* **29**, 636 (1980).

33. W. K. Soderstrum, Z. R. Freedman, and A. Lernmark, *Diabetes* **28**, 397 (1979).

34. T. Dyberg, A. F. Nakhooda, S. Baekkeskov, A. Lernmark, P. Poussier, and E. B. Marliss, *Diabetes* **31**, 228 (1982).

35. A. A. Like, A. A. Rossini, D. C. Guberski, M. C. Appel, and R. M. Williams, *Science* **206**, 142 (1979).

36. A. F. Nakhooda, A. A. F. Sima, P. Poussier, and E. B. Marliss, *Endocrinology* **109**, 2264 (1981).

37. P. Poussier, A. F. Nakhooda, A. A. F. Sima, and E. B. Marliss, *J. Exp. Med.* **4**, 35B (1981).

38. P. Poussier, A. F. Nakhooda, J. A. Falk, C. Lee, and E. B. Marliss, *Endocrinology* **110**, 1825 (1982).

39. G. F. Jackson, N. Rassi, T. Crump, B. Haynes, and G. S. Eisenbarth, *Diabetes* **30**, 887 (1981).

40. R. Lendrum, G. Walker, and D. R. Gamble, *Lancet* **1**, 880 (1975).

41. W. J. Irvine, C. G. McCallum, R. S. Gray, G. J. Campbell, and L. J. P. Duncan, *Diabetes* **26**, 138 (1977).

42. G. F. DelPrete, A. Tiengo, G. Bersani, R. Nosadini, C. Garroti, and A. Trisotto, *Horm. Metabol. Res.* **8**, 49 (1976).

43. G. F. Bottazzo, J. I. Mann, M. Thorogood, J. D. Baum, and D. Doniach, *Brit. Med. J.* **2**, 165 (1978).

44. W. J. Irvine, C. J. McCallum, R. S. Gray, and L. J. P. Duncan, *Lancet* **1**, 1025 (1977).

45. G. F. Bottazzo and D. Doniach, *Ric. Clin. Lab* **8**, 29 (1978).

46. M. Sensi, P. Pozzilli, A. N. Gorsuch, G. F. Bottazzo, and A. G. Cudworth, *Diabetologia* **20**, 106 (1981).

47. P. Pozzilli, U. Dimario, and D. Andreani, *Acta Diabetol. Lat.* **19**, 295 (1982).

48. E. R. Richens, J. Quilley, and M. Hartog, *Acta Diabetol. Lat.* **19**, 329 (1982).

49. P. Pozzilli, M. Sensi, B. Dean, A. N. Gorsuch, and A. G. Cudworth, *Acta Diabetol. Lat.* **17**, 119 (1980).

50. R. Pujol-Borrell, E. L. Khoury, and G. F. Bottazzo, *Diabetolgia* **22**, 89 (1982).

51. A. Lernmark, B. R. Högglöf, Z. Freedman, J. W. Irvine, J. Ludvigsson, and G. Holmgren, *Diabetologia* **20**, 471 (1981).

52. W. F. Barllinger and P. E. Lacy, *Surgery* **73**, 175 (1972).

53. G. F. Bottazzo, B. M. Dean, A. N. Gursuch, A. G. Cudworth, and D. Doniach, *Lancet*, March 29, 668 (1980).

54. J. Wigzell and I. B. Tailjedal, *Transplantation* **3**, 423 (1965).

55. A. Lernmark, J. Sehlin, I. B. Tailjedal, H. Kromann, and J. Nerup, *Diabetologia* **14**, 25 (1978).

56. A. J. Böyum, *J. Clin. Lab. Invest.* **21**, 77 (1968).

57. A. I. Ly and R. I., Mishell, *J. Immunol. Methods* **5**, 239 (1974).

58. N. T. Berlinger, C. Lopez, M. Lipkin, J. E. Vogel, and R. A. Good, *J. Clin. Invest.* **59**, 761 (1977).

59. S. Gupta, S. A. Schwartz, and R. A. Good, *Cell. Immunol.* **44**, 242 (1979).

60. T. Timonen and E. Saksela, *J. Immunol. Methods.* **36**,285 (1980).

61. P. Perlmann and H. Perlmann. *Cell. Immunol.* **1**, 300 (1970).

62. B. S. Handwerger and H. S. Koren, *Clin. Immunol. Immunopathol.* **5**, 319 (1976).

B

CHARACTERIZATION OF IMMUNE COMPLEXES FROM PLASMA OF PATIENTS WITH INSULIN-DEPENDENT DIABETES MELLITUS

MOHAMMAD ALI GHALAMBOR, SUMER BELBEZ PEK, STANLEY A. SCHWARTZ, AND DALE L. OXENDER
The University of Michigan, Departments of Biological Chemistry, Internal Medicine, Pediatrics, and Epidemiology, Ann Arbor, Michigan

1. INTRODUCTION

In various autoimmune disorders specific antibodies (Ab) are formed against potential host antigens (Ag) (1–5). Repeated exposure of the Ag to Ab results in the formation of Ag–Ab complexes (immune complexes). Circulating immune complexes (ICs) are normally removed by the reticuloendothelial system. However, certain characteristics of the ICs (valences of Ag and Ab, stability in solution, etc.) may lead to deposition of these complexes in the vascular system and in other tissue sites. This may be followed by tissue injury and interference with humoral and cellular immune mechanisms (6, 7). The possibility that ICs play a role in the pathogenesis of autoimmune disorders is supported by immunological evidence and by data from experimental animal models (8, 9). Increased levels of circulating ICs have been reported in the sera of patients with IDDM at the onset of the disease and in treated patients (10–15).

The role of ICs in cell-mediated immunity and their relationship to the pathogenesis of IDDM have been investigated (6). It has been observed that K cell activity is enhanced in newly diagnosed IDDM patients due to the attachment of ICs to K cells, thereby altering the cytotoxic activity of these cells. In addition, IC-induced aggregation of platelets has been detected in IDDM patients. This phenomenon may account for the abnormality in platelet function encountered in diabetic patients (10).

Regarding the chemical nature of the constituent Ab and Ag molecules of ICs, IgG-containing ICs have been identified in patients with rheumatoid arthritis and diabetes (4, 10). However, there are no data available on the nature of the antigenic component of ICs.

In this chapter isolation and purification of ICs from the plasma samples of diabetic patients and partial characterization of their constituent Ab and Ag components are presented.

2. PURIFICATION OF IMMUNE COMPLEXES

2.1. Materials

Phosphate-buffered saline, 0.05 M phosphate buffer in 0.90 percent NaCl, pH 7.3 (PBS).

Saturated ammonium sulfate solution: 70 g/1000 mL distilled water, adjusted to pH 7.0 with 2 N NaOH.

2 N NaOH.

Na-borate buffer, pH 8.0, 0.04 M.

Polyethylene glycol (PEG): 15 g/100 mL of 0.04 M Na-borate buffer, pH 8.0 (Siegfried Zotingen, Switzerland).

Acetate buffer, 0.10 M, pH 4.6.

Ultrogel AcA-34: A slurry of 10 g/100 mL distilled water (LKB Instruments Co., Rockville, MD).

Radioiodinated plasma pools from normal (nondiabetic) and IDDM patients. 2×10^8 cpm/μg protein/mL (prepared as described in this series).

Nonradioactive plasma pools from normal and IDDM patients, diluted with PBS to a final concentration of 40 mg protein/mL.

Various techniques have been used for detection and isolation of ICs from sera or plasma samples based on the ability of ICs to bind with adsorbents such as Concanavalin A–Sepharose, RAJI cells, C_1q, protein A–Sepharose, and charcoal (16–20) or its precipitation in the presence of polyethylene glycol and ammonium sulfate (21, 22). The procedure used in our studies is a combination of several precipitation steps, followed by column chromatography.

2.2. Procedure

Radioiodinated plasma samples from normal and IDDM patients (5 mL containing 2×10^8 cpm/μg protein/mL) are diluted with 5 mL of nonradioactive plasma, equivalent to 200 mg of protein, to yield a solution with a final protein concentration of 20 mg/mL and a specific activity of 5×10^3 cpm/mg protein. The plasma solutions are subjected to the sequential steps of precipitation with 40 percent ammonium sulfate and isoelectric precipitation of the residual albumin by dialysis of the samples against 0.10 M acetate buffer, pH 4.6, followed by 7 percent PEG precipitation of IgG and ICs (in the acetate buffer retentate) using the procedures described in this series. The IgG and IC-rich fractions thus obtained are further purified by chromatography on Ultrogel AcA-34 according to the procedures described previously. Two peaks, Peak I and Peak II, resolved by Ultrogel chromatography, are partially characterized by several criteria to be discussed. In our experience, the chromatographic elution profile of the PEG-ppt on Ultrogel invariably shows two peaks for each IDDM and control plasma. Peak I, which is excluded from the column, has a molecular weight of > 300,000 and is comprised partially of ICs. Peak II has a molecular weight estimated at 150,000 and is eluted from the gel in the same position as human IgG and contains immunoglobulins of the IgG class.

3. CHARACTERIZATION OF ULTROGEL PEAKS

3.1. Demonstration of IgG in Peaks I and II of Ultrogel

3.1.1. MATERIALS

Staphylococcus aureus (Cowan I strain) formalin-fixed cells suspended in PBS containing 0.02 percent NaN$_3$ (Bethesda Research Laboratories, Gaithersburg, MD).
Peaks I and II fractions, or their pooled eluates.
PBS.
2 N NaOH.
NCS tissue solubilizer (New England Nuclear, Boston, MA).

3.1.2. PROCEDURE

Aliquots (10–100 μL containing 2–20 μg protein and 10^4–10^5 cpm) from Peaks I and II are mixed with 100–190 μL of PBS. Then 100 μL of 10 percent

S. aureus cell suspension are added and the mixture is incubated at 24°C for 30 min, followed by 1 hr at 4°C. Mixtures are centrifuged at 1000g for 5 min at 24°C and cell pellets are washed with two 500 μL portions of PBS. Pellets are dissolved in 200 μL of NaOH, incubated at 37°C for 5 min, and assayed for radioactivity. Triplicate tubes are used for each sample along with two sets of triplicate control tubes: (i) tubes containing PBS instead of plasma and (ii) tubes receiving 100 μL of PBS in lieu of *S. aureus* suspension. These tubes are used as blanks for the radioactivity assay and for estimating total radioactivity, respectively. *S. aureus*-free controls also allow for detection of possible changes in samples resulting from experimental manipulations other than adsorption to *S. aureus* cells. Data are expressed as mean values of counts of each triplicate set (on the ordinate) against the protein content of the same set (on the abscissa). When an excess of *S. aureus* cell suspension is used, a linear relationship between the ^{125}I adsorbed by *S. aureus* and ^{125}I content of the peak materials (used as a source of IgG or IgG-containing immune complexes) is obtained. Both Peaks I and II contain IgG. Under the experimental conditions described, a minimum of 500 μg of IgG are routinely adsorbed by 1 mL of 10 percent *S. aureus* cell suspension.

3.2.   Immunoreactivity of Ultrogel Peaks with Islet Cells

3.2.1.   MATERIALS

Islet cell suspension in PBS, pH 7.3 (50,000 cells/mL).

Peaks I and II containing 2×10^6 cpm/mL.

L-Glutamine, 0.10 M, pH 7.3.

Bovine serum albumin (BSA) 20 g/mL with PBS (Calbiochem, Los Angeles, CA).

Dithiothreitol (DTT), 0.10 M, pH 7.3 (Calbiochem, Los Angeles, CA).

Ethylenediaminetetraacetate (EDTA), 5 mM in PBS (Sigma Chemical Co., St. Louis, MO).

Penicillin-streptomycin solution, 50,000 U/mL and 5 mg/mL (Pen-strep) (Grand Island Biological Co., Grand Island, NY).

Assay mixture: 1 mL of glutamine, 20 mL BSA, 1 mL DTT, 1 mL EDTA, and 1 mL of Pen-strep and 26 mL PBS are mixed.

3.2.2.   PROCEDURE

Aliquots of Peaks I and II eluates (containing 2000–16,000 cpm, 1–8 μg protein) are diluted with 20–90 μL of PBS. Then 100 μL of assay mixture and 50 μL of islet cell suspension are added. Reaction tubes are incubated at 37°C for 1 hr, followed by 1 hr at 4°C. Tubes are centrifuged at 1000g for 5 min, and cell pellets are washed with 500 μL aliquots of PBS. The pellets are dissolved in 250 μL of 2 N NaOH at 37°C for 5 min and assayed for radioactivity.

Triplicate diabetic and normal plasma Peaks I and II are used along with triplicate samples of normal and IDDM Ultrogel Peaks with a 20-fold excess of unlabeled PEG-ppt in order to reduce the specific activity of radioiodinated samples (nonspecific binding controls). All data are expressed as mean counts of experimental tubes minus mean counts of corresponding nonspecific control tubes. When sufficient numbers of cells are used against an appropriate range of IgG or total immunoglobulins, a linear relationship is established between immunoglobulin and IgG concentration versus ^{125}I counts bound to islet cells as illustrated in Figure 1. As shown, the IgG-rich Peak II reacted with islet cells to an appreciable extent, whereas Peak I, which contains immune complexes, was relatively inactive. The lack of significant reactivity of Peak I is due to the fact that the antigen binding sites of immunoglobulin molecules are occupied by the specific antigens.

4.   DETERMINATION OF MOLECULAR WEIGHTS OF PEAKS I AND II

4.1.   Materials

Radioiodinated Peaks I and II.
PBS.

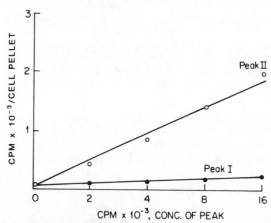

Effect of Concentration of Peaks I and II from Ultrogel Column On Their Reactivity With Islet Cells

FIGURE 1.   Immunoreactivity of radioiodinated Ultrogel peaks I and II with rat islet cells. Increasing concentrations of the peaks (2–16 × 10^3 cpm) were incubated with 5 × 10^3 islet cells, and the cell-bound ^{125}I assayed as described. Reaction of diabetic peak I (●—●—●) after correction for the normal peak I is compared with the activity of diabetic peak II (uncomplexed IgG) (O—O—O) corrected for its corresponding peak II from the normal control plasma. Data are shown as mean values of cpm in triplicate determinations.

Sucrose, 3.42 mg/mL.

Na-Borate buffer, 0.04 M, pH 8.0.

Blue dextran, 1 mg/mL (Pharmacia Fine Chemicals, Piscataway, NJ).

Human IgG, 1 mg/mL (Bethesda Research Laboratories, Rockville, MD).

Protein standards: 1 mg each of crystalline cytochrome c, ovalbumin, and bovine serum albumin (BSA) in 1 mL of PBS, pH 7.3.

4.2. Procedure

A column (110 × 1.4 cm) of Ultrogel is prepared and equilibrated with 0.04 M Na borate buffer, pH 8.0, as described previously in this series. The column is calibrated with blue dextran for measurement of the void volume (Vo). For this purpose, 1 mL of blue dextran is applied to the column, allowed to absorb to the gel, washed with 5 mL of Na-borate buffer (elution buffer), and the eluate is collected in two 2.5 mL portions. Then the column is attached to the reservoir-containing elution buffer, and 2.5 mL fractions are collected in an LKB model 7000 Ultrarac fraction collector at 23°C. The position of the blue dextran is determined by measurement of absorbance at 600 nm in a spectrophotometer. The $^A600$ nm is plotted against eluate volume in milliliters, or the fraction number. The void volume is the volume of fraction number 1 through the fraction with the highest $^A600$-nm value (i.e., number of fractions × 2.5 mL. Then the column is calibrated with standard proteins (cytochrome c, ovalbumin, BSA, and IgG, with molecular weights of 13,800, 45,000, 68,000, and 150,000, respectively). Blue dextran is used for the determination of the void volume and sucrose for the determination of the elution end point. One milliliter of protein standards is mixed with 0.5 mL of blue dextran solution and 0.5 mL of sucrose solution, applied to the column, and treated as described. Fractions (2.5 mL) are collected and assayed for protein by measurement of $^A280$ nm. The elution position of blue dextran is established by measurement of the blue color at $^A600$ nm, and the position of sucrose is determined by quantitative measurement of sucrose by the anthrone procedure (23). The $^A280$, $^A600$, and $^A660$ nm as measures of protein, blue dextran, and sucrose, respectively, are plotted on the ordinate versus the effluent volume in milliliters on the abscissa. The elution volume of each compound is determined by measurement of the volume between the first fraction and the fraction with the highest absorbance for the same compound, being equal to the number of tubes times 2.5 mL. The same chromatograph procedure is then carried out, including 2 × 10⁷ cpm each of Peaks I and II, and the elution position of the peaks is determined by measurement of radioactivity. The elution volume of the peaks is determined and a standard curve for molecular weight determination is constructed by plotting the elution volume of each material divided by the void volume (Ve/Vo) on the ordinate, versus the log mol wt of the corresponding material on the abscissa. The molecular weight of each unknown is determined using the Ve/Vo value for extrapolation. Using these procedures, the molecular weights of Peaks I and II are determined to be > 300,000 and equivalent to 150,000, respectively. Peak I is eluted in the void volume with blue dextran, and Peak II in the same elution position as authentic human IgG. The same column should be used in all of the procedures described to yield reproducible and reliable results. After each run the column is washed with 300 mL of the elution buffer and at the termination of the experiment should be protected against bacterial and fungal contamination by placing 3 mL of 2.5 N NaOH on top of the column and closing the outlet and inlet stopcocks. The standardization of Ultrogel column with proteins of known molecular weight is illustrated in Figure 2.

5.   CHARACTERIZATION OF IMMUNE COMPLEXES IN PEAK I

5.1.   Dissociation of Immune Complexes into Antigen and Antibody

5.1.1.   MATERIALS

Peak I, immune complexes after rechromatography on Ultrogel column, 1×10^7 cpm in 4 mL of PBS.
HCl solution, 0.10 N.
NaOH, 2.5 N.
Glycine-HCl buffer, 0.3 M, pH 2.3.
Sephadex G-50 (Pharmacia Co., Piscataway, NJ).

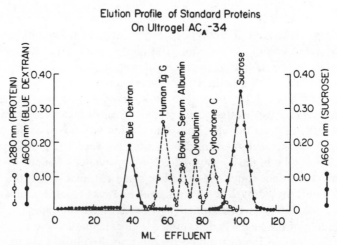

Elution Profile of Standard Proteins
On Ultrogel AC_A-34

FIGURE 2.   Estimation of the molecular weights of components of peak I and peak II. Determination of the molecular weights of peaks I and II was carried out by chromatography with standard proteins on an Ultrogel column. Absorption of blue dextran at 600 nm (●—●—●), protein determination at ^{A}280 nm (O---O---O), and sucrose determination at ^{A}660 nm (●---●---●).

5.1.2. PROCEDURE

Peak I (2 mL, 6×10^6 cpm/mL) is adjusted to pH 2.3 by the addition of 0.10 N HCl. One milliliter of 0.3 M glycine-HCl buffer, pH 2.3, is added. The mixture is incubated at 4°C for 20 min and then chromatographed on a column (45 × 0.77 cm) of Sephadex G-50 equilibrated with 0.10 M glycine-HCl buffer, pH 2.3. The column is eluted with 0.10 M glycine-HCl buffer at a flow rate of 10 mL/hr. Fractions (1 mL) are collected in a fraction collector in 100 × 12 mm plastic tubes at a rate of 10 mL/hr. The pH of the eluate in the tubes is adjusted immediately to 7.3 by the addition of 2.5 N NaOH (using phenol red as an indicator) and the entire contents of the tubes assayed for radioactivity. Two peaks emerge from the column. Peak Ia is excluded from the column in the void volume and Peak Ib, with a considerably smaller molecular weight, is retained by the column. Peak Ia is characterized as the antibody (Ab) component and Peak Ib as the antigen moiety (Ag) of the immune complexes, by the criteria to be described.

The chromatographic elution profile of the dissociated Ag and Ab components of Ics on Sephadex G-50 is illustrated in Figure 3. Peak Ia with a molecular weight of 150,000, which is excluded from the column, is the antibody moiety and under the experimental conditions described emerges from the gel in fractions 4–8. Peak Ib is retained by the column, has a smaller molecular weight than the Ab, and is characterized as the antigenic moiety by various criteria. Comparison of Peaks Ia and Ib derived from the diabetic sample with the corresponding peaks obtained from the control demonstrates that Peaks Ia and Ib of the diabetic sample contain four- to fivefold more radioactivity than Peaks Ia and Ib dissociated from ICs derived from the control.

6. CHARACTERIZATION OF THE ANTIBODY MOIETY OF ICs

6.1. Specific Reactivity with *S. aureus* Cells

6.1.1. MATERIALS

Sephadex G-50 column fractions ([^{125}I] labeled peaks Ia and Ib).
S. aureus suspension, 10 percent in PBS.
PBS.
HBSS.
NaOH, 2 N.

Duplicate aliquots (100 μL) of each of the Sephadex G-50 column fractions are treated with *S. aureus* cell suspension by the procedure described. The amount of ^{125}I adsorbed by *S. aureus* cells per fraction is plotted on the ordinate versus the corresponding fraction number on the abscissa. Comparison of the

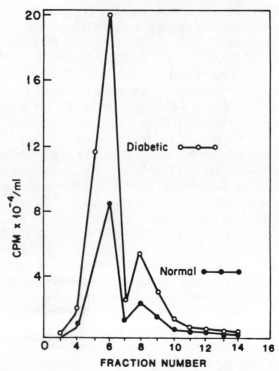

FIGURE 3. Chromatographic elution profile of acid-dissociated radioiodinated IC on Sephadex G-50. Total cpm ^{125}I in fractions obtained from the diabetic sample (O—O—O) are compared with total content of ^{125}I per fraction of the normal (●—●—●). The ^{125}I content of the entire volume of each fraction was counted and mean cpm/fraction is plotted against fraction number.

plots obtained with the chromatographic elution profile of the dissociated ICs on a Sephadex G-50 column demonstrates that only Peak Ia, containing antibody of the IgG isotype, reacts with *S. aureus* cells (Fig. 4, panel A). Furthermore, the amount of ^{125}I adsorbed by *S. aureus* for Peak Ia from the diabetic ICs is much greater than that of Peak Ia derived from ICs obtained from normal plasma.

6.2. Immunoreactivity with Islet Cells

6.2.1. MATERIALS

Sephadex G-50 column fractions.
Rat islet cells.
Assay mixture.

PBS.

HBSS.

NaOH, 2 N.

Duplicate aliquots (100 µL) from each of the Sephadex G-50 fractions are incubated with 10^4 islet cells under the experimental conditions described. Islet cell pellets obtained by centrifugation are washed with PBS, dissolved in 2 N NaOH, and assayed for radioactivity. The quantity of islet-cell-bound ^{125}I per fraction is plotted on the ordinate against the corresponding fraction number on the abscissa (Fig. 4, panel B). Similar to adsorption of IgG by S. *aureus* cells, fractions corresponding to Peak Ia reacted with islet cells significantly; no reactivity was observed in fractions corresponding to Peak Ib, the Ag moiety of dissocated IC.

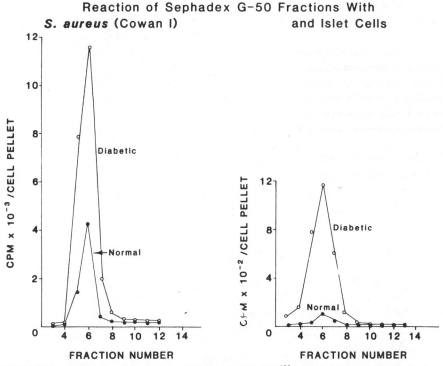

FIGURE 4.   Reactivity of S. *aureus* and islet cells with the [^{125}I]-labeled Ag and Ab components separated on a Sephadex G-50 column. Left panel: Adsorption of IgG present in peak Ia with S. *aureus* testing an aliquot (100 µL) from each fraction including fractions corresponding to peak Ib. Reactivity of the diabetic sample (O—O—O) is compared with the nondiabetic sample (●—●—●). Right panel: Immunoreactivity of IC components with rat islet cells. An aliquot (150 µL) from each fraction was incubated with 2.5 × 10^3 islet cells, and the cell-bound [^{125}I] content determined as described. The islet cell-bound [^{125}I] from diabetic samples (O—O—O) is comapred to nondiabetic samples (●—●—●). Data are presented as mean values cpm of duplicate samples.

6.3.   Specific Adsorption by Protein A

6.3.1.   MATERIALS

Antibody component of IC, $1.5-2.0 \times 10^5$ cpm/mL, total of 5 mL.
Protein A–agarose: 5 mL (Bethesda Research Laboratories).
Acetic acid, 0.5 N in distilled water.
Phosphate buffer, 0.10 M, pH 7.2.
Phenol red indicator solution: 1 mg/100 mL.
2.5 N NaOH.

6.3.2.   PROCEDURE

A plastic column (10 × 0.5 cm) is packed with 5 mL of a slurry of protein A–agarose and equilibrated with 0.10 M phosphate buffer, pH 7.2. The entire radioiodinated Peak Ia from the Sephadex column (the Ab moiety of dissociated ICs, $7-10 \times 10^5$ cpm) is applied to the column and eluted with the same phosphate buffers. The initial eluate is collected in 1 mL fractions in 100 × 12-mm capped plastic tubes, and the entire contents of the tubes are assayed for radioactivity. Tubes 7 and 8 of the phosphate buffer eluate should contain less than 1000 cpm/mL at which point the column is eluted with 0.5 N acetic acid in distilled water, and sixteen 1-mL fractions are collected. Fractions are immediately neutralized to pH 7.3 by the addition of NaOH, capped, and assayed for radioactivity. Most (80–90 percent) of the radioactivity is eluted in the first five tubes of acetic acid eluate, indicating that the majority of the ^{125}I is retained by the column. Since protein A specifically adsorbs IgG (24, 25), the Ab component of the ICs is identified as an immunoglobulin of the IgG isotype.

6.4.   Immunoreactivity with Islet Cell Subcomponents

6.4.1.   MATERIALS

Unlabeled Peak I from Ultrogel column.
Glycine-HCl buffer, 0.10 M, pH 2.3.
Sephadex G-50 column.
[^{3}H]Leucine-labeled rat islet cells.
[^{3}H]Leucine-labeled rat islet cell subcomponents prepared as described in this series.
Radioiodinated Peak I from Ultrogel column.
Unlabeled rat islet cells.
Unlabeled rat islet cell subcomponents.
2 N NaOH.

Phenol red indicator.

Assay mixture.

PBS.

A sample of unlabeled immune-complex-rich material (Peak I from Ultrogel column) is dissociated at pH 2.3 in 0.10 M glycine-HCl buffer as described for [^{125}I] labeled IC-rich samples. The dissociated Ag and Ab are separated by chromatography on a Sephadex G-50 column, and Peak Ia (Ab) and Peak Ib (Ag) are pooled and tested for their immunoreactivity with 5×10^4 cpm of [^{3}H]leucine-labeled islet cells or islet cell subcomponents by the procedures previously described in this series. Another variation of the incubation mixture is used to determine the reactivity of radioiodinated Peak Ia obtained by chromatographic separation of the dissociated Ab and Ag moieties of ICs using a Sephadex G-50 column. Fifty-microliter aliquots of Peak Ia, equivalent to 2×10^4 cpm/10 μg of radioiodinated Peak Ia, are incubated with 5×10^4 unlabeled islet cells or subcomponents derived from an equal number of cells. The incubations are carried out as described and the washed pellets are assayed for radioactivity. Results are presented as the mean of triplicates per assay and the specific activities of islet cells and their subfractions are expressed as cpm per microgram of protein. Table 1 summarizes the comparison of the reactivity of purified Peak Ia (Ab component of ICs) with whole islet cells and their subcomponents. As indicated, in both variations of the incubation mixture the membrane fraction has the highest degree of reactivity with the Ab component of ICs.

6.5. Specificity of IgG (Ab component of ICs) for Islet Cells

6.5.1. MATERIALS

Rat cell types: liver, lung, spleen, erythrocytes, and islet cells prepared from autologous rats as described in this series.

Ab moiety of ICs (36,000 cpm/10 μg protein) from diabetic and normal samples.

Assay mixture.

Rat islet cells.

Ficoll-Hypaque.

PBS and HBSS.

NaOH, 2 N.

6.5.2. PROCEDURE

Lung, liver, and spleen cells are prepared from the corresponding tissues, and erythrocytes are separated from the blood of autologous rats from which the islets of Langerhans are isolated. [^{125}I] labeled Ab moiety of ICs (100 μL = 10 μg protein containing 36,000 cpm) is mixed with 100 μL of assay mixture

TABLE 1. Comparison of Reactivity of IgG from Diabetic Plasma with Islet Cells and Their Subcomponents

Experiment[a] No.	Fractions[b]	Protein[c] (μg)	cpm[d]	Specific[e] Activity
			^{125}I	
I	Nuclei	10	1,130	113
	Granules	18	2,230	124
	Mitochondria	20	2,660	112
	Membrane	11	3,800	345
	Whole cells	158	5,500	31
			^3H	
II	Nuclei	10	7,400	740
	Granules	18	12,000	667
	Mitochondria	20	13,200	660
	Membrane	11	17,200	1537
	Soluble fraction	100	25,900	259
	Whole cells	158	18,600	118

[a] Experiment I: 10μg (40,000 cpm) of [^{125}I]–labeled IgG purified from dissociated immuno complexes of diabetic plasma (pool 1) were incubated with 5×10^4 whole rat islet cells or the subcellular fractions derived from an equivalent number of islet cells. Experiment II: 10 μg of unlabeled IgG from diabetic plasma (pool 2) purified as above were incubated with 5×10^4 [^3H]–labeled islet cells, or the subcellular fractions derived therefrom. Radioactivity bound to the differentially sedimented fractions was determined by solubilization of radioactive pellets in NCS prior to the addition of scintillation fluid.

[b] Whole islet cells or their subcellular fractions were prepared as described in materials and methods.

[c] Protein content of each fraction was measured by solubilization in 3 percent SDS, 4 percent urea, 0.1 M Tris-HCl, pH 7.5, at 100°C for 5 min, followed by Lowry protein determination. Standards were assayed simultaneously under identical conditions.

[d] Values (cpm) are the mean of triplicate determinations minus corresponding controls. Controls consist of all of the ingredients of the incubation of mixture plus an additional 100 μg of unlabeled diabetic IgG to compete for specific binding; the residual counts are designated as nonspecific and subtracted from the experimental counts. As an additional control for nonspecificity, IgG from pooled normal plasma is incubated with islet cells and subfractions exactly as described for diabetic IgG; these counts are also subtracted from the experimental counts.

[e] Specific activities are expressed as cpm per μg microgram of protein.

This experiment has been performed twice as presented in Table 1. In addition, the reaction of subcellular materials with other sources of IgG [e.g, Peak II (IgG-rich fraction)] of Ultrogel obtained from diabetic pools 1 and 2, total immunoglobulin fraction from diabetic pools 1 and 2, and individual fractions collected from Sephadex column corresponding to IgG from diabetic pools 2 and 3 gave similar results.

and 50 μL of cell suspension containing 2×10^4 of one type of cell. The mixtures are incubated at 37°C for 60 min, followed by 3 hr at 4°C, and centrifuged at 1000g for 5 min. Pellets are dissolved in 250 μL of 2 N NaOH and assayed for radioactivity as described. The immunoreactivity of the various cell types with the Ab moiety of ICs is compared with the islet cells. The percent immunoreactivity of a cell type is calculated by dividing ^{125}I counts bound to the cells by the counts bound to the islet cells, times 100. Comparison of the reactivity of various cell types is illustrated in Table 2. As indicated, only islet cells demonstrated significant reactivity with the Ab; other cell types were relatively inactive.

7. CHARACTERIZATION OF THE ANTIGEN MOIETY OF ICs

7.1 Immunoreactivity with Islet-Cell-Specific Ab

7.1.1. MATERIALS

Total Ig from diabetic and normal plasma (pool 2).

Peak II from Ultrogel: unlabeled IgG-rich fraction (pool 2).

Peak Ia from Sephadex G-50 column: Unlabeled Ab moiety of ICs obtained from pools of diabetic and normal plasma (pools 2 and 3).

Ag moiety of ICs, [^{125}I]–labeled (4×10^6 cpm/mg protein).

Assay mixture.

2 N NaOH.

TABLE 2. Organ Specificity of Purified IgG from Diabetic Plasma

Cell Source[a]	Cell-Bound ^{125}I[b] (cpm)	Percent Activity[c]
Liver	360	7.7
Lung	200	4.3
Spleen	350	7.5
RBC	570	12.2
Islet Cells	4660	100.00

[a] Single cell suspensions were prepared from autologous organs and 2×10^4 cells were incubated with 36,000 cpm of [^{125}I]–labeled purified IgG equivalent to 10 μG of protein from diabetic (pool 1) and normal plasma.
[b] ^{125}I bound to the cell pellet represents the net counts of the diabetic samples minus the nonspecific binding of normal donor IgG. The mean of triplicate determinations was recorded.
[c] Percent activity is calculated as ^{125}I counts per nonislet cell pellet divided by ^{125}I counts in the islet cell pellet ($\times 100$).
   This experiment has been performed twice on pool 1 and once on pool 2 and similar results have been obtained.

Peak Ia purified by protein A–agarose chromatography.

PBS.

7.1.2. PROCEDURE

Aliquots of $[^{125}I]$-labeled Ag (50 μL equivalent to 5 μg of protein with 20,00 cpm) are mixed with 100 μL of assay mixture and 100 μL (10 μg) of one of the Ab preparations mentioned above. The mixtures are incubated at 37°C for 60 min, followed by 3 hr at 4°C. After centrifugation at 20,000 for 10 min, the pellets are washed in 5 mL PBS, solubilized in 250 μL NaOH, and counted. Results presented in Table 3 demonstrate that the Ag moiety of ICs (Peak Ib of the Sephadex column) derived from the IDDM samples consistently shows significant reactivity with islet-cell-specific Ab in various preparations, whereas Peak Ib (Ag component of ICs) from the control samples tested under the same conditions is relatively inactive. As seen, the reactivity of the Ag moiety of ICs with an IgG preparation derived from the same immune complex-rich material (purified by protein A–agarose chromatography) is maximal as compared to antibodies present in the less purified preparations such as total Ig and Peak II from the Ultrogel column.

7.2. Reconstitution of Immune Complexes

7.2.1. MATERIALS

Unlabeled IgG (Ab component dissociated from ICs) from the diabetic plasma.

TABLE 3.   Reaction of Small Molecular Weight Component Dissociated from Immune Complexes from Diabetic Plasma with Islet-Specific Ab

Ab Preparations	cpm ^{125}I		percent ^{125}I Incorporated[a]	
	Diabetic[b]	Normal[c]	Diabetic	Normal
Total Ig	1460	210	7.3	1.05
Peak II (Ultrogel)	1660	302	8.3	1.51
Peak Ia (Sephadex)	2080	430	10.4	2.15
Peak Ia (Sephadex, plasma pool #3)	1910	395	9.6	1.97
Peak Ia (Sephadex, purified)	4160	710	20.8	3.8

[a] 20,000 cpm $[^{125}I]$–labeled antigen equivalent to 5 μg protein was used in each incubation mixture and the mean of triplicate determinations was recorded.

[b] Unless otherwise noted, Ab were derived from IDDM plasma (pool 2); 10 μg protein was used in each reaction mixture.

[c] Ab from normal plasma reacted against the small component dissociated from diabetic ICs.

Ag component of the same IC preparation from diabetic sample, 8×10^5 cpm/mg protein.

PEG, 10 percent in Na-borate buffer, 0.04 M, pH 8.0

PBS.

Assay mixture.

Na-Borate buffer, 0.08 M.

PEG, 5 percent in 0.04 M Na-borate buffer, pH 8.0.

PEG, 10 percent in 0.08 M Na-borate buffer, pH 8.0.

Assay mixture.

PBS.

2 N NaOH.

Unlabeled IgG from the plasma of diabetic patients purified by protein A–agarose chromatography as described in this series.

7.2.2. PROCEDURE

Varying concentrations (2.5–25 μg in 5.0–50 μL) of the [^{125}I] labeled Ag moiety of ICs (Sephadex Peak Ib) containing $2-20 \times 10^3$ cpm are mixed with 100 μL of assay mixture and 50–95 μL of PBS and 50 μL of the unlabeled IgG (Ab component of the same ICs) containing 10 μg protein and incubated at 37°C for 60 min, followed by 4 hr at 4°C. A 10 percent solution (250 μL) of PEG is added to each incubation mixture, mixed, and incubated at 4°C for 4 hr. Following centrifugation at 3000g at 4°C for 10 min, the pellets are washed in 10 mL of cold (4°C) 5 percent PEG solution and centrifuged at 3000g for 10 min at 4°C. The washed pellets are dissolved in 200 μL of 2 N NaOH and assayed for radioactivity. As illustrated in Figure 5 the reactivity of Ag with its specific Ab derived from the same IC preparation followed first-order kinetics. The Ag–Ab complex thus obtained was indistinguishable from the ICs from which the Ag and Ab had been initially derived on the basis of their cochromatography on Ultrogel AcA-34 column, precipitation with 5 percent PEG, and dissociation at pH 2.3.

7.3. Effect of Insulin

7.3.1. MATERIALS

[^{125}I]–labeled Ag component of ICs.

Unlabeled IgG (Ab component of ICs).

Assay mixture.

Rat insulin, 1000 ng/mL (Novoterapeutisk Labs, Copenhagen, Denmark).

PBS.

$S.$ $aureus$ cell suspension, 10 percent in PBS containing 0.02 percent NaN_3.

NaOH, 2 N.

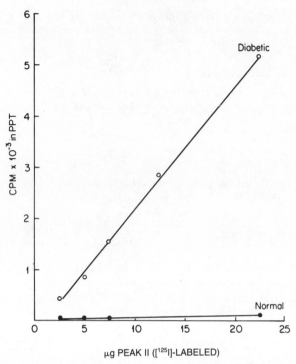

Reaction of Peak II (Sephadex) with Unlabeled Peak I (Sephadex)

FIGURE 5.   Reactivity of peak Ib from Sephadex G-50 column with IgG moiety of IC obtained from diabetic plasma. Varying concentrations of [^{125}I]-labeled peak Ib from Sephadex G-50 chromatography of dissociated IC are incubated with unlabeled peak Ia (IgG) dissociated from another aliquot of the diabetic sample. The Ag-Ab complexes formed are adsorbed by *S. aureus* cells. The pellets are washed with PBS, dissolved in NaOH, and assayed for radioactivity. Data are expressed as the mean values of cpm of duplicate aliquots from the diabetic samples (O—O—O) compared with the corresponding nondiabetic samples (O—O—O).

7.3.2.   PROCEDURE

Two different aliquots, 2.5 and 5.0 μg (25–50 μL, containing 1–2 × 10^4 cpm) of [^{125}I]–labeled antigenic components of ICs are mixed with 15–75 μL of insulin solution. Then 100 μL of assay mixture, 25–110 μL PBS, and 50 μL of unlabeled Ab moiety of ICs (5 μg protein) are added, mixed, and incubated at 37°C for 60 min, followed by 4 hr at 4°C. *S. aureus* cell suspension (100 μL) is added to each tube, mixed, incubated at 25°C for 30 min, followed by 2 hr at 4°C. After centrifugation of the samples at 1000*g* for 5 min at 23°C, the pellets are washed with two 2 mL portions of PBS, dissolved in NaOH, and assayed for radioactivity. Duplicate tubes for each concentration of insulin with IDDM samples are carried out simultaneously with duplicates of each

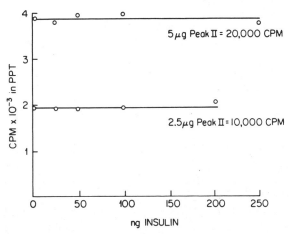

The Effect of Insulin on the Reaction of Peak II
from Sephadex (Ag) with Unlabeled IgG
(Peak I from Sephadex)

FIGURE 6. Effect of rat insulin on the reaction of peak Ia with peak Ib from the dissociated IC. Increasing quantities of rat insulin are added to incubation mixtures containing unlabeled IgG (Ab) and mixed. Then 2.5 or 5.0 μg of dissociated peak Ib containing 10,000-20,000 cpm ^{125}I are added, mixed, and processed as described. The resulting Ag-Ab complex is precipitated with protein A and the radioactivity in the washed pellets is counted. Data represent the mean values of duplicate determinations for diabetic samples.

aliquot of [^{125}I]–labeled Ag and the arithmetic mean value of the counts is recorded. Results obtained in our experiments indicate that rat insulin did not cause any detectable inhibition of the reaction of Ag with Ab components of ICs, confirming the premise that these Ag-Ab systems are distinct from the insulin–anti-insulin system (Fig. 6).

REFERENCES

1. F. J. Dixon, *J. Invest. Dermatol.* **59**, 413 (1973).

2. H. G. Kunkel and E. M. Tan, *Adv. Immunol.* **4**, 351 (1964).

3. A. C. Maccich and W. J. Irvine, *Clin. Endocrinol. Metabol.* **4**, 435 (1975).

4. H. G. Kunkel, H. J. Muller-Eberhard, and H. H. Fundenberg, *J. Clin. Invest.* **40**, 117 (1961).

5. M. B. A. Oldstone, *J. Natl. Cancer Inst.* **54**, 223 (1972).

6. P. Pozzilli, U. DiMario, and D. Andreani, *Acta Diabet. Lat.* **19**, 295 (1982).

7. E. R. Richens, J. Quiley, and M. Hartog, *Acta Diabet. Lat.* **19**, 329 (1982).

8. M. A. Mannik, O. Haakenstand, and W. P. Arend, *Prog. Immunol. II* **5**, 91 (1974).

9. C. G. Cochrane and D. Koffler, *Adv. Immunol.* **16**, 185 (1973).

10. J. M. Kilpatrick and G. Virella, *Acta Diabet. Lat.* **19**, 107 (1982).

11. W. J. Irvine, B. F. Clarke, and L. Scarth, *Lancet* **2**, 163 (1970).

12. W. J. Irvine, U. DiMario, K. Guy, C. M. Feek, R. S. Gray, and L. P. J. Duncan, *J. Clin. Lab. Immunol.* **1**, 183 (1978).

13. W. J. Irvine, S. F. Al-Kateeb, U. DiMario, C. M. Feek, R. S. Gray, B. Edmond, and L. P. J. Duncan, *Clin. Exp. Immunol.* **30**, 16 (1977).

14. W. J. Irvine, U. DiMario, K. Guy, and D. Q Borsey, *J. Clin. Lab. Immunol.* **4**, 87 (1980).

15. U. DiMario, M. Iavicoli, and D. Andreani, *Diabetologia* **19**, 89 (1980).

16. R. Heimer and G. Klein, *Inter. J. Cancer* **18**, 310 (1976).

17. A. N. Theofilopoulos, R. A. Eisenberg, and F. J. Dixon, *J. Clin. Invest.* **61**, 1570 (1978).

18. F. C. Hay, I. J. Nineham, and I. M. Roitt, *Clin. Exp. Immunol.* **24**, 396 (1976).

19. F. Chenais, G. Virella, C. C. Patrick, and H. H. Fundenberg, *J. Immunol. Methods* **18**, 183 (1977).

20. W. D. Odel, in *Methods in Enzymology*, H. van Vunakis and J. J. Langone (eds.), Vol. 70, Academic Press, New York, 1980, p. 274.

21. W. D. Creighton, P. H. Lambert, and P. A. Meischer, *J. Immunol* **III**, 1219 (1973).

22. T. Chard, in *Methods in Enzymology*, H. van Vunakis and J. J. Langone (eds.), Vol. 70, Academic Press, New York, 1980, p. 280.

23. T. A. Scott and E. H. Melvin, *Anal. Chem.* **25**, 1656 (1953).

24. J. J. Langone in *Methods in Enzymology*, H. van Vunakis, and J. J. Langone (eds.), Vol. 70, Academic Press, New York, 1980, p. 356.

25. C. C. Patrick and G. Virella, *Immunochemistry* **15**, 137 (1978).

C

ISLET-CELL-SPECIFIC ANTIBODIES IN PLASMA OF PATIENTS WITH INSULIN-DEPENDENT DIABETES MELLITUS

MOHAMMAD ALI GHALAMBOR,
STANLEY A. SCHWARTZ, SUMER BELBEZ PEK,
AND DALE L. OXENDER

The University of Michigan, Departments of Biological Chemistry, Pediatrics, Internal Medicine, and Epidemiology, Ann Arbor, Michigan,

1. INTRODUCTION

The presence of several types of islet-cell-specific antibodies (ICA) in sera from patients with insulin-dependent diabetes mellitus (IDDM) has been documented immunologically and also demonstrated in experimental animal models (1–14). As a consequence of a normal immunologic reaction, some of these antibodies (Ab) combine with islet cell antigens to form antigen–antibody complexes (15). However, a number of ICA remain free in circulation and may be detected by immunochemical techniques (2, 3, 6, 8, 11, 13, 15). Anticytoplasmic and complement-fixing ICA have been detected by indirect immunofluorescence techniques on frozen sections of pancreas (16, 17). Cytotoxic ICA have been shown in the sera of patients with IDDM by measurement of ^{51}Cr released from ^{51}Cr labeled islet cells following their complement-mediated lysis (14, 18, 19). Cytotoxic ICA specific for β cells of islets of Langerhans have been detected in the sera of patients with IDDM (14, 19, 20). Islet-cell-surface-specific antibodies have been demonstrated in up to 87 percent of the sera from patients with IDDM by immunofluorescence techniques (3, 6). These findings were confirmed using $[^{125}I]$–labeled protein A ($[^{125}I]$-PA) as an immunoadsorbent in a rat islet cell anti-rat cell system (8, 13, 14). Similar results were obtained when plasma samples from experimental diabetic BB rats were used against dispersed islet cells prepared from normal homologous animals (13). The presence of antibodies specifically directed against the surface antigenic moieties of α, δ, and β cells have been demonstrated in sera of patients with recent onset of IDDM by immunofluorescent and cytochemical characterization of ICS-Ab bound to cells (21). Complement-dependent cytotoxic islet cell surface antibodies have also been shown to be present in the sera of IDDM patients (18, 19, 22–25).

This chapter describes procedures for demonstration and characterization of ICA directed toward intact islet cells and their subcomponents. Special emphasis is placed on the use of radioligand assay procedures developed in our laboratory.

2. PREPARATION OF ISLET CELLS AND THEIR SUBCOMPONENTS

2.1. Preparation of Single Islet Cells

2.1.1. MATERIALS

Sprague-Dawley rats.

D-Glucose solution, 0.139 M in distilled water.

L-Glutamine solution, 0.20 M in distilled water.

Dithiothreitol solution (DTT), 0.20 M in distilled water.

Penicillin-streptomycin, 100,000 U/mL and 10 mg/mL, respectively (Pen-strep).

Ethylenediaminetetraacetate (EDTA), 0.10 M, pH 7.3.

Bovine serum albumin (BSA), 20 percent in distilled water.

Fetal calf serum (FCS).

RPMI 1640 culture medium (Grand Island Biological Co., Grand Island, NY).

Hanks' balanced salt solution (HBSS), Ca^{2+}, MG^{2+}-free.

Medium supplement: 10 mL each of glucose, DTT, glutamine, and pencillin-streptomycin solutions are mixed and sterile filtered.

Islet medium: 4 mL of the medium supplement and 96 mL of RPMI 1640 medium are mixed aseptically.

Dispase, 10,000 μ/vial (Gono Shusei, Tokyo, Japan).

2.1.2. PROCEDURE

Rat islets isolated by the collagenase method of Lacy and Kostianovsky (26) are dispersed by controlled digestion with Dispase (27) as follows: 1000 islets are washed in HBSS and suspended in 1 mL of islet medium containing 10 percent FCS. EDTA solution (10 μL) is added to the suspension, mixed gently, and incubated for 7 min at 24°C. The islets are sedimented by centrifugation at 500g for 2 min, washed with 5 mL of HBSS, and resuspended in 0.5 mL of HBSS. Then 0.5 mL of a Dispase solution containing 1000 U/mL HBSS is added, mixed, and the suspension is incubated in a 37°C water bath for 8–10 min with gentle constant shaking. The suspension is removed from the water bath and allowed to settle at 24°C for 1 min. The supernate is withdrawn with a Pasteur pipette, diluted with 10 mL of cold HBSS, and centrifuged at 500g for 3 min. The pellet containing single islet cells is washed with two 5 mL portions of HBBS, resuspended in 1 mL of islet medium (with 4 percent BSA), and counted in a hemocytometer. Trypan blue dye exclusion test is used to determine percent cell viability. The yield is 600–1800 islet cells per islet with 80–90 percent viable cells.

2.2. Islet and Islet Cell Culture

Islets or single islet cells are suspended in islet medium at a concentration of 1000 islets or 10^6 islet cells/5 mL and incubated at 37°C for a period of 1–14 days in a humidified 5 percent CO_2/95 percent air incubator. At 24 hr intervals islets or islet cell suspensions are centrifuged, the islet or islet cells resuspended in fresh medium containing 10 percent FCS, and the culture supernates are assayed for insulin and prostaglandin content. The islet or islet cells routinely retain their ability to secrete insulin and prostaglandins up to 2 weeks.

3. LABELING AND FRACTIONATION OF ISLET CELLS

3.1. MATERIALS

L-leucine-free minimal essential medium (MEM).

L-Leucine [3,4,5,-^{3}H], specific activity (S.A.) > 100 Ci/mmol, diluted to 1 Ci/mL with distilled sterile water.

L-Leucine-free islet medium: Mix 1 mL each of glucose, DTT, glutamine, and Pen-strep and 10 mL of FCS with 86 mL of MEM aseptically.

Sodium bicarbonate solution, 1 M, sterilized by filtration.

NaOH, 2.5 N.

Saturated ammonium sulfate (SAS), pH 7.0: Dissolve 700 g of crystalline ammonium sulfate in 800 mL of distilled water, adjust to pH 7.0 by addition of 2.5 N NaOH and dilute to 1000 mL with distilled water.

Phosphate-buffered saline (PBS): Mix 1 L of 0.05 M phosphate buffer, pH 7.3, with 1 L of 1.8 percent NaCl and sterilize by autoclaving.

HEPES buffer, 0.01 M, pH 7.3: Dissolve 2.383 g of 4-(2-hydroxymethyl)-1-piperazineethane-sulfonic acid (HEPES) in 600 mL of PBS, adjust the pH to 7.3 by the addition of 2.5 N NaOH, dilute to 1000 mL with PBS, readjust the pH, and sterilize by filtration.

Sucrose solution, 5 M in distilled water.

Tris-HCl, 0.40 M, pH 7.3.

Tris-sucrose solution: Mix equal volumes of Tris-HCl and sucrose solution.

NCS Tissue solubilizer (New England Nuclear, Boston, MA).

Hydrofluor scintillation fluid (New England Nuclear, Boston, MA).

3.2. Procedure

Islet cells ($1-5 \times 10^6$) are suspended in leucine-free MEM at a concentration of 2×10^6 cells/mL. [^{3}H]leucine solution (250 μL = 0.25 mCi) is added to the suspension using a sterile microsyringe and the pH is adjusted to 7.4 by the addition of sodium bicarbonate solution. The cell suspension is incubated at 37°C for 4 hr, and the pH adjustment is repeated at hourly intervals. Cells are harvested by centrifugation at 500g for 2 min, washed with two 10 mL portions of HBSS, resuspended in HBSS (10^6 cells/mL) and assayed for radioactivity as follows: 5 μL of the cell suspension are added to a tube containing 495 μL of HBSS and mixed thoroughly. Triplicate aliquots of 25 μL of the 1:100 dilution of islet cell suspension thus obtained are placed in scintillation vials, and 100 μL of a tissue solubilizer reagent such as NCS (New England Nuclear) is added and mixed on a vortex shaker. Then scintillation fluid (Hydrofluor) is added and the radioactivity is determined in a Beckman LS-7000 spectrometer. Total counts of the cell suspension is calculated from the average counts per 25 mL sample as follows:

$$\text{Total counts} = 1000/25 \times \text{dilution factor} \times \text{volume of the cell suspension}$$

To determine the efficiency of incorporation of [^{3}H]leucine in islet cells, a constant parameter such as cpm per cell, or cpm per mg protein is used.

Islet cells ($1-5 \times 10^6$) are suspended in 4 mL of Tris-sucrose solution and disrupted with sonic oscillation by four 30 sec cycles with intermittent cooling in ice. The disrupted cell suspension is fractionated by differential centrifugation according to the method of Taratakoff and Jameison (28) as follows: The suspension is centrifuged at 300g for 10 min in a Sorvall RC-2 centrifuge at 4°C. The pellet (cell debris) is suspended in 250 μL of PBS and the supernatant fluid (S_1) is centrifugated at 600g for 10 min. The granules present in the pellet are saved, and the supernatant (S_2) is centrifuged at 1000g for 10 min to sediment the nuclei. The supernate from this step (S_3) is centrifuged at 9000g for 20 min, the pellet (mitochondria) is saved, and the supernatant fluid (S_4) is centrifugated at 100,000g for 70 min in a Beckman L2-65-B ultracentrifuge and the pellet obtained is designated as the membrane fraction. The supernatant fluid is dialyzed against 1 L of saturated ammonium sulfate for 16 hr at 4°C, the retentate centrifuged at 15,000g for 15 min and the supernate is discarded. The pellet obtained is dissolved in 0.8 mL of HEPES buffer and dialyzed against 2 L of HEPES containing 0.02 percent NaN$_3$ at 4°C for 24 hr. The content of the dialysis bag is centrifuged at 15,000g for 15 min and the sediment discarded. The volume of the supernatant solution (soluble fraction) is adjusted to 1 mL. Each of the islet cell subcomponents (granules, nuclei, mitochondria, and the membranes) is suspended in 250 μL of PBS and all of the fractions are assayed for radioactivity as follows: A 1:10 dilution of the cell debris and each of the islet cell subcomponents is prepared by adding 10 μL of each to 90 μL HBSS. The soluble fraction is diluted 1:100 by adding 10 μL of this fraction to 990 μL of HBSS. Triplicate 25 μL aliquots of each fraction are

TABLE 1. **Distribution of [³H]Leucine in Various Subfractions of the Rat Islet Cells**

Cell Fractions[a]	Total CPM[b]	Percent Total[c]
Cell debris	1.8×10^6	0.351
Nuclei	3.0×10^5	0.058
Granules	2.8×10^5	0.054
Mitochondria	1.1×10^5	0.021
Membrane	2.3×10^7	4.290
Soluble material[d]	4.9×10^8	95.205

[a] Rat islet cells were dispersed by sonic oscillation in 0.25 M sucrose, 0.10 M Tris-HCl, pH 7.5, medium and subjected to differential centrifugation as described in methods.
[b] CPM represents the average of two sets of duplicate samples of different concentrations. Each sample was counted three times, for 1.0, 5, and 10 min.
[c] Percentages are based on the total CPM recovered at the end of the experiment; possible losses during the experiment were not considered.
[d] The soluble fraction was concentrated by dialysis against a solution of saturated ammonium sulfate, pH 7.0, followed by centrifugation. The pellet was dissolved in PBS and dialyzed against PBS; the retentate was centrifuged and the supernate (soluble) was saved as described in methods.

assayed for ^{3}H content as described previously and the total cpm per fraction are calculated from the mean counts per 25 μL as described above. A representative pattern of the distribution of [^{3}H]leucine among the various islet cell fractions is shown in Table 1.

4. RADIOIODINATION OF PROTEIN SAMPLES

4.1. Materials

Phosphate buffer, 0.5 M, pH 7.2 (PB).

Sodium iodide, Na [125]I (New England Nuclear, Boston, MA) diluted to 100 mCi/mL

Iodination beads, IODO-BEADS, N-chloro-benzenesulfonamide (sodium salt): derivatized uniform nonporous polystyrene beads (Pierce Chemical Co., Rockford, IL).

Chloramine-T solution: 1 mg/mL of 0.5 M phosphate buffer, pH 7.2.

Sodium metabisulfite solution: 1 mg/mL PBS (MB).

Thimerosal: 1.0 percent in water.

Diabetic plasma: individual samples or pools.

Normal control plasma: individual samples or pools.

Diabetic and normal plasma solutions: pooled plasma samples are centrifuged at 10,000g for 10 min at 4°C, and the supernatant fluids are diluted to yield 200 mg protein/mL.

Diluted plasma pools: plasma solutions obtained above are diluted to 1 mg/mL with PBS.

BSA, 5 percent in 0.10 M phosphate buffer, pH 7.2.

Bio-Gel P-60 (Pharmacia, Piscataway, NJ).

Sodium thiosulfate, saturated solution.

4.2. Procedure

To a 1 mL crimped vial are added 10 μL of plasma protein solution, 65 μL of PB, 20 μL of Na ^{125}I, and 5 μL of chloramine-T solution. The mixture is stirred on a vortex mixer for 5 min at 4°C. The 5 μL of MB solution are added, followed by 100 μL of albumin solution. The radioiodinated proteins are isolated by column chromatography as follows: a 1 × 15 cm borosilicate glass tube is connected to Tygon tubing, and the outlet equipped with a Teflon stopcock. The column is packed with a slurry of Bio-Gel P-60 to a 10 cm height and treated with 15 mL of BSA solution, allowed to drain, and equilibrated with 0.10 M phosphate buffer, pH 7.2, containing 0.01 percent thimerosal. The top of the column is capped with a rubber septum, with a 1 mL tuberculin syringe and needle plunged in the septum to function as a vent. The syringe is filled with charcoal sandwiched between two thin layers of cotton. The radioiodinated sample is introduced on top of the column (with the stopcock closed) via a 1 mL syringe and needle plunged in the septum. The reaction vial is washed with 500 μL of PBS, using the same syringe, and added to the column. The stopcock is opened and 500 μL fractions are collected in closed crimped 2 mL vials via a syringe fitted to the stopcock. After collection of seven 500 μL fractions, a 20 mL crimped serum vial containing 10 g of Kaolin pellet ("Speedy-Dry") and 1 mL of saturated sodium thiosulfate solution is used to collect 7 mL of eluate and the vial is discarded as solid waste. The fractions are assayed for ^{125}I content in a Capintec Dose Calibrator Model CRC-44 Spectrometer, or fixed-well γ counter. In our studies the efficiency of iodination has been higher than 90 percent. The peak fractions are combined, diluted with PBS containing 4 percent BSA and 0.01 percent Thimerosal to 0.2 mCi/μg protein/mL, and stored at 4°C. Under these conditions, the radioiodinated proteins are stable for 3–4 weeks. Radioiodination using IODO-BEADS is initiated by adding a bead to the mixture of Na ^{125}I and protein solution, followed by a 5 min incubation. The reaction is terminated by removing the bead. Using 1000 beads, up to 95 percent protein recovery and quantitative iodination has been achieved.

5. FRACTIONATION OF POOLED PLASMA

5.1. Materials

[^{125}I]–labeled plasma pools: 0.2 mCi/μg protein/mL (total of 9.0 mL).

Plasma pool solutions: 200 mg protein/mL of PBS.

Radioiodinated plasma samples used for fractionation: 2.5 mL of [^{125}I]-labeled protein sample is mixed with 1 mL of the pooled plasma solution, or total Ig containing 200 mg of protein (samples diluted with distilled water to yield 200 mg protein/mL) and 6.5 mL of PBS to yield a solution containing 20 mg protein/mL and 5×10^3 cpm/mg protein.

Na-borate buffer, 0.04 M, pH 8.1.

Polyethylene glycol (PEG): dissolve 15 g of PEG (DBA-7, mol wt. 6000) in 80 mL of 0.06 M Na-borate buffer, pH 8.1, and make up to 100 mL with same.

Blue dextran solution, 1 mg/mL distilled water.

Human IgG, 1 mg/mL in phosphate-buffered saline, pH 7.3.

Protein standards: 1 mg each of crystalline cytochrome c, ovalbumin, human IgG, and bovine serum albumin dissolved in 1 mL PBS.

5.2. Procedure

STEP 1. Ten milliliters each of radioiodinated pooled IDDM and normal plasma are incubated at 56°C for 30 min to inactivate the serum complement.

The samples are cooled to 4°C, centrifuged at 10,000g for 15 min at 4°C, and the pellets are discarded. The supernatants are adjusted to 15 mL by the addition of PBS. Saturated ammonium sulfate (10 mL) is added dropwise while mixing the samples on a magnetic stirrer for 30 min. The resultant suspensions are stored at 4°C for 3–6 hr and then centrifuged at 15,000g for 10 min at 4°C. The supernates are dialyzed against HEPES buffer for 16 hr at 4°C. The volume of retentate of each sample is adjusted to 5 mL with HEPES buffer. The final preparations are designated as total immunoglobulins (Ig) hereafter. The recovery at the end of this step is routinely 45–55 percent of the starting plasma protein.

STEP 2.   An aliquot (5 mL containing about 100 mg protein and $1–2 \times 10^8$ cpm) of each of the total Ig fractions is mixed with 5 mL of Na-borate buffer and 10 mL of 15 percent PEG, stirred for 10 min at 24°C, and incubated at 4°C for 16 hr. The turbid suspensions are centrifuged at 15,000g for 15 min at 4°C and the supernates discarded. Each pellet is suspended in 10 mL of 7.5 percent PEG, cooled to 4°C, centrifuged at 4°C for 10 min, and the supernate is discarded. The washed pellets are dissolved in 5 mL of PBS and stored at −20°C. This preparation is referred to as PEG-ppt henceforth. The recovery at the end of this step is 45–50 percent for the diabetic samples and 25–30 percent for the control samples.

STEP 3.   The PEG-ppt is chromatographed on a 120×1.4 cm column of Ultrogel AcA-34 as follows: 200 mL of the slurry of Ultrogel are mixed with 200 mL of 0.04 Na-borate buffer. With the outlet of the column closed, 50 mL of borate buffer are run down the column, and 20 mL of the slurry is slowly added with a pipette held against the wall of the column and allowed to settle. The outlet is opened and the buffer is allowed to drain dropwise until 5 cm of the column length is packed with gel particles. The addition of the slurry is repeated as described until 110 cm of the column length is packed with the gel with 2 cm of column length buffer solution on top. The column is inspected thoroughly for possible disruption of the gel due to the presence of air bubbles as well as horizontal lines indicating separate layer of the gel. In either case the column should be emptied, washed, and repacked. The top of the column is connected to a 1 L aspirator bottle (buffer reservoir) via Tygon tubing and the column is washed with 500 mL of the buffer. The sample of PEG ppt (5 mL equivalent to $1.25–2.0 \times 10^8$ cpm) is added to the column, the outlet is opened, and the sample and the buffer are allowed to penetrate into the gel. About 3 mL of buffer are added to the column and allowed to drain. The reservoir is connected to the top of the column again and the column is eluted with Na borate buffer at a rate of 20 mL/hr. Fractions (2.5 mL) are collected in an LKB 7000-Ultrarac fraction collector. Duplicate 50 μL aliquots from each fraction are used for assay of protein content by measurement of $^A280$ nm and duplicate 50 μL aliquots used for assay of ^{125}I content. The column should be calibrated with blue dextran for the determination of the void volume (Vo) and protein standards. Under the experimental conditions described, Vo = 37.5–40 mL. Two peaks are resolved: Peak I in the elution position of blue dextran, indicating the exclusion of the materials from the column, and Peak II in the elution position of authentic human IgG, with a molecular weight of 150,000. Analyses to be described in this series demonstrate that Peak I is comprised partially of immune complexes with an approximate molecular weight > 300,000 and Peak II contains IgG-rich compounds.

5.3. Comments

The efficiency of PEG to precipitate immune complexes (ICs) and free immunoglobulins depends on various criteria such as the pH of the solution, ionic strength, temperature, and protein concentration. Therefore, it is important to determine the optimum concentration of PEG in order to precipitate immunoglobulins and IC. For this purpose, varying quantities of PEG are added to a constant protein concentration, mixed, and incubated at 4°C for 3–6 hr. The mixtures are centrifuged at 2000g for 20 min at 4°C, and the pellets are washed with cold solutions of the corresponding PEG concentration. The pellets are dissolved in the same volume of PBS (approximately 1–2 mg protein/mL) and assayed for protein concentration using the method of Lowry et al. (29). The percent total protein precipitated is plotted versus percent PEG concentration. The optimum concentration of PEG for precipitation of IC or immunoglobulins is determined from the percent PEG. Figure 1 illustrates the dependence of the extent of precipitation versus PEG concentration under the experimental conditions described. Peak fractions are pooled and concentrated to 2 mL each by ultrafiltration using an Amicon 52 cell with a PM-10 ultrafilter. To determine the immunoreactivity of Peaks I and II, equal aliquots of Peak I and Peak II are incubated with islet cells and the cell-bound radioactivity is measured by the procedure that will be described.

Results show that Peak II contains immunoglobulins that react with islet cells, whereas Peak I is minimally active. The lack of significant reactivity in Peak I material is presumed to be due to the fact that in Ag–Ab complexes (immune complexes) the majority of binding sites of the Ab molecules are occupied by its specific Ag molecules.

6.   MEASUREMENT OF IgG IN IMMUNOGLOBULIN FRACTIONS

6.1.   Materials

Staphyllococcus aureus (Cowan I strain), 10 percent suspension in PBS containing 0.02 percent NaN$_3$. (Bethesda Research Laboratories, Rockville, MD).

Normal and IDDM plasma or their purified fractions.

Phosphate-buffered saline, pH 7.3 (PBS).

NaOH, 2 *N*.

Comparison of Reactivity of Islet Cell Subfractions with Purified IgG

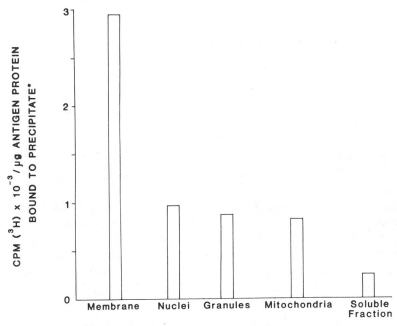

*All values have been corrected for the normal IgG controls

FIGURE 1.   Effect of concentration of PEG on the precipitation of Ig. Aliquots (250 μg in 250 μL) of total Ig were treated with 250 μL of varying concentrations of PEG; the precipitate formed was isolated by centrifugation and the percent protein of the total Ig in the PEG-ppt was determined by the method of Lowry. Mean values of triplicate determinations of the diabetic samples (O—O—O) are compared with the normal samples (●—●—●).

6.2.   Procedure

S. aureus protein A reacts selectively with the IgG isotype of immunoglobulins and is widely used as a specific immunoadsorbent for detection and quantitation of IgG in immunoglobulin preparations (30, 31). To 200 μL of a 10 percent suspension of *S. aureus*, 25–250 μg of immunoglobulin protein from normal or IDDM plasma are added and the volume of the mixture is adjusted to 500 μL with PBS. The mixtures are incubated at 24°C for 30 min, followed by 60 min at 4°C. The suspensions are centrifuged at 1000*g* for 5 min at 24°C, pellets are washed with two 500 μL portions of PBS, and supernatant fluids and PBS washings combined. A blank and a control tube are included which contain the following: Blank tube—200 μL of *S. aureus* suspension mixed with 300 μL of PBS; Control tube—25—250 μL of protein from plasma samples mixed with 475–250 µL of PBS to yield a final volume of 500 µL. The blank tube is used to adjust the spectrophotometer to zero for measurement of absorbance of the sample tubes at 280 nm, and the control tube is used for the total protein determination using a reagent blank for measurement of the ^A750 nm (Lowry's protein determination). The percent total protein adsorbed by *S. aureus* cells is calculated as follows:

$$\text{Percent protein adsorbed} = \frac{(\text{total protein}) - (\text{supernate protein})}{(\text{total protein})} \times 100$$

The same procedure is used for estimation of IgG in [^{125}I]–labeled IgG-containing samples from IDDM or normal plasma or purified fractions derived therefrom. The cell pellets are suspended in 200 µL of 2 *N* NaOH, heated at 80°C for 5 min, cooled to 24°C, and assayed for ^{125}I content. All assays must be performed in triplicate and results recorded as the arithmetic mean values of cpm. As the amount of *S. aureus* required varies with IgG content samples, to assure maximum adsorption, at least two concentrations (e.g., 100 and 200 µg/tube) of *S. aureus* should be used. If percent total protein adsorbed in the above tubes is linear with *S. aureus* concentration, the amount of *S. aureus* should be

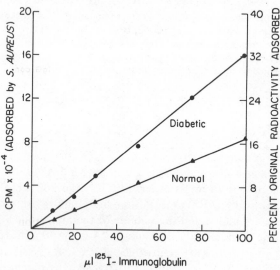

FIGURE 2. Adsorption of [^{125}I]-labeled total Ig with *S. aureus*. Varying aliquots (10–100 µL) of [^{125}I]-total Ig containing 10^5–10^6 cpm and 50–500 µg protein were treated with 200 µL of a 10 percent *S. aureus* suspension as described. The [^{125}I]-Ig adsorbed from the diabetic sample (O—O—O) and normal sample (●—●—●) are recorded as mean values of triplicate determinations.

increased. It is recommended that an *S. aureus* dose–response curve be constructed for the assay of IgG in plasma, or total Ig samples and the optimal concentration of *S. aureus* be determined (Fig. 2).

7. IMMUNOLOGICAL ASSAY PROCEDURES

7.1. Immunofluorescence Techniques

7.1.1. MATERIALS

Diabetic and normal Ig.

Rat islet cells.

Islet medium.

Phosphate-buffered saline, pH 7.3 (PBS).

BSA, 4 percent in PBS (Calbiochem., Los Angeles, CA).

Fluorescein isothiocyanate (FITC)–protein A conjugate (Bethesda Research Labs, Gaithersburg, MD).

7.1.2. PROCEDURE

Aliquots (20 µL) of diluted diabetic or normal Ig, equivalent to 600 µg protein, are mixed with $5-50 \times 10^5$ islet cells suspended in the islet medium containing 4 percent BSA in a final volume of 250 µL. The mixtures are incubated at 37°C for 30 min, followed by 15 min at 23°C, and centrifuged at 500g for 5 min. Cell pellets are washed twice with 700 µL portions of the islet medium, and washed cells suspended in 50 µL of the same medium. The 50 µL of a 1:10 dilution of FITC–protein A conjugate is added to the cell suspensions. The mixtures are incubated at 23°C for 30 min, followed by 70 min at 4°C. The suspensions are washed twice with 700 µL portions of the islet medium and then centrifuged at 500g for 5 min. Washed pellets are suspended in 25 µL of islet medium and examined under an epi-fluorescence microscope (Carl Ziess Model) equipped with a built-in camera. Photographs are taken under both light microscopic and epi-fluorescent illumination.

Two controls are included: (i) normal control—cells incubated with pooled normal plasma, followed by FITC–protein A as described and (ii) islet cell controls: islet cells carried out through the entire procedure without treatment with Ig and FITC–protein A conjugate. The latter is included to show the possible changes in the cells due to experimental manipulations. In many experiments cells treated with Ig from IDDM plasma show intense fluorescent staining, while the reaction of islet cells with pooled normal plasma Ig treated with FITC–protein A conjugate does not display any detectable fluorescence. Islet cell controls show a normal morphology under the light microscope.

7.2.   Reaction of ICA with Islet Cells

7.2.1.   MATERIALS

Immunoglobulin preparations: 1 mg/mL.

Phosphate-buffered saline: 0.05 M phosphate buffer in 0.9 percent NaCl (PBS).

BSA, 10 percent in PBS.

Assay mixture: 1.0 mL of each of 0.2 M glutamine, 0.2 M DTT, 0.10 M EDTA, and penicillin-streptomycin solution are mixed with 36 mL of PBS, dispensed in 5 mL tubes and stored at $-20°C$.

7.2.2.   PROCEDURE

5–50 μL (12–20 mg) of immunoglobulin with ICA activity containing 10^4–10^5 cpm are diluted with PBS to 100 μL and mixed with 100 μL of assay mixture. Fifty microliters of islet cell suspension (10^4 cells) are then added, contents of tubes are mixed gently, and incubated for 60 min at 37°C, followed by 2 hr at 4°C. The incubation mixtures are centrifuged at 500g for 5 min at 23°C and pellets are washed with two 500 μL portions of PBS. Washed pellets are dissolved in 250 μL of NCS and assayed for ^{125}I content. Routinely, triplicate aliquots of IDDM plasma samples are assayed simultaneously with triplicate normal plasma samples containing identical amounts of radioiodinated plasma protein plus a 20-fold excess of the same Ig preparation which has not been radioiodinated. Control tubes are used for estimation of "nonspecific binding" (NSB) of ^{125}I to islet cells (NSB controls). Another control without islet cells is run in duplicate along with the IDDM samples to account for any changes occurring in the Ig protein due to experimental manipulations. Mean values of cpm in these tubes is taken as total cpm per incubation mixture. All data are presented as the mean value of the counts in triplicate experimental tubes minus the mean value of the counts in the corresponding triplicate NSB control tubes. When purified Ig preparations are used, invariably the counts in the NSB controls of the normal plasma samples are equal to the NSB controls of the IDDM plasma samples within ±2 percent. In these cases the NSB controls may be omitted. When comparison of the ICA activity of different plasma samples is desired, at least two different-sized aliquots (e.g., 25 and 50 μL of a 1:30 dilution of plasma) are assayed in duplicate and the mean cpm bound to islet cells per milliliter of undiluted plasma are calculated as follows:

$$\text{Undiluted plasma} = \frac{1000 \text{ μL}}{2} \times \frac{(\text{cpm}/A_1 + \text{cpm}/A_2)}{2 \times 25}$$

$$+ \frac{(\text{cpm}/B_1 + \text{cpm}/B_2)}{2 \times 50} \times 30 \quad (\text{cpm/mL})$$

where A_1 and A_2 are duplicate tubes containing 25 μL of the diluted plasma and B_1 and B_2 are tubes containing 50 μL of the diluted plasma sample. By pilot experiments it is possible to find a range of immunoglobulin concentration that gives a linear response with a constant number of islet cells.

7.3. Comparison of the Immunoreactivity of Islet Cell Subcomponents with ICA

7.3.1. MATERIALS

[^{3}H]Leucine-labeled islet cell subcomponents.

S. aureus suspension, 10 percent in PBS.

S. aureus protein A, 1 mg/mL of PBS.

Unlabeled total Ig.

Assay mixture.

Phosphate-buffered saline, pH 7.3 (PBS).

7.3.2. Procedure

Unlabeled total Ig or other purified fractions from normal or diabetic plasma samples (100 μL) are incubated with 5–50 μL (10^4–10^5 cpm) of [^{3}H] labeled islet cell subcomponents and mixed with 100 μL of the assay mixture and adjusted to 250 μL with PBS. The reaction mixtures are incubated at 37°C for 1 hr, followed by 3 hr at 4°C. Five microliters of protein A solution (5 μg) and 45 μL of PBS are added to tubes containing subcellular particulate matter (membranes, mitochondria, nuclei, and granules), and 50 μL of a 10 percent suspension of *S. aureus* are added to the tubes containing the soluble fraction. All tubes are incubated at 24°C for 30 min, followed by 4 hr at 4°C. Tubes are centrifuged as follows: the tubes containing the soluble fraction at 1000*g* for 10 min at 24°C, the tubes containing nuclear, granules, and mitochondria at 300*g*, 400*g*, and 5000*g* for 10 min at 24°C, respectively. The membrane-containing tubes are centrifuged at 20,000*g* for 30 min at 4°C. Pellets are resuspended in 500 μL PBS, mixed on a vortex mixer for 1 min, and centrifuged as described above. Pellets are suspended in 250 μL of NCS tissue solubilizer at 37°C for 5 min and assayed for radioactivity using Hydrofluor scintillation fluid. Control tubes are included for each subfraction as described previously. Triplicate tubes containing only [^{3}H]–labeled islet cell subcomponents and PBS are included simultaneously with the experimental tubes for determination of the total ^{3}H content. After correction of the counts for controls, the specific activity of each fraction is calculated on the basis of the protein content as follows:

$$\text{Specific activity} = \frac{\text{net cpm per experimental tubes}}{\text{μg protein per aliquot used}}$$

The reactivity of islet cell subcomponents with ICA present in total Ig is shown in Figure 3. Particulate fractions tend to aggregate upon storage at 4°C after 2–3 days, or at −20°C after a week with repeated freezing and thawing. If particulate suspensions appear to be nonhomogeneous, a 1 percent Triton X-100 solution is added to a final concentration of 0.10 percent and the mixture shaken vigorously on the vortex. If the particles do not dissolve by this treatment, the suspension is homogenized in a glass homogenizer equipped with a Teflon pestle until complete solubilization of the particulate matter is achieved.

Effect of PEG Concentration on Precipitation of Immune Complexes from Total Immunoglobulin

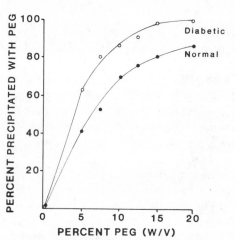

FIGURE 3. Comparison of the immunoreactivity of islet cell subcomponents. 10 µg of unlabeled purified IgG dissociated from IC were incubated with 100,000 cpm of [³H]leucine-labeled islet cell subcomponents under the experimental conditions described. The amount of cell-bound radioactivity using the diabetic IgG was measured and corrected for the corresponding normal control tested simultaneously. Protein content of each fraction was measured by solubilization in 3 percent SDS, 4 percent urea, 0.1 M Tris-HCl pH 7.5, at 100°C for 5 min, followed by the Lowry protein determination. Results are expressed as mean values of counts minus corresponding controls. Controls consist of all the ingredients of the incubation mixture plus an additional 100 µg of unlabeled diabetic IgG to compete with specific binding; the residual counts are designated as nonspecific and subtracted from the counts in the experimental tubes. As an additional control, IgG from pooled normal plasma is incubated with islet cell subfractions as described for diabetic IgG, and these counts are also subtracted from the experimental counts. Specific activities are expressed as cpm/µg protein of islet cell subcomponent. This experiment has been performed twice as represented in the figure with similar results.

8. SPECIFICITY OF ICA FOR ISLET CELLS

8.1. Preparation of Cells from Various Rat Organs

8.1.1. MATERIALS

Rat islet cells.

Spleen, liver, lung, and blood of autologous rats.

Ficoll-Hypaque (Pharmacia Co.) 5 g/100 mL, 10 g/100 mL, and 20 g/100 mL in PBS.

Tris-HCl, 0.10 M, pH 7.5.

Urea, 8 M in 0.10 M Tris-HCl, pH 7.5.

Sodium dodecyl sulfate, 6 percent in Tris-HCl, 0.10 M, pH 7.5 (SDS).

Urea–SDS–Tris-HCl solution: 100 mL of urea solution are mixed with 100 mL of SDS solution.

Phosphate-buffered saline, pH 7.3 (PBS).

8.1.2. PROCEDURE

Spleen, lung, and liver of the same rats from which islet cells are isolated are excised, washed several times with PBS, minced into small pieces, and suspended in PBS at a concentration of 1 g/2mL. Suspensions are very gently homogenized in a 10 mL glass homogenizer equipped with a Teflon pestle using three strokes to minimize cell breakage. Homogenates are freed from unbroken tissues and connective tissues by filtration through cheese cloth. Five mL of heparinized blood from the same animals are obtained and centrifuged, and erythrocytes (RBC) are washed in two 5 mL portions of PBS and suspended in PBS at a concentration of 10^6 RBC/mL. Spleen, lung, and liver homogenates are centrifuged for 5 min at 24°C. The pellets are taken up in 2 mL of PBS and layered gently over a discontinuous density gradient of 2.5 mL aliquots of 5, 10, and 20 percent Ficoll-Hypaque solution in 10 mL plastic tubes. The tubes are centrifuged at $500g$ for 10 min at 24°C and the bands corresponding to each cell type, except erythrocytes which are sedimented to the bottom of the tubes, are withdrawn with a Pasteur pipette. The cells are added to tubes containing 7 mL of PBS, mixed, and centrifuged. The cells are again washed with 7 mL of PBS, counted in a hemocytometer, and adjusted to a concentration of 10^6 cells/mL.

8.2. Reaction of ICA with Various Rat Cells

8.2.1. MATERIALS

Cell suspensions from various rat organs.

[^{125}I]–labeled Ig fraction from normal and diabetic plasma.

Assay mixture (Section 7.2).

Phosphate-buffered saline, pH 7.3 (PBS).

NCS tissue solubilizer.

An aliquot (50 μL) of [^{125}I]–labeled total Ig derived from normal or diabetic plasma pools equivalent to 20 μg of protein (containing 3.6×10^4 cpm) is mixed with 100 μL of the assay mixture, followed by 40–80 μL of cell suspension ($4—8 \times 10^4$ cells), and PBS to a final volume of 250 μL. The mixtures are incubated at 37°C for 1 hr, followed by 3 hr at 4°C. The cell suspensions are washed with PBS as described, and the washed pellets are dissolved in NCS and assayed for radioactivity. For each cell type triplicate tubes are used for diabetic and normal IgG samples and the mean value of the counts for each set is used to determine percent activity as follows:

1. Net counts for a given cell type = mean cpm per diabetic Ig − mean cpm per normal Ig.

2. Percent activity = $\dfrac{\text{net cpm for any cell type}}{\text{net cpm for islet cell}} \times 100.$

Table 2 demonstrates the results obtained in a prototype experiment. As the size of the cells varies from one cell type to another, an absolute parameter such as protein content should be used for accurate comparison of the reactivity of ICA with different cell types in lieu of the cell number. For this purpose, the cell pellets are dissolved in 200 μL of urea–SDS–Tris-HCl solution in a boiling water bath for 3 min. Tubes are cooled to room temperature and their protein content is determined by the method of Lowry, and the specific activity (S.A.) of each cell type is calculated as follows:

1. S.A. in cpm/μg protein of a given cell type =

    $\dfrac{\text{cpm/protein content of the aliquot}}{\text{μg protein in the aliquot}}.$

2. Percent S.A. = $\dfrac{\text{cpm/μg protein of a cell type}}{\text{cpm/μg protein of islet cells}} \times 100.$

The difference between expression of specific activity based on the number of cells and protein content are are illustrated by the data shown in Table 3. The specific activity of the reaction of human islet cells with diabetic Ig as compared with rat islet cells based on cell number is a maximum of 1.5, whereas, when they are compared on a protein basis, the specific activity of human islet cells is as high as 11 times that of the rat islet cells. This is primarily due to the

TABLE 2. Specificity of Ig from Diabetic Plasma for Rat Islet Cells

Experiment[a] No.	Cell Suspensions[b]	$[^{125}I]$-Ig-Bound[c] (cpm)	Percent Activity[d]
	Islet cells	6850	100.0
	RBC	1190	17.0
I	Spleen	610	9.0
	Liver	530	7.7
	Lung	370	5.4
	Islet cells	5750	100.0
	RBC	700	12.2
II	Spleen	450	7.8
	Liver	450	7.8
	Lung	350	6.1

[a] For experiment I: 8×10^4 of the designated cells were incubated with an aliquot of $[^{125}I]$–labeled total Ig derived from diabetic plasma pool 1 yielding 36,000 cpm (equivalent to 20 μg protein). For experiment II: 4×10^4 of the indicated cells were incubated as described for experiment I.

[b] Cells were obtained from rat tissues autologous to the islet cell source.

[c] $[^{125}I]$-labeled Ig was incubated with unlabeled islet cells and the radioactivity was measured in the pellet by the procedure described in methods. The cpm represent the average of triplicate samples per experiment after correction for the corresponding normal controls run simultaneously under the same conditions.

[d] Percent activity was calculated as the ratio of ^{125}I counts per cell pellet divided by ^{125}I counts in the islet cell pellet × 100.

TABLE 3. Comparison of the Activity of ICA with Human and Rat Islets[a]

Total Cells	Specific Activity (cpm/1000 cells)[b]		Specific Activity (cpm/μg) protein[c]	
	Human	Rat	Human	Rat
5,000	350	282	2540	275
10,000	292	252	2230	237
20,000	267	199	2112	192
30,000	243	183	1972	173
40,000	226	171	1871	164

[a] Human and rat islet cells were prepared by the collagenase and Dispase method. Varying aliquots of cell suspensions were incubated with 40,000 cpm of diabetic or normal total Ig fraction as a source of ICA and assayed by the procedure described.

[b] Mean value of triplicates of diabetic and normal samples carried out simultaneously. Data are expressed as mean values of diabetic samples minus corresponding normal control values.

[c] Protein concentration was determined by the method of Lowry et al. for duplicate aliquots of each cell suspension following solubilization of cell pellets in 4 M urea, 3 percent SDS, 0.10 M tris-HCl, pH 7.5, for 3 min in a boiling water bath.

177

fact that the human islet cells are much smaller than the rat islet cells, thus posessing a smaller cell surface area for the binding of antibodies.

9.   EFFECT OF INSULIN ON THE REACTIVITY OF ICA WITH ISLET CELL ANTIGENS

As anti-insulin antibodies and insulin–anti-insulin complexes may be present in the plasma of IDDM patients who have received insulin therapy, it is important to show that ICA is distinct from anti-insulin antibody by inhibition studies using insulin in the reaction mixtures containing ICA and islet cell antigens.

9.1.   Materials

[^{3}H]Leucine labeled rat islet cells and islet cell subcomponents, 2×10^6 cpm/mL.

Unlabeled total IgG, or purified fractions derived from normal and diabetic plasmas, 1 mg/mL.

S. aureus cell suspension, 10 percent in PBS.

Assay mixture (Section 7.2).

PBS, 0.05 *M* phosphate-buffered saline, pH 7.3.

Rat insulin (Terapeutisk Laboratorum, Copenhagen, Denmark).

1 μg/mL of PBS.

S. aureus protein A solution, 1 mg/mL (Bethesda Research Laboratories, Rockville, MD).

9.2.   Procedure

[^{3}H]leucine-labeled islet cell subcomponents (e.g., membranes and soluble fraction) and 100 μL containing $1-2 \times 10^5$ cpm are mixed with 100 μL of assay mixture, and 5, 10, 20, or 25 μL of the rat insulin solution corresponding to 20–100 ng of insulin and PBS are added to a 230 μL final volume and mixed. Then 20 μL of unlabeled total Ig, or purified IgG solution containing 20 μg of protein, are added to each tube, mixed, and incubated as described previously. The ^{3}H islet cell subcomponent–ICA complex is selectively separated from the free islet cell subcomponents by specific adsorption to *S. aureus* cell, or protein A. To tubes containing the soluble fraction, 100 μL of *S. aureus* cell suspension are added; to tubes containing the membrane fraction 10 μL of protein A solution are added. Tube contents are mixed, cooled to 4°C, and centrifuged at 1000*g* for 10 min at 23°C and 20,000*g* for 20 min at 4°C, respectively. Pellets are washed with 5 mL of PBS, and washed pellets obtained following centrifugation are dissolved in 250 μL NCS and assayed for radioactivity as described. All experiments are carried out in triplicate and mean

TABLE 4. Effect of Insulin on the Immunoreactivity of IgG from Diabetic Plasma with [³H]Leucine-labeled Islet Cell Subfractions[a]

Insulin Concentration (ng/mL)	IgG-Bound [³H]Leucine[b] (cpm)	
	Soluble[c]	Membrane[d]
0	25,300	43,100
20	26,450	42,950
40	24,500	43,650
80	25,400	43,900
100	23,970	43,100

[a] Unlabeled IgG (20 μg) from IDDM plasma, pool 2, was incubated with 200,000 cpm of [³H]leucine-labeled islet cell subcellular fractions and the [³H]leucine bound in the resultant complex was measured as described in methods. Insulin was mixed with IgG where indicated prior to the addition of subcellular fractions.
[b] Data presented are mean values of triplicate determinations, corrected for nonspecific binding using IgG from pooled normal donor plasma. This experiment has been repeated three times with two different IDDM plasma pools yielding similar results.
[c] Corresponds to 200 μg protein/incubation mixture.
[d] Corresponds to 10 μg protein/incubation mixture.

values of the counts are recorded. A control set of triplicates containing no insulin is included. All data are presented as the net values (cpm per diabetic sample minus cpm per corresponding normal plasma tube). In our experiments the reactivity of purified IgG obtained from Ig with islet cell subcomponents was not inhibited in the presence of insulin (Table 4).

REFERENCES

1. G. F. Bottazzo, A. Florin-Christensen, and D. Doniach, *Lancet* **2**, 1979 (1974).

2. R. Lendrum, G. Walker, and D. R. Gamble, *Lancet* **1**, 880 (1975).

3. N. K. MacLaren, S. W. Huang, and J. Fogh, *Lancet* **1**, 997 (1975).

4. W. J. Irvine, C. J. McCallum, M. Campbell, J. W. Farquhar, H. Vaughan, and P. J. Morris, *Diabetes* **26**, 138 (1977).

5. G. F. Bottazzo and D. Doniach, *Ric. Clin. Lab.* **8**, 29 (1978).

6. A. Lernmark, Z. R. Freedman, C. Hofmann, A. H. Rubenstein, D. F. Steiner, R. L. Jackson, R. J. Winter, and H. S. Traisman, *N. Engl. J. Med.* **229**, 375 (1978).

7. G. F. Bottazzo, J. I. Mann, M. Thorogood, J. D. Baum, and D. Doniach, *Brit. Med. J.* **2**, 165 (1978).

8. A. Lernmark, T. Kanatsuñsa. C. Patzelt, K. Diakoumis, R. Carrol, A. H. Rubenstein, and D. F. Steiner, *Diabetologia* **19**, 445 (1980).

9. A. Lernmark and S. Baekkeskov, *Diabetologia* **21**, 431 (1981).

10. A. Lernmark, B. Hägglöf, Z. R. Freedman, W. J. Irvine, J. Ludvigsson, and G. Holmgren, *Diabetologia* **20**, 471 (1981).

11. R. Pujol-Borrel, E. L. Khoury, and G. F. Bottazzo, *Diabetologia* **22**, 89 (1982).

12. S. Baekkeskov, J. H. Nielsen, B. Marner, T. Bilds, J. Ludvigson, and A. Lernmark, *Nature* **298**, 167 (1982).

13. T. Dyrberg, A. F. Nakhooda, S. Baekkeskov, A. Lernmark, P. Roussier, and E. B. Marliss, *Diabetes* **31**, 278 (1982).

14. T. Dyrberg, S. Baekkeskov, and A. Lernmark, *J. Cell Biol.* **94**, 472 (1982).

15. A. N. Theofilopoulos and F. J. Dixon, *Adv. Immunol.* **28**, 89 (1979).

16. Z. R. Freedman, C. M. Feek, J. W. Irvine, and A. Lernmark, *Trans. Assoc. Amer. Physicians* **96**, 64 (1979).

17. R. Lendrum, G. Walker, and D. R. Gamble, *Lancet* **1**, 880 (1975).

18. H. G. Rittenhouse, D. L. Oxender, S. B. Pek, and D. Ar, *Diabetes* **29**, 317 (1980).

19. M. J. Dobersen, J. E. Scharff, F. Ginsberg-Fellner, and A. L. Notkins, *N. Engl. J. Med.* **303**, 1493 (1980).

20. M. J. Dobersen and J. R. Scharff, *Diabetes* **31**, 459 (1982).

21. M. van De Winkel, G. Smets, W. Gepts, and D. Pipeleers, *J. Clin. Invest.* **70**, 41 (1982).

22. G. F. Bottazzo, B. M. Dean, A. N. Gorsuch, A. G. Cudworth, and D. Doniach *Lancet* **1**, 668 (1982).

23. W. K. Soderstrum, Z. R. Freedman, and A. Lernmark, *Diabetes* **28**, 397 (1979).

24. J. Ilonen, A. Mustonen, K. H. Akerblom, and N. P. Huttunen, *Lancet* **2**, 805 (1980).

25. M. A. Charles, M. Suzuki, N. Waldeck, L. E. Dodson, L. Slater, K. Ong, R. A. Kerashnak, B. Buckingham, and M. Golden, *J. Immunol.* **130**, 1189 (1983).

26. P. E. Lacy and M. Kostianovsky, *Diabetes* **16**, 35 (1976).

27. J. Ono, R. Kakaki, and M. Fukuma, *Endocrinol. Japan.* **24**, 265 (1977).

28. A. M. Taratakoff and J. D. Jameison, in *Methods in Enzymology*, Vol. 31, S. Fleisher and L. Packer (eds.), Academic Press, New York, 1974, p. 41.

29. O. H. Lowry, N. J. Rosenbrough, L. A. Farr, and R. J. Randall, *J. Biol. Chem.* **193**, 265 (1951).

30. E. Premakumar-Reddy, S. K. Devare, R. Vasudev, and P. S. Sarma, *J. Natl. Cancer Inst.* **48**, 1859 (1977).

31. S. W. Kessler, *J. Immunol.* **115**, 1617 (1975).

D

IMMUNOLOGICAL INVESTIGATIONS
Islet Cell Antibodies

**BIRGITTE MARNER, CAJ KNUTSSON,
ÅKE LERNMARK, JØRN NERUP, AND THE HAGEDORN
STUDY GROUP**
*Hagedorn Research Laboratory and the Steno Memorial Hospital,
Gentofte, Denmark*

1. INTRODUCTION

Immunocytochemical methods are widely used in cellular analyses and localization of antigens by means of specific antibodies conjugated with a fluorescent
label introduced by Coons (1). The fluorescent antibody is added directly to
sections or preparations of living cells and, after separating antigen-bound
from free antibodies, the former are identified in a fluorescence microscope.
Improvements in protein chemistry and in the preparation of fluorescent labels
or peroxidase-conjugated antibodies (2) later permitted the detection and localization of a variety of tissue antigens. Introduction of fluorescent antibodies
directed against immunoglobulin from different species, including man, to be
used in a sandwich composed of a first layer of antibody bound to antigen and
detected by a second layer of fluorescent antibody proved to represent a major
improvement. First, the sensitivity was markedly increased. Second, it became
possible to determine antibody types. Third, antibodies including autoantibodies
which had reacted with cells or tissue components could be detected. Fourth,
it allowed identification and localization of tissue antigens. Immunohisto-
chemical analysis therefore permitted the detection of antibodies deposited in
tissues (e.g., immune complexes in glomerulonephritis) or the presence of
circulating autoantibodies (e.g., antibodies against thyroglobulin in thyroiditis)
or the demonstration of microbial antigens (e.g., virus) (2). The Ploem epi-
illumination system (1967) was a major improvement in increasing the sensitivity
and specificity of immunofluorescence microscopy. Since then, the list of
antibodies, detected in man as well as in other species, reacting with a variety
of tissue antigens is steadily growing (2).

Members of the Hagedorn Study Group include G. Bille, I. Gerling, A. M. Olesen, H. Richter-
Olesen, L. Lyngsie, S. Bækkeskov, and J. H. Nielsen. Caj Knutsson is a Research Fellow from
the Department of Pathology, University of Lund, Lund, Sweden

We acknowledge samples from diabetic children treated with plasmapheresis kindly donated by
Dr. Johnny Ludvigsson, Linköping, Sweden. C.K. acknowledges a fellowship from the University
of Lund, Lund, Sweden. The preparation of these methods has been supported in part by the
National Institute of Health (Grant AM 26190).

Immunofluorescence methods, previously applied to several organ-specific disorders of autoimmune character, were successfully used in detecting antibodies in serum samples from diabetic patients, reacting with pancreatic islet cells in sections of frozen human pancreas (3, 4). These islet cell antibodies, which will be referred to as islet cell cytoplasmic antibodies (ICCA), were found to be present among the majority of patients with newly diagnosed insulin-dependent diabetes mellitus (IDDM) (5, 6).

The Ploem fluorescence illumination system, combined with phase-contrast microscopy, permitted specific and sensitive immunofluorescence analysis of living cells. This system, applied either to suspensions of living, dispersed human insulinoma cells (7) or to normal mouse or rat islet cells (8, 9), also allowed detection of islet cell surface antibodies. These antibodies, in many patients which were specific against the pancreatic β cells (10) and reactive with human fetal β cells in monolayer cultures (11), were likewise found primarily among recently diagnosed IDDM patients (12). Dispersed, living cells are not permeable to immunoglobulin (8). Antibodies recognizing determinants expressed in the plasma membrane are detected in the indirect immunofluorescence test, and the diabetes-associated antibodies are therefore referred to as islet cell surface antibodies (ICSA).

The immunofluorescence tests for ICCA and ICSA are widely utilized to study their presence in relation to the progression either of an already diagnosed IDDM (5, 13–15) or of individuals at risk of developing IDDM (16, 17). ICCA may be of predictive value for IDDM (16, 17), however, rigorous tests of long-term assay reproducibility and precision will be needed before present immunofluorescence tests are applicable to prospective analyses, perhaps lasting for several years. This chapter describes, first, the tests for ICCA with sections of frozen human pancreas and, second, the test for ICSA by indirect immunofluorescence on dispersed, viable rat islet cells. ICCA and ICSA in human and experimental IDDM have been discussed in several reviews (18–23).

2. QUANTITATION OF ISLET CELL CYTOPLASMIC ANTIBODIES

The present method (24), based on previous reports (3, 4, 25) is an indirect immunofluorescence assay with cryostat sections prepared from pancreas of blood group O donors.

2.1. Assay Reagents

2.1.1. SAMPLES

Plasma or serum samples are stored ($-20°C$) in aliquots to avoid repeated freezing and thawing. The present approach also allows the detection of, for example, human–human monoclonal IgM antibody, B6 (26) reactive with human pancreatic α cell cytoplasmic antigens or of mouse monoclonal human proinsulin antibodies (27). Control experiments comparing serum with plasma obtained from the same individual and with immunoglobulin purified by poly-ethyleneglycol (12.5 percent, w/v) precipitation and a subsequent standard DEAE-Sephadex (Pharmacia, Uppsala, Sweden) chromatography showed that there was no difference in the individual ICCA titres of 10 IDDM patients.

2.1.2. PANCREATIC SPECIMENS AND SECTIONING

Blood group O normal pancreatic tissue (25) is obtained either from patients undergoing abdominal surgery or from brain-dead kidney donors. The major part (80–90 percent) of the source of pancreatic tissue is from the latter category (24). In Denmark respiratory functions of a potential donor are maintained artificially, and after switching off the respirator it takes about 20 min before heart function ceases. During this agonal phase, the blood and oxygen supply to the internal organs will decrease. The surgeon removes organs after the heart function has ceased, and at least 15 min will pass before the pancreas is removed since priority is given to the kidneys. This time of warm ischemia is associated with a complete arrest of blood circulation, and attempts are made to prevent ischemic damage by the previous injection of chlorpromazine and heparin to permit facilitated perfusion of organs with cold physiological salt solutions. The donors of pancreatic tissue have in general no systemic or major vascular disease. All individuals are typed for HLA-A, B, C and DR antigens.

Immediately upon removal of the pancreas, usually leaving part of the head attached to the duodenum to avoid rupture of the intestine, the pancreatic tissue is cut with a knife into 0.5-cm^2 pieces. The pieces are frozen directly in a container with melting isopentane ($-160°C$). After freezing, the pancreatic specimens are put into airtight polyethylene-coated aluminum bags (Otto Niel-sens Emballage, Lyngby, Denmark) and stored at $-70°C$.

2.1.3. PREPARATION OF SECTIONS

The pancreatic specimens are transferred on dry ice to a cryostat, which is operated at $-24°C$. The tissue block is mounted onto the metal holder with Tissue-Tek (Lab-Tek Products, Division of Miles Laboratories, Naperville, IL) and allowed to freeze while kept in the cryostat. The tissue block is cut into 3-μm thick sections which are collected on 76 × 26-mm glass microscope slides, previously cleaned in concentrated RBS 35 overnight and then rinsed in running tap water first for 6 hr and then twice in distilled water for 1 hr each before being dried at 60°C–80°C. The sections are melted onto the glass slide inside the cryostat and dried at room temperature for 30 min to 3 hr. Roughly, 60 sections/hr are prepared. The sections are either used directly or packed on top of each other and stored at $-70°C$. Sections have been kept for more than 1 year without deterioration of immunofluorescence reactivity.

2.1.4.   INDIRECT IMMUNOFLUORESCENCE ASSAY

1. Sections kept at $-70°C$ are first placed on a tray and then air dried under a fan for 30 min at room temperature.

2. Place slides in a moist chamber (a standard household polystyrene plastic box with wet paper towels at the bottom is used).

3. Pipette 30–50 μL of plasma or serum onto sections [dilute with PBS (Table 1) for determination of titer] and incubate at room temperature for 30 min.

4. Remove the drop of serum/plasma from the slides.

5. Transfer the slides to slide racks (max. 16 in each) and place these in Ziehl Neelsen standard glass jars containing PBS. Wash three times each for 5 min in 200 mL PBS.

6. Remove PBS around tissue with filter paper and place slides in the moist chamber.

TABLE 1.   Phosphate-Buffered Saline, pH 7.2 (PBS)

KH_2PO_4	15.3 g
Na_2HPO_4, $2H_2O$	46.7 g
NaCl	68.0 g

Add double-distilled H_2O to a final volume of 10.0 liters.
Check pH, which should be 7.10–7.15.

FITC-conjugated Rabbit Anti-Human IgG

The second fluorescent antibody is routinely purchased from Dakopatts A/S, Copenhagen, Denmark, with the following specifications: fluorescein-conjugated rabbit immunoglobulins to human IgG (β chains), code F202, kept in 0.01 M PBS containing 15 mM NaN_3, pH 7.2. Dakopatts A/S claims that the fluorescein–protein ratio measured as the extinction ratio E495nm/E278nm is 0.65 ± 0.05 for all preparations, corresponding to a molar F/P ratio of 2.3. The undiluted FITC-conjugated rabbit anti-human IgG is stored at 4°C for 6–8 months. The working solution is prepared once a week at a working dilution of 1:5–1:20 in PBS. This solution is filtered through 0.45-m Millipore filter (Millex, Millipore) and immediately added to the tissue sections. Different preparations of FITC-conjugated antisera from other suppliers are treated similarly. Each new batch is carefully titrated to find the optimal dilution for reactivity with the quality control samples.

Mounting medium

Make a 0.05 M Tris-HCl buffer, pH 8.4. Mix 20 mL of glycerol (*pro analysi*) with 80 mL of Tris-HCl buffer. Store at 4°C.

7.   While the tissue is still moist, pipette onto sections 30–50 µL of FITC-conjugated rabbit anti-human IgG (Table 1) and incubate at room temperature for 30 min in the dark.

8.   Remove FITC antibody and wash the slide as in steps 4 and 5.

9.   Remove PBS from back of slide and around the tissue with filter paper and mount sections in 20 percent glycerol buffered with 50 mmol/L Tris-HCl (pH 8.4). (Table 1).

10.   The samples are coded and evaluated by two independent observers.

11.   The samples are read in a fluorescence microscope equipped with epi-illumination. The samples are kept at 4°C no longer than 2–3 days, while being independently evaluated by the observers.

2.1.5.   ASSAY PROTOCOL AND EVALUATION OF IMMUNOFLUORESCENCE

In each experiment slide 1 represents a ICCA-positive quality control serum, slide 2 an ICCA-negative quality control serum sample, and slide 3 the ICCA-positive sample diluted 1:9. After that, unknown samples are mixed with the positive and the negative control samples both undiluted and diluted 1:3, 1:27, and 1:81 in PBS.

Each blinded sample is tested on duplicate slides in two different assays. The dilutions are increased, if necessary, in the second assay to permit a determination of the end-point titer for each sample being positive in the first assay.

The evaluation of the immunofluorescence reaction is standardized by allowing the observers to know that the first and third slides to evaluate are always positive and that the second slide is always negative. All subsequent slides are kept unknown to each observer. The observers are not to confer with each other and the scores are summarized by a third person.

Each slide is evaluated only for the purpose of determining whether there is an immunofluorescent reaction in the islets or not. A sample is considered positive if at least three to seven islets in a section show immunofluorescence (Fig. 1a). If the islet immunofluorescence cannot be distinguished from fluorescence in the exocrine tissue, the preparation is considered negative (Fig. 1b). Hence, the end-point titer of each sample is assigned only by entering a positive or negative score in the assay protocol.

2.1.6.   ASSAY QUALITY CONTROLS

Several pancreatic specimens should be evaluated (24) to determine whether they are useful in routine ICCA determinations. In this analysis, which is carried out for each pancreas, *sensitivity* is defined as the number of times the ICCA-positive quality control sample is read positive divided by the number of times the sample is tested, while *specificity* is defined as the number of

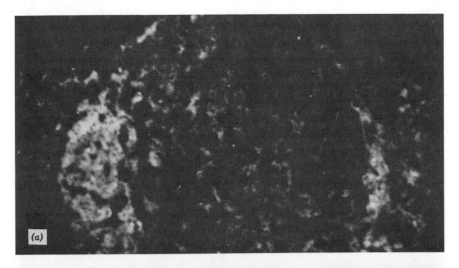

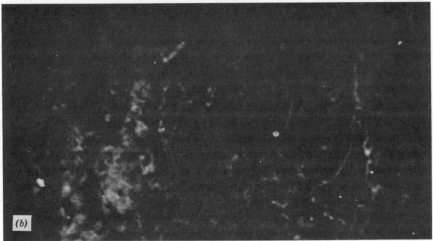

FIGURE 1.   Indirect immunofluorescence reaction in frozen sections of a human blood group O pancreas. The sections were incubated with either a serum sample from an insulin-dependent diabetic patient (*a*) showing cytoplasmic fluorescence in pancreatic islet or a sample from a healthy control (*b*). Note the vessel structure in the right part of the figure. × 150.

times the ICCA-negative quality control sample is read negative divided by the number of times the sample is tested. Our analysis of pancreatic specimens obtained from seven different donors revealed that the *specificity* varied only between 79–100 percent while the *sensitivity* varied between 23–99 percent. Only pancreatic specimens with 80–100 percent sensitivity and specificity should be used in routine analyses of ICCA. Parameters of assay precision and reproducibility in recent determinations are summarized in Table 2.

TABLE 2. Parameters of Islet Cell Cytoplasmic Antibody Assay Precision and Reproducibility

Parameter	Definition	Results	Percent
Sensitivity	Number of times a positive control sample is read positive by the total number of times this sample was tested.	1249/1362	91.7
Specificity	Number of times a negative control sample is read negative divided by the total number of times this sample was tested.	721/757	95.2
False negative score	Number of samples found negative in the first assay but proved positive in two to three subsequent assays.	10/195	5.1
False positive	Number of samples found positive in the first assay but proved negative in two to three subsequent assays.	6/165	3.6

3. QUANTITATION OF ISLET CELL SURFACE ANTIBODIES

The method presented, based on previous studies (8, 12), is an indirect immunofluorescence assay with dispersed, living islet cells prepared from normal rats. The present approach is also useful for cells prepared from other tissues and species.

3.1. Assay Reagents

3.1.1. SAMPLES

Samples of plasma or serum are obtained from IDDM patients and healthy controls. All samples are heat inactivated (30 min at 56°C) and centrifuged (100,000g for 10 min) at 4°C to remove protein precipitates. A crude immunoglobulin fraction is prepared from 0.3–1 mL of sample by either ammonium sulfate (8, 10) or polyethylene glycol precipitation. In the latter method the sample is first centrifuged (100,000g for 60 min) to remove lipids, which will float, and nonsoluble material, which will be pelleted. The supernatant fluid is mixed with an equal volume of 25 percent polyethylene glycol (PEG) 6000 (analytical grade should be used) and mixed on a vortex mixer. The immunoglobulin precipitate is collected by centrifugation at 4°C (20 min at 1200g) and, following careful removal of the supernatant, finally redissolved in the same type of medium that is used for the dispersed cells (see below). It is advisable to allow the immunoglobulin precipitate to dissolve slowly (leave overnight in a refrigerator) rather than to try to dissolve it by vigorous vortexing. In assays with living cells ammonium sulfate as well as PEG-precipitated immunoglobulin preparations are dialyzed against the type of medium used for the cells.

3.1.2. PREPARATION OF CELLS

Dispersed islet cells are prepared as described in detail in Vol. IC, IVE (28). Briefly, pancreatic islets, isolated by the methods outlined in other chapters (29, 30), are transferred to a tissue culture medium supplemented with 1 percent BSA and 1–2 mM EGTA. The islets are disrupted by mild mechanical treatment either by a micromixer (31) or by forcing the islets through a pipette with a blunt-ended tip (32). The dispersed cells are centrifuged through tissue culture medium supplemented with 4 percent BSA and the pellet of cells resuspended in a desired volume of the same type of medium. The cells are kept on ice or at 4°C throughout the experiment. Culture of islet cells after they have been dispersed into single cells often results in extensive reaggregation and formation of pseudoislets, which are less suitable for the cell surface immunofluorescence assay.

3.1.3. ISLET CELL SURFACE IMMUNOFLUORESCENCE ASSAY

1.   Add 100 µL dispersed cells (0.2–1.0 × 10^6 cells/mL) to a 12–15 mL tapered plastic centrifuge test tubes previously coated and rinsed once in the same type of medium (Table 3) as used for the cells. Keep the tubes on ice.

2.   Add a 100 µL sample representing diluted heat-activated plasma or

TABLE 3.   Medium for Cell Surface Antibody Determination of Dispersed Islet Cells

1. Add 10 mL of 1 M HEPES, pH 7.4, to 450 mL of double-distilled water in 500 mL medium flasks with screw caps. Autoclave at 121°C for 20 min. Allow the flasks to cool.
2. Add the following sterile solutions:
   (a). 50 mL of RPMI-1640 10X (Flow Laboratories of Gibco).
   (b). 2.4 mL of 7.5 percent sodium bicarbonate solution.
   (c). 10 mL of 5000 IU/mL penicillin/5000 µg/mL streptomycin solution (Flow Laboratories).
   (d). 5 mL of 200 mM L-glutamine.
3. Adjust pH, if necessary, to pH 7.4 with sterile 1 M HCl. Keep at 4°C and use within 2 weeks. If albumin (bovine serum albumin) is added, the medium is adjusted to pH 7.4 and then filtered through 0.45 µm Millipore filter.

serum or preferably an immunoglobulin preparation dissolved in and dialyzed against the same type of medium as used for the cells.

3.   Mix the cells with the sample by gently tapping the tube. Islet cells are very fragile and excessive mechanical treatment is avoided.

4.   Incubate the cells for 60 min either on ice or in a refrigerator (4°C).

5.   Add 10 mL of medium supplemented with 4 percent BSA to each tube and centrifuge at 4°C for 15 min at $50g$.

6.   Remove the entire supernatant, the first 9.5 mL with a Pasteur pipette connected to a water pump, the remainder with a 100–250 µL constriction pipette. It is imperative to leave the cell pellet in as small a volume of medium as possible.

7.   Add 100 µL fluoresceinisothiocyanate conjugated anti-human immunoglobulin diluted 1:20 in medium supplemented with 4 percent BSA. Immediately before addition, the second fluorescent antibody is filtered through 0.45 µm Millipore filter.

8.   Resuspend the cells gently by tapping the tube and incubate for 60 min in the dark either on ice or in a refrigerator.

9.   Add 10 mL of medium supplemented with 4 percent BSA and pellet the cells by centrifugation ($50g$ for 10 min). Remove the supernatant and resuspend the cell pellet carefully in a total volume of 200 µL of medium containing 4 percent BSA.

10.   Add 3 mL of 4 percent formaldehyde in 10 mM HEPES containing 140 mM NaCl and 1 percent BSA (prepare fresh from stock solutions of 8 percent formaldehyde and 2 percent BSA, respectively, and filter through a 0.45-µm Millipore filter before use) and allow the cells to fix (30 min at 4°C is sufficient).

11.   Collect the cells by centrifugation ($50g$ for 10 min) and wash once by centrifugation in 5 mL of medium buffered with 10–20 mM HEPES and supplemented with 4 percent BSA. After the last wash, the entire supernatant is removed leaving the cell pellet in a maximum of 15 µL medium.

12.   Resuspend the cells vigorously without forming foam with the aid of a 15 µL coated constriction pipette, rinsed several times in medium with 4 percent BSA. Place the 15 µL droplet with the cell suspension on a clean slide. Gently place a coverslip on top of the droplet and seal the coverslip. Evaluate the slides in a fluorescence microscope.

3.1.4.   Assay Protocol and Evaluation of Immunofluorescence

The yield of islet cells, which varies depending on the number of islets isolated, determines the number of unknown sera that can be tested in each assay. Samples shown to be positive and negative, respectively, in several subsequent assays are included among the unknown samples. All slides are coded and the fluorescence reaction evaluated by two independent readers. It is possible to keep the fixed cells at 4°C for 1–2 days before evaluation of fluorescence.

The fluorescence reaction is evaluated by inspecting 50–100 intact cells. Each cell is first identified by phase-contrast microscopy (preferably using an X100 oil immersion objective) (Fig. 2a) and then inspected for the fluorescence reaction (Fig. 2b). A cell is denoted positive if the fluorescence reaction results in either a ring-shaped cell surface reaction or a minimum of 20–25 fluorescent dots on the surface. Dead cells often accumulate the second fluorescent antibody in their cytoplasm. Clumps of more than four cells are excluded from the evaluation. The fluorescence intensity between cells varies, and it is often

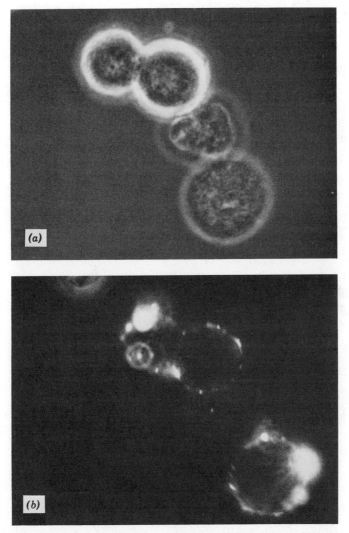

FIGURE 2. Indirect immunofluorescence reaction in living, dispersed rat islet cells incubated in serum from an insulin-dependent diabetic patient. The cells are first inspected in phase contrast (a) before their cell surface immunofluorescent reaction is evaluated. × 260.

necessary to score a sample positive or negative only using the differential count to guide the final decision. Positive samples are titrated and reanalyzed in repeated assays.

3.1.5. ABSORPTION OF SAMPLES

Human pancreatic islet cells or purified human β cells are yet to be made available in sufficient numbers for routine testing of islet cell surface antibodies. In a xenogenic approach it is necessary to test whether human immunoglobulin preparations contain antibodies which react with rodent determinants, present· on other cell types as well. Such heterophilic antibodies are not unusual among laboratory workers who often donate blood as controls (33). Heterophilic antibodies are removed by extensive absorptions, for example, to tissue powder prepared as described in ref. 34 from liver and kidney of the strain serving as the source of pancreatic islets.

4. DISCUSSION AND CONCLUSIONS

The presence of autoantibodies can be estimated in a semiquantitative manner by determining islet cell antibodies by indirect immunofluorescence either in sections of frozen human pancreas or in dispersed islet cells. Both methods have been found useful in several laboratories to determine the prevalence of islet cell antibodies in defined populations. However, the usefulness of the indirect immunofluorescence test in long-term follow-up studies of either patients

TABLE 4.   Islet Cell Cytoplasmic (ICCA) and Surface (ICSA) Antibodies in Newly Diagnosed Diabetic Children

Sample	Age/Sex	Days of IDDM	ICCA Titer	ICSA (percent positive cells)[a]
1	13/F	2	1:1	20
2	12/M	4	1:3	43
3	15/M	5	1:27	21
4	14/M	7	neg	49
5	11/F	6	1:27	23
6	10/F	7	1:27	3
7	16/M	7	1:27	20
8	12/F	9	1:3	39
9	12/M	6	1:3	34
10	13/M	5	1:3	24

[a] Tests of normal sera showed 20 percent fluorescent cells to be considered as the upper level of a negative sample.

or individuals at risk of developing diabetes remains to be determined. Routine use of the immunofluorescence test is assisted by the introduction of, for example, defined criteria for evaluation of the immunofluorescence reaction, titration of samples, blind evaluation by several independent readers, and the use of antibody positive and negative samples to be included in each assay. The observations of islet cell antibodies in samples from 10 newly diagnozed diabetic children are summarized in Table 4. These patients were treated with plasmaphoresis, and plasma is available in large quantities to permit long-term use as assay quality control samples. Until specific islet cell antigens have been identified (35) and isolated in sufficient amounts to permit the development of sensitive, accurate, and objective assays for islet cell antibodies, the present immunofluorescence techniques offer a semiquantitative approach to the determination of autoantibodies against the pancreatic islet cells.

REFERENCES

1. A. H. Coons, H. J. Creech, R. N. Jones, and E. Berliner, *J. Immunol.* **45**, 159 (1942).

2. A. Kawamura, *Fluorescent Antibody Techniques and Their Applications*, University of Tokyo Press, Tokyo, 1977.

3. G. F. Bottazzo, A. Florin-Christensen, and D. Doniach, *Lancet* **ii**, 1279 (1974).

4. A. C. MacCuish, J. Jordan, C. J. Campbell, L. J. P. Duncan, and W. J. Irvine, *Lancet* **II**, 1529 (1974).

5. R. Lendrum, G. Walker, and D. R. Gamble, *Lancet* **i**, 880 (1975).

6. W. J. Irvine, C. J. McCallum, R. S. Gray, G. J. Campbell, L. J. P. Duncan, J. W. Farquhar, H. Vaughan, and P. J. Morris, *Diabetes* **26**, 138 (1977).

7. N. K. MacLaren, S.-W. Huan, and J. Fogh, *Lancet* **i**, 997 (1975).

8. Å. Lernmark, Z. R. Freedman, C. Hofmann, A. H. Rubenstein, D. F. Steiner, R. L. Jackson, R. J. Winter, and H. S. Traisman, *N. Engl. J. Med.* **299**, 375 (1978).

9. Å. Lernmark, B. Hägglöf, Z. R. Freedman, W. J. Irvine, J. Ludvigsson, and G. Holmgren, *Diabetologia* **20**, 471 (1981).

10. M. van den Winkel, G. Smets, W. Gepts, and D. G. Pipeleers, *J. Clin. Invest.* **70**, 41 (1982).

11. R. Pujol-Borrell, E. L. Kouhry, and G. F. Bottazzo, *Diabetologia* **22**, 89 (1982).

12. Å. Lernmark, T. Kanatsuna, C. Patzelt, K. Diakoumis, R. Carroll, A. H. Rubenstein, and D. F. Steiner, *Diabetologia* **19**, 445 (1980).

13. S. Madsbad, G. F. Bottazzo, A. G. Cudworth, B. Dean, O. K. Faber, and C. Binder, *Diabetologia* **18**, 45 (1980).

14. A. Mustonen, M. Knip, and H. K. Åkerblom, *Diabetes* **32**, 743 (1983).

15. B. Marner, T. Agner, C. Binder, Å. Lernmark, and J. Nerup, *Diabetologia* **25**, 179 (1983) (abstr.)

16. A. N. Gorsuch, K. M. Spencer, J. Lister, J. M. McNally, B. M. Dean, G. F. Bottazzo, and A. G. Cudworth, *Lancet* **ii**, 1363 (1981).

17. S. Srikanta, O. Gunda, G. Eisenbarth, and J. S. Soeldner, *N. Engl. J. Med.* **308**, 322 (1983).

18. D. Doniach, and G. F. Bottazzo, *Pathobiol. Annu.* **7**, 327 (1977).

19. G. F. Bottazzo, R. Pujol-Borrell, and D. Doniach, *Clin. Immunol. Allergy* **1**, 139 (1981).

20. W. J. Irvine, *Recent Progr. Horm. Res.* **26**, 509 (1980).

21. Å. Lernmark and S. Baekkeskov, *Diabetologia* **21**, 431 (1981).

22. G. K. Papadopoulos and Å. Lernmark, "The Spectrum of Islet Cell Antibodies," in *Autoimmune Endocrine Disease*, Terry F. Davies (ed.), Wiley, New York, 1983.

23. C. H. Brogren and Å. Lernmark, *Clin. Endocrinol. Metab.* **11**, 409 (1982).

24. B. Marner, Å. Lernmark, J. Nerup, J. L. Molenaar, C. W. Tuk, and G. J. Bruining, *Diabetologia* **25**, 93 (1983).

25. R. Lendrum and J. G. Walker, *Gut* **16**, 365 (1975).

26. G. S. Eisenbarth, A. Linnenbach, R. Jackson, R. Scearce, and C. M. Croce, *Nature* **300**, 264 (1982).

27. O. D. Madsen, R. M. Cohen, F. W. Fitch, A. H. Rubenstein, and D. F. Steiner, *Endocrinology*, **113**, 2135 (1983).

28. Å. Lernmark, T. Dyrberg, J. H. Nielsen, and the Hagedorn Study Group, in *Methods in Diabetes Research*, J. Larner (ed.), in press.

29. J. Brunstedt, J. H. Nielsen, Å. Lernmark, and the Hagedorn Study Group, in *Methods in Diabetes Research*, J. Larner (ed.), in press.

30. J. H. Nielsen, B. Marner, T. Bilde, and the Hagedorn Study Group, in *Methods in Diabetes Research*, J. Larner (ed.), in press.

31. Å. Lernmark, *Diabetologia* **10**, 431 (1974).

32. T. Dyrberg, A. F. Nakhooda, S. Baekkeskov, Å. Lernmark, P. Poussier, and E. B. Marliss, *Diabetes* **31**(3), 278 (1982).

33. H. Jahr, S. Marx, W. Besch, and K.-P. Ratzmann, *Acta Biol. Med. Germ.* **41**, 1099 (1982).

34. A. H.-J. Huen, M. Haneda, Z. Freedman, Å. Lernmark, and A. H. Rubenstein, *Diabetes* **32**, 460 (1983).

35. S. Baekkeskov, J. H. Nielsen, B. Marner, T. Bilde, J. Ludvigsson, and Å. Lernmark, *Nature* **298**, 167 (1982).

E

ANTI-ISLET CELL MONOCLONAL ANTIBODIES

S. SRIKANTA AND G. S. EISENBARTH

Joslin Diabetes Center, Research Division, Brigham and Women's Hospital, Harvard Medical School, Boston, Massachusetts

1. INTRODUCTION

The "hybridoma" technique (1) of fusing myeloma cells with antibody-secreting lymphocytes to generate monoclonal antibodies with predefined specificity has contributed greatly to several fields of biomedical research. The genetic information in the myeloma cell line confers immortality to the antibody-producing lymphocyte. By utilizing a parent myeloma line deficient in the enzyme hypoxanthine–guanine phosphoribosyl transferase (HGPRT) and a selective medium known as HAT (hypoxanthine, aminopterin, and thymidine), only hybrid cells can be selected to grow in culture. Aminopterin blocks the main biosynthetic pathway for the synthesis of nucleic acids, and the myeloma cells are not able to utilize hypoxanthine in the salvage pathway because of their HGPRT deficiency. Normal lymphocytes contribute the enzyme HGPRT, and thus the fused cells can grow. The hybrids are then screened for the production of desired antibodies and the positive ones are cloned and frozen (2).

In this chapter we describe the production, characterization, and some applications of monoclonal antibodies directed toward antigens on the islet cells (3–6). While the general methodology for the production of murine monoclonal antibodies is relatively simple (though requiring 6–8 months of cell culture, assays, and biochemical analyses), production of human monoclonal antibodies is more difficult, although improvements in methodology are anticipated.

We have obtained monoclonal anti-islet antibodies from four sources:

1. Screening of selected monoclonal antibodies which initially were produced to another cell type, such as neurons (A2B5, 3G5) (7, 8) or malignant cell lines (9).

2. Murine monoclonal antibodies produced following immunization of mice with rat islet cells (A4A11) or a rat islet-cell tumor line (5D6, A1D2) (3, 10).

3. Murine anti-human islet antibodies produced following immunization of mice with human islets or insulinoma cells (HISL 1 to 22).

4) Human monoclonal autoantibodies produced by fusing circulating lymphocytes from patients with Type I diabetes with a human myeloma line (B6) (4).

2. MATERIALS

2.1. Media and Reagents

Dulbecco's modified Eagle's medium (DMEM) with high glucose (4.5 g/L) or Roswell Park Memorial Institute (RPMI) medium is used as our base medium. A week prior to fusion 5 L of medium (DMEM or RPMI; Gibco, Grand Island, NY) is prepared with deionized double-distilled water. This assures a fresh standardized medium for the entire procedure.

Concentrated (100×) stocks of medium supplements should be prepared and frozen ($-20°C$) in convenient aliquots.

HAT solutions (selective reagents: hypoxanthine, aminopterin, thymidine): 100× HT: 136 mg hypoxanthine (Sigma, St. Louis, MO) and 38.7 mg thymidine (Sigma) are prepared in 75 mL of distilled water and adjusted to pH 10.0 with NaOH before bringing final volume to 100 mL. Solution is sterilized by Millipore filtration and stored in 5 mL aliquots at $-20°C$ (final 100× molar concentrations: hypoxanthine = $10^{-2} M$, thymidine = $1.6 \times 10^{-3} M$). 100× aminopterin: 4.4 mg aminopterin (Sigma) is added to 75 mL of distilled water and adjusted to pH 9.8 before bringing final volume to 100 mL (final 100× molar concentration: aminopterin = $10^{-4} M$). Sterilize by Millipore filtration and pipette into 5 mL aliquots. Aminopterin can be frozen at $-20°C$ or stored in the dark at 4°C. Care should be observed when handling aminopterin powder and concentrated aminopterin stock because of its toxicity.

100× bovine insulin: (final concentration 2000 microunits). Stock insulin is in crystalline form and should be solubilized in 5 mL of a 1:500 dilution of concentrated HCl in water before bringing to final volume. Insulin should also be stored at $-20°C$ in 5-mL aliquots after sterile filtration.

The remaining supplements can be bought commercially as 100× stock solutions. MEM sodium pyruvate solution: 100× 100 mM (Gibco); MEM nonessential amino acids: 100× (Gibco); L-glutamine: 100× (Gibco). NCTC-109 is offered as a supplement (MA Bioproducts, Walkersville, MD).

Selection medium formula (Super HAT): Freshly prepared DMEM/RPMI is used for preparing 4 L of Super Base. Super Base lacks HAT selective supplements and can be used to grow hybrid cells when selection has occured or can be used for selection with the addition of HAT. Add 40 mL of $100\times$ stock solutions of insulin, sodium pyruvate, nonessential amino acids, and L-glutamine and 400 mL of NCTC-109 to 3.36 L of DMEM to prepare Super Base. Super Base should be sterilized by Millipore filtration and stored in 500 mL sterile bottles. To prepare selective medium (Super HAT) from Super Base, add 5 mL of $100\times$ HT and 5 mL of $100\times$ aminopterin stock to 500 mL Super Base. Twenty percent heat-inactivated fetal calf serum (HIFCS) (56°C for 30 min) is used throughout the procedure for fusing, routine passaging, and cloning. Once a new hybridoma line has been cloned and safely frozen, the hybrid cells may be adapted to 10 percent HIFCS.

We have found that with proper sterile techniques and appropriate precautions no antibiotics are necessary.

2.2. Equipment and Supplies

Disposable, individually wrapped plastics are used when possible to reduce the risk of contamination. Essential equipment includes a fully humidified 37°C incubator with a controlled atmosphere of 5 or 10 percent CO_2 in air (depending on the medium), a laminar flow sterile hood equipped with pipette aid (Fisher Scientific), a centrifuge and a liquid nitrogen tank for cell storage. We keep approximately 1 in. of distilled water with 1 percent sodium dodecyl sulfate in the bottom of the incubator.

3. PARENTAL MYELOMA LINES

We have had success with three of the available HAT-sensitive mouse myeloma lines, P3X63-Ag8, NS1-Ag4-1 (11), and P3X63-Ag8·653 (12). P3X63-Ag8 (P3) expresses immunoglobulin with chain composition of a γ-heavy chain and K chains and P3X63-Ag8·653 (653), a subclone of P3, does not express heavy or light chain immunoglobulin. For human fusions we have used the following human myeloma cell lines: GM15006TG-2 (13) and GM4672 (14) (Cell Repository, Camden, NJ). It is recommended that several lines be used with fusions, and, regardless of the line used, it is essential that it be in its log phase of growth for a successful hybridization. It is best to obtain the cell line from an investigator who has successfully performed fusions with the line, to develop a large stock of frozen cells and use cells for fusion after only a limited number of passages.

4. IMMUNIZATION

Immunization methods and schedules vary tremendously depending on the antigens and the investigator. A major advantage of the monoclonal antibody system is the ability to immunize with only partially purified antigens (e.g., whole cells). An important parameter is that the fusion be performed 3–5 days after the last antigen injection.

We use female Balb/c mice 6–12 weeks old. Soluble antigens are normally injected subcutaneously, first with complete, and subsequently with incomplete, Freund's adjuvant. When making monoclonal antibodies to cellular antigens, whole cells or dissociated cellular stroma can be used. Cells (2×10^7) are suspended in PBS and are injected intravenously and intraperitoneally on day 0, and intraperitoneally only on days 7 and 14. The final injection should not employ adjuvant. Splenocytes are fused on day 17. We usually continue immunizations of other mice at 7-day intervals until the results of an initial fusion are clear. If the first fusion is not successful, another mouse is sacrificed and splenocytes fused.

After several immunizations the mouse can be test-bled and the serum assayed for circulating antibody. Checking for serum antibody at this point serves two important purposes:

1. By performing serial serum dilutions, the screening assay can be tested for sensitivity and last minute technical problems can be worked out before fusing.
2. A mouse that has no serum antibody against an antigen is unlikely to produce specific hybrids. If no antibodies are produced, changing the strain of mice immunized may result in the generation of serum antibodies.

5. FUSION PROTOCOL

5.1. Materials

1, 5, 10, and 25 mL individually wrapped sterile pipettes (Costar, Cambridge, MA).

15 mL sterile centrifuge tubes (Falcon).

50 mL sterile centrifuge tubes (Falcon).

96 well flat-bottom microtiter plates (Linbro, Flow Labs, Hamden, CT).

24 well plates (Costar).

25 cm^2 flask (Corning, Fisher Scientific).

75 cm^2 flask (Corning, Fisher Scientific).

Petri dishes, 60 × 15 mm (Falcon).

Two sets of sterile scissors and forceps.

Dulbecco's PBS: 8 g/L NaCl, 0.2 g/L KCL, 1.15 g/L Na$_2$PO$_4$, 0.2 g/L KH$_2$PO$_4$, 0.1 g/L MgCl$_2$·6H$_2$O, and 0.1 g/L CaCl$_2$.

70 percent alcohol: 250 mL in a 500 mL beaker.

DMEM with 20 percent HIFCS.

Super HAT with 20 percent HIFCS.

50 percent polyethylene glycol 1000 (PEG; J. T. Baker Chemical Co., Phillipsburg, NJ); autoclave 5 g and allow to cool to 50°C before adding 5 mL DMEM.

Feeder spleen cells: Normal spleen cells are prepared as described in the following protocol and frozen as described in Section 8. Ten frozen vials of cells are prepared from each spleen, yielding approximately 1×10^7 normal spleen cells per vial.

5.2. Procedure

1. An immunized mouse is sacrificed by cervical dislocation and dipped immediately in 70 percent ethanol for 1 min.

2. The spleen is aseptically removed using one set of sterile instruments to incise the skin, another to incise the peritoneum, and another to remove the spleen.

3. The spleen is placed in 5 mL of Dulbecco's PBS in a Petri dish, and fat remnants are carefully removed.

4. Intact spleen is then transferred to another Petri dish with 5 mL of cold PBS and minced with fine scissors.

5. Triturate minced spleen four to five times with a 10 mL pipette and transfer to a 15 mL centrifuge tube.

6. While the spleen clumps are settling, 2×10^7 myeloma cells in 40 mL of DMEM containing 20 percent HIFCS are transferred to a 50-mL centrifuge tube.

7. Suspended spleen cells are carefully removed, not disturbing the gravity-sedimented tissue, and added directly to the myeloma cell centrifuge tubes with the myeloma cells.

8. Combined cells are pelleted ($600g$) for 7 min at room temperature.

9. Supernatant is discarded, and pellet is gently disrupted by tapping at the bottom of the tube.

The following steps are performed at 37°C:

10. 0.8 mL of 50 percent PEG is slowly added with a 1 mL pipette over a period of 1 min, while swirling the suspension.

11. After an additional minute of swirling, 1 mL of DMEM is added over a 1 min period.

12. While continuing to swirl, 20 mL of DMEM is added over a 5 min period to slowly dilute the PEG.

13. Suspension is centrifuged ($600g$) for 7 min and supernatant is discarded.

14. Pellet is disrupted by tapping the bottom of the tube and is resuspended in 2 mL of DMEM; 1 mL is transferred to another centrifuge tube and 40 mL Super HAT containing 20 percent HIFCS is added to both centrifuge tubes.

15. 1×10^7 normal spleen cells from a frozen vial in 1 mL of DMEM are added to the fused cells.

16. Two drops from a 10 mL pipette ($\sim$100 μL) are added to each well of ten 96 well plates.

17. Plates are taped with cellophane tape to prevent accidental opening when handled, and placed in a humidified 10 percent CO_2 incubator at 37°C.

18. After 7 days, plates are fed with an additional 1 drop of Super HAT containing 20 percent HIFCS.

19. Visible colonies should be apparent in $\sim$14 days. When visible colonies (covering $\sim$ one quarter of bottom of well) are present, supernatant is removed for assay.

6. ANTIBODY SCREENING ASSAY

Selection of an appropriate assay to detect specific antibody in supernatants should be given careful consideration. The assay must be sensitive, yet flexible enough to screen rapidly hundreds of samples (15). The following are examples of some of the assays we have used to screen specific monoclonal antibody production.

6.1. Radioimmunoassay for Anti-Cell-Surface Antibodies (e.g., monoclonal antibodies to RIN cells) (3)

1. RIN (rat insulinoma) cells are cultured as monolayers in RPMI 1640 medium supplemented with 10 percent heat-inactivated fetal calf serum (FCS).

2. Cells are removed from flasks by incubation in Dulbecco's phosphate-buffered saline in the absence of Ca^{2+} and Mg^{2+} (PBS).

3. $1-5 \times 10^5$ cells/well are added to 96-well V-bottomed microtiter plates (Cooke Laboratory Products, Alexandria, VA).

4. Cell suspensions are incubated with antibody (supernatant) at room temperature for 30 min.

5. Plates are centrifuged at $500g$ and then inverted onto a utility wipe to remove unreacted antibody.

6. Either [^{125}I]-F(ab')$_2$ affinity-purified anti-mouse IgG ($\sim$10,000 cpm) or [^{125}I]staphylococcal protein A (sp. act. = $2-12 \times 10^4$ cpm) in PBS,

0.1 percent gelatin, and 1 percent albumin (Amersham-Searle Company, Arlington Heights, IL) are incubated with cells.

7. Cells are washed twice with PBS-1 percent albumin.

8. Individual wells are cut from microtiter plate and counted.

6.2. Cytotoxicity Assay (^{51}Cr release using RIN cells) (3)

1. RIN cells are cultured overnight as a monolayer in 96-well microculture plates with 0.1 mL RPMI medium containing heat-inactivated FCS and 7.5×10^4 cpm of ^{51}Cr in each well.

2. Before assay, invert plate onto utility wipe, and wash well three times with 200 µL of RPMI.

3. Incubate cells with 50 µL of the antibody (supernate) and 5 µL of rabbit complement for 20 min at 37°C.

4. Centrifuge plate at 500g; 75 µL from each well are counted to determine ^{51}Cr release as an index of cytotoxicity.

6.3. Indirect Immunofluorescence

6.3.1. MATERIALS

Glass slides, coplin jar: 75×25 mm 1.0 mm (American Scientific Products, Charlotte, NC).

Coverslips: 22×44 mm, number 1 (American Scientific Products).

Sqeeze bottle.

Moist chamber: 150×15-mm Petri dish (Falcon #1058) with a moist towel.

Acetone.

Dulbecco's phosphate-buffered saline (PBS) with 0.02 percent Na sodium azide.

30 percent glycerol: 30 mL glycerol in 70 mL PBS containing 0.02 percent azide.

FITC goat anti-mouse IgG (TAGO, Burlingame, CA).

DMEM with 2 percent bovine serum albumin (BSA): 2 g BSA/100 mL DMEM.

6.3.2. PROCEDURE

1. Frozen sections are cut with a cryostat from tissue that was quickly frozen in liquid nitrogen or on dry ice and placed two per slide.

2. Sections on slides are fixed in cold acetone (-70°C) for 5 min.

3. Allow slides to air dry. Note: At this point slides can be stored in a slide box at -70°C until needed.

4. In a moist chamber incubate 25 μL of monoclonal antibody supernate on the tissue sections for 30 min at room temperature.

5. Rinse antibody with a squeeze bottle of PBS and place slide into a rinse coplin jar containing PBS at 4°C for 5 min. Transfer to a second similar container for 5 min and then to a third for an additional 5 min.

6. After final PBS rinse, gently dry slide surrounding the tissue.

7. Add to section goat anti-mouse IgG, FITC conjugated, diluted 1:100 in DMEM with 2 percent BSA.

8. Incubate 30 min at room temperature.

9. Repeat step 5.

10. After final PBS wash, rinse by briefly dipping slide into a coplin jar containing distilled water.

11. Add two drops of 30 percent glycerol to the slide and seal with a coverslip and nail polish.

12. Store slides at 4°C in the dark until they are to be examined with a fluorescent microscope.

7. CELL EXPANSION, CLONING, AND FREEZING

When a desirable antibody is detected with the screening assay, the hybrid cells are transferred to 0.5 mL cultures in 24 well plates using a 0.1 mL pipette. When these wells become 50 percent confluent (4–5 days), a sample of supernatant is assayed. Positive colonies are then transferred to 25 cm^2 flasks containing 5 mL of media, and the initial well is refed with 1 mL of medium. At this point it is very important to clone positive colonies to ensure a homogeneous culture, thus preventing overgrowth by hybrid cells not producing the desired antibody. Then confluent cells from the 25 cm^2 flask should be frozen in dimethylsulfoxide containing medium to assure a permanent stock of antibody-producing cells. After the initial freeze, cells from the 25 cm^2 flasks should be expanded to 75 cm^2 flasks and large densities of cells should be grown to harvest supernatant and to develop frozen stocks of cells. If a cell line should stop producing antibody, it can be retrieved from an early freeze and recloned. No lines should be discontinued until a frozen vial is thawed, grown up in culture, and its supernatant assayed.

7.1. Cloning by Limiting Dilution

7.1.1. Materials

15 mL centrifuge tubes.

Super HAT with 20 percent HIFCS medium containing 1×10^7 normal spleen cells/50 mL.

1 and 10 mL pipettes.

96 well flat-bottom plates.

Ten milliliters Super HAT containing 20 percent HIFCS is added to a centrifuge tube and 9 mL to an additional three tubes labeled 2, 3, and 4. One hundred microliters of cells from a confluent hybrid culture is added to the first centrifuge tube and mixed thoroughly. One milliliter of mixed suspension is taken from the first tube and added to tube 2, and, after several aspirations, 1 mL is taken from tube 2 and added to tube 3 and similarly to the fourth tube from each dilution. Two drops are added to each of 24 wells of 96 well plates (2 drops/well) with a 10 mL pipette. Plates are taped and placed in a 37°C incubator with 10 percent CO_2. In 1–2 weeks colonies will be visible. Several colonies may appear in a single well in the lower diluted wells. Five to ten supernatant samples for assaying should be taken from the highest dilution wells with one visible colony per well. Several of the positive colonies should be expanded, frozen, and recloned. Recloning should continue until all resulting clones are positive.

7.2. Freezing and Thawing Hybridoma Cells

7.2.2. Materials

Freezing vials (Nunc, Gibco).

$2 \times$ freezing medium: 85 mL Super HAT with 20 percent HIFCS + 15 mL dimethylsulfoxide (DMSO; Malinckrodt Paris, Kent) Sterilized by Millipore filtration.

DMEM with 20 percent FCS.

Polystyrene box: 2 cm thick walls.

25 cm^2 flask.

1, 5, and 10 mL pipettes.

Approximately 1×10^6 cells in log phase are pelleted by centrifugation at 600g for 5 min. The supernatant is removed and the pellet is resuspended in 0.5 mL of DMEM with 20 percent FCS. Slowly add 0.5 mL of $2 \times$ freezing medium and transfer mixture to Nunc vial. Vial is placed in a polystyrene box and stored at -70°C overnight. The following day the vial is transferred directly into liquid nitrogen for storage.

Frozen vials should be thawed quickly by swirling in a 37°C water bath. When thawed, centrifuge 5 min (600g) and sterilely aspirate the supernatant. Resuspend the pellet with 1 mL of Super HAT with 20 percent HIFCS using a 1 mL pipette and transfer to an additional 4 mL in a 25 cm^2 flask. Cell viability usually ranges from 60–80 percent.

8. HIGH-TITERED ANTIBODY IN MICE

As an alternative to growing large volumes of monoclonal antibody by circulating cells, high-titered antibody in ascites form can be obtained by injecting viable cells into pristane (2,6,10,14 tetramethylpentadecane; Aldrich Chemical, Milwaukee) primed Balb/c mice (0.25 mL pristane injected 1–7 days prior to hybrid cells). Hybridoma cells *in vitro* produce from 10 to 50 μg/mL of monoclonal antibody, whereas ascites fluid often contains as much as 20 mg/mL of antibody. Occasionally, even a contaminated hybrid culture can be rescued by growth as an ascites tumor in Balb/c mouse.

8.1. Procedure

Inject $1–10 \times 10^6$ viable cells in 0.5 mL PBS intraperitoneally into the lower abdomen of the pristane-treated mouse. Ascites fluid should begin to accumulate 7–14 days after inoculation (the mouse develops a tense, large abdomen). Ascites is removed by inserting a 19-gauge 1-in. needle into the abdomen and allowing the fluid to drain into a centrifuge tube. Cells are separated from the fluid by centrifuging $600g$ for 5 min. Ascites fluid should be aliquoted and stored at $-20°C$ to minimize repeated freezing and thawing. Ascites cells can be frozen using the same procedure as for cultured hybrid cells. An assay should be performed using various dilutions to determine the saturating titer of the ascites antibody. Some ascites containing monoclonal antibody can be diluted as much as 1:100,000 without loss in binding activity, but when added undiluted no binding is detected. We recommend screening ascites at a 1:100 initial dilution.

9. HUMAN × HUMAN FUSIONS

Several attempts have been made to immortalize autoantibody-producing human B lymphocytes from patients with various autoimmune diseases including Type I diabetes (4, 14, 16). The basic principles of producing human–human hybridomas are essentially similar to mouse fusions; some salient features are summarized:

1. Human myeloma cell line GM 1500 6TG-2 and GM 4672 (HGPRT deficient; HAT sensitive) have been used as fusion partners.
2. Peripheral blood lymphocytes (PBL) are isolated by Ficoll–Hypaque gradient.
3. After multiple washings in serum-free medium, the myeloma cells and lymphocytes are mixed (1:5; 1:10 ratio) and pelleted.
4. Fusion is effected with 50 percent polyethylene glycol (PEG) 1540.
5. Fusion products are plated in 96 or 24 well plates in Super HAT medium with irradiated (2000R) human peripheral blood lymphocytes as feeder cells ($10–15 \times 10^3$ cells/well).
6. Cells are fed with RPMI Super HAT as required.

TABLE 1. Anti-Islet Monoclonal Antibodies

Monoclonal Antibody	Type	Antigen	Cells	Target
A2B5[a]	Mouse	GQ ganglioside	Islet, neuron, and neuroendocrine	Murine, human, rat, bovine, etc.
3G5 (Akeson)	Mouse	Ganglioside	Islet, neuron, and neuroendocrine	Murine, human, rat, bovine, etc.
Tetanus toxin + 3D8	Mouse	GD,GT ganglioside	Islet, neuron, neuroendocrine, and thyroid	Murine, human, rat, bovine, etc.
4F2[a]	Mouse	80K:40K glycoprotein	Islet, monocyte, activated T cell	Human
LC7/2 (Levine)	Mouse	80K:40K glycoprotein	Tumor lines, monocyte, islet	Human
A4All	Mouse	Unknown	Islet	Rat
5D6	Mouse	Unknown	Islet, fibroblast	Rat
A1D2	Mouse	24K glycoprotein	Islet	Rat
B6	Human	Unknown	A cells	Human
A1G12	Rat-mouse	Unknown	"Nuclear" islet	Rat, human
BB-TECS	Rat-mouse	Unknown	Thymic endocrine, islet	Rat, human
HISL 1 to 22 (except 19)	Mouse	Unknown	Islet	Human
HISL 19	Mouse	Unknown	Islet	Human, bovine, porcine

[a] Donated to the American Type Culture Collection, Rockville, MD.

206

7. When hybridomas have grown to confluence (4–8 weeks), the supernatant fluids are screened for antibody production and positive hybrids are cloned by limiting dilution and frozen.

10. MONOCLONAL ANTIBODY AVAILABILITY

As the use of monoclonal antibodies increases, more companies are marketing media, reagents, and devices for making monoclonal antibodies. Many hybridoma lines along with parent myeloma lines are available through the American Type Culture Collection (Rockville, MD) and the Human Genetic Mutant Cell Repository (Camden, NJ). Monoclonal antibody supernatants and ascites are also available from Accurate Chemical and Scientific Corporation (Westbury, NY), Pel-Freeze (Rodgers, AK), Becton-Dickenson (Sunnyvale, CA), Ortho Diagnostics (Raritan, NJ) and many other companies. Many investigators will share their monoclonal antibodies or even cell lines, and existing monoclonals can be useful to characterize screening assays.

Table 1 summarizes the library of monoclonal anti-islet antibodies that we have developed. These monoclonal antibodies have been utilized to characterize islet-cell surface antigens—glycoproteins and gangliosides (7, 8, 10)—to positively identify pancreatic islets by double immunofluorescence during screening human sera for islet cell antibodies (9), to isolate rat and human islet cells using plates coated with anti-mouse antibody (17) or, using a fluorescence-activated cell sorter, to detect by external scanning insulinoma tumors in rats (using [^{125}I]-labeled monoclonal antibodies) (18, 19). Further applications of these anti-islet monoclonal antibodies remain to be explored.

REFERENCES

1. G. Kohler and C. Milstein, *Nature* **256**, 495 (1975).
2. G. S. Eisenbarth and R. Jackson, *Endocr. Rev.* **3**, 26–39 (1982).
3. G. S. Eisenbarth, H. Oie, A. Gazdar, W. Chick, J. A. Schultz, and R. M. Scearce, *Diabetes* **30**, 226–230 (1981).
4. G. S. Eisenbarth, A. Linnenbach, R. A. Jackson, R. Scearce, and C. Croce, *Nature* **300**, 264–267 (1982).
5. G. S. Eisenbarth, R. A. Jackson, S. Srikanta, A. C. Powers, J. B. Buse, A. Rabizadeh, and H. Mori, "Utilization of Monoclonal Antibody Techniques to Study Type I Diabetes Mellitus," in *Immunology of Diabetes*, U. DiMario (ed.) in press.
6. R. M. Scearce and G. S. Eisenbarth, "Production of Monoclonal Antibodies Reacting with the Cytoplasm and Surface of Differentiated Cells," in *Methods in Enzymology: Neuroendocrine Peptides*, Vol. 103, S. P. Colowick and N. O. Kaplan (eds.), Academic Press, New York, 1983, pp. 459–469.
7. G. S. Eisenbarth, K. Shimizu, M. A. Bowring, and S. Wells, *Proc. Natl. Acad. Sci. USA* **79**, 5066–5070 (1982).

8. A. C. Powers, A. Rabizadeh, R. Akeson, and G. S. Eisenbarth, *Endocrinology*, **114**(4), 1338–1343 (1984).

9. S. Srikanta, R. Dolinar, and G. S. Eisenbarth, *Diabetes* **31**(2), 19A(76) (1982).

10. M. A. Crump, R. Scearce, M. Dobersen, W. J. Kortz, and G. S. Eisenbarth, *J. Clin. Invest.* **70**, 659–666 (1982).

11. G. Kohler, S. C. Howe, and C. Milstein, *Eur. J. Immunol.* **6**, 292 (1976).

12. J. F. Kearney, A. Radbruch, B. Leisegang, and K. Rajewsky, *J. Immunol.* **123**, 1548 (1979).

13. C. M. Croce, A. Linnenbach, W. Hall, Z. Steplewski, and H. Koprowski, *Nature* **288**, 488–489 (1980).

14. Y. Shoenfeld, S. C. Hsu-Lin, J. E. Gabriels, L. E. Silberstein, B. C. Furie, B. Furie, B. D. Stollar, and R. S. Schwartz, *J. Clin. Invest.* **70**, 205–208 (1982).

15. G. Galfre and C. Milstein, "Preparation of Monoclonal Antibodies: Strategies and Procedures," in *Methods in Enzymylology*, Vol. 73, Academic Press, New York, 1981, pp. 3–46.

16. J. Sotoh, B. S. Prabhakar, M. V. Haspel, F. G. Fellner, and A. L. Notkins, *N. Engl. J. Med.* **309**, 217–220 (1983).

17. W. J. Kortz, T. H. Reiman, R. Bollinger, and G. S. Eisenbarth, *Surg. Forum* **33**, 354–356 (1982).

18. D. Reintgen, K. Shimizu, E. Coleman, G. S. Eisenbarth, W. Briner, and H. F. Siegler, *Surg. Forum* **33**, 431–434 (1982).

19. K. Shimizu, D. Reintgen, R. Rowley, E. Coleman, W. Briner, H. Seigler, and G. S. Eisenbarth, *Hybridoma* **2**(1), 69–77 (1982).

IV

TISSUE, CELL, AND CULTURE PREPARATIONS

A

PERFUSED WORKING RAT HEART FOR METABOLIC STUDIES

HOWARD E. MORGAN AND DANIEL L. SIEHL

Department of Physiology, The Milton S. Hershey Medical Center, The Pennsylvania State University, Hershey, Pennsylvania

1. ADVANTAGES AND DISADVANTAGES OF THE PERFUSED RAT HEART

The isolated, perfused rat heart has been used extensively for studies of cardiac metabolism. Both the Langendorff preparation (1, 2) and the working heart (3–5) have advantages and disadvantages in these studies. Both preparations share the following advantages:

1. The muscle cells are intact and substrates and hormones reach the cells via the normal capillary bed.

2. Viability of the preparations can be easily monitored by measuring heart rate, coronary flow, and intraventricular pressure development.

3. The preparations are stable for periods of 2–6 hr, depending upon substrate availability and the magnitude of ventricular pressure development.

4. The heart can be perfused in a NMR spectrometer for continuous monitoring of energy metabolism (6).

5. The tissue can be frozen rapidly at the termination of the experiment for estimation of metabolite content. Freezing can be gated to specific phases of the cardiac cycle to follow cyclical changes in metabolites (7).

The disadvantages of both preparations are as follows:

1. Extrapolation of the results obtained *in vitro* to the intact animal is uncertain.

2. The hearts are perfused with low-viscosity buffer, a situation that results in rates of coronary flow that are several-fold greater than found *in vivo*.

3. The perfusate is oxygenated with gas mixtures containing 95 percent oxygen; this procedure leads to effluent oxygen tensions (150–250 mm Hg) that are three- to fivefold greater than found *in vivo* (4, 5).

The particular advantages of the working heart preparation are as follows:

1. The effects of hormones, drugs, substrate availability, and metabolic and hormonal status of the animal donor on mechanical function and metabolism can be easily assessed.

2. Effects of preload (left atrial pressure) and afterload (aortic pressure) can be varied; this property allows for a comprehensive evaluation of cardiac function of normal and diseased hearts (8, 9).

The major disadvantages of the working heart is the inability to vary independently ventricular volume, ventricular pressure, and aortic pressure. This

Supported by grants from NIH (HL-18258 and HL-20388).

disadvantage is of importance because stretch of the ventricular wall appears to be an important determinant of several metabolic processes including oxygen consumption (10, 11), glucose and pyruvate utilization (12), and rates of protein synthesis (11, 13).

Advantages of the Langendorff preparation also should be noted.

1.   The preparation is technically easy to use.
2.   Ventricular pressure development can be varied from 50 to 140 mm Hg by elevation of aortic pressure (4).
3.   Aortic pressure can be dissociated from intraventricular pressure development by insertion of a ventricular drain (10–12).
4.   Effects of aortic pressure on cardiac metabolism can be studied in arrested-drained hearts by elevation of the potassium concentration or addition of tetrodotoxin (10–12).

A disadvantage of the use of this preparation for studies of the relationship between aortic pressure and oxygen consumption is the inability to use aortic pressures higher than approximately 140 mm Hg due to overdistension of the left ventricle and edema of the ventricular wall (11).

Two methods for perfusion of the isolated rat heart will be described: (i) the working heart preparation in which the aorta and left atrial appendage are cannulated and perfusate is introduced into the left atrium, pumped by the left ventricle, and either passes through the coronary bed or is ejected through a resistance pathway (3–6) and (ii) the Langendorff preparation (1, 2) in which the aorta is cannulated and the coronary vessels are perfused by introducing perfusate into the aorta. Perfusion by the second method precedes perfusion of rat hearts as working preparations.

2.   PERFUSION MEDIUM

A modified Krebs–Henseleit bicarbonate buffer, pH 7.4, is generally used (14). Final concentrations of buffer components (in mM) are: NaCl, 117.4; KCl, 4.7; CaCl$_2$, 3.0; MgSO$_4$, 1.2; KH$_2$PO$_4$, 1.2; EDTA, 0.5; NaHCO$_3$, 24.7; and bathocuproine disulfonate, 50 μM. Na$_2$EDTA and bathocuproine disulfonate are added to chelate heavy metals that are present in the reagents (3, 4, 15–17). Oxidizable substrates and amino acids are added as desired. When long-chain fatty acids are provided as substrate, addition of bovine serum albumin (3–4 percent) is required. The perfusion medium must be prepared each day and must be continuously equilibrated with O$_2$–CO$_2$ (95:5) throughout the day to prevent precipitation of calcium salts. Dry reagents are weighed out each day; all of the reagents except for NaHCO$_3$ are dissolved in a volume of water somewhat less than the desired final volume and the pH adjusted to 7.4. This solution is thoroughly gassed with O$_2$–CO$_2$ and the NaHCO$_3$ added. Gassing with 5 percent CO$_2$ lowers the pH and prevents precipitation of calcium salts when NaHCO$_3$ is added. The fatty acid albumin complex is prepared by dissolving the fatty acids in absolute ethanol (minimum volume), adding a slight molar excess of K$_2$CO$_3$ (to form the potassium salt) and about 2 mL of H$_2$O. Ethanol is evaporated by carefully warming the mixture on a hot plate. The aqueous solution is added to a warm albumin solution (10 percent) to give a clear solution which is dialyzed overnight against at least 10 volumes of Krebs–Henseleit buffer. The dialyzed albumin is added to fresh buffer to give the desired final concentration and passed through a Millipore filter (0.8 μM). Buffer that does not contain albumin also is filtered prior to use.

3. PREPARATION OF THE HEART

Rats of the Sprague-Dawley strain weighing 150–350 g are either fed *ad libitum* or fasted for the desired period before use. Heparin sodium (2.5 mg) is injected intraperitoneally 30–60 min before the rats are killed. The rat is anesthetized with Nembutal (30 mg/rat, i.p.) and the abdomen is opened by making a transverse incision with scissors. The diaphragm is transected and lateral incisions are made along both sides of the rib cage. The anterior chest wall is folded back. The pericardium and other filamentous tissues of the mediastinum are pulled away with the fingers. The heart is picked up and the lungs and other chest contents pushed toward the back. The point at which the pulmonary veins join the left atrium is identified, and the heart is removed by making a single cut with the scissors through the pulmonary veins and on through the other vessels arising from the heart (5 mm of aorta should remain). The heart is dropped into a beaker containing 0.9 percent sodium chloride chilled in ice water. It is important that the removal of the heart occur expeditiously; approximately 20 sec should suffice to transfer the heart to cold saline once the chest is opened.

The heart is picked up by the aorta using fine-tipped forceps, and any connective tissue, thymus, or lung that may be removed is pulled away. The aorta is slipped about 3 mm onto a grooved perfusion cannula (Fig. 1) and held with a small serrafine clamp. Retrograde perfusion down the aorta is begun immediately from a reservoir 75 cm above the heart as soon as the heart is positioned with the serrafine clamp. The heart is secured with a ligature. If the heart is to be perfused as a Langendorff preparation, no further cannulation is required. If a working preparation is desired, the openings into the left atrium are positioned to receive the second perfusion cannula. The left atrium is slipped onto this cannula and tied; the accuracy and competence of the cannulation is tested by unclamping the tube leading from the oxygenator to the left atrium and observing filling of the left atrium. Commonly, a preliminary perfusion as a Langendorff preparation lasts for 10 min, a period sufficient to cannulate the left atrium. In some experiments the preliminary perfusion period is extended for periods up to 70 min. In these cases the heart is suspended in a 250-mL Erlenmeyer flask to prevent cooling. The preliminary perfusion

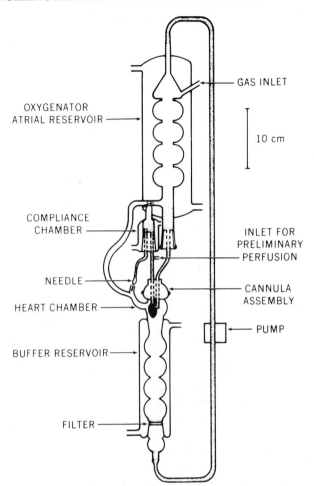

FIGURE 1. Modified apparatus for perfusion of working rat hearts. Components are described in the text. Reproduced from Morgan et al. (5) with permission of the *American Journal of Physiology*.

serves to remove all blood, to equilibrate the substrate concentration in the medium with those in the extracellular space, to increase the dependence of the heart of the exogenous substrate supply, and to adapt the heart to perfusion with a lower mean aortic pressure. When oxygen consumption is to be measured, the pulmonary artery is carefully freed from connective tissue down to its base. A third cannula is inserted into the rubber stopper or Teflon ball joint that supports the left atrial and aortic cannulae, and the pulmonary artery is slipped onto this cannula and tied. Approximately 90 percent of the coronary flow is ejected via the pulmonary artery. Samples of effluent from the pulmonary artery cannula are collected in 5-mL gas-tight syringes and used for estimation of oxygen tension (4, 5, 11).

4. PERFUSION APPARATUS FOR WORKING HEARTS

The apparatus that was described earlier (3, 4) was modified (5) to reduce circulating volume and to facilitate oxygenation of albumin-containing buffer (Fig. 1). The apparatus consists of six major parts (Kontes Glass Co., Vineland, NJ): (i) cannula assembly, (ii) aortic compliance chamber, (iii) combined oxygenator and left atrial reservoir, (iv) heart chamber, (v) buffer reservoir and filter, and (vi) peristaltic pump. The cannula assembly is mounted in a size 35 ball joint made of Teflon. Two stainless steel cannulae (outside diameter, 0.134 in.) are grooved to accommodate ligatures. A tip of 0.109-in. outside diameter tubing is soldered into the aortic cannula and a side arm is attached for preliminary perfusion. The atrial cannula terminates in a short horizontal segment to carry perfusate directly into the left atrium. The compliance chamber consists of the female portion of a 14/35 standard taper joint (waterjacketed). Male plugs made of Teflon and fitted with neoprene "O" rings are used to hold inlet and outlet tubes. The top of the compliance chamber is closed by a short piece of Tygon tubing that is clamped with a hemostat. Outflow from the compliance chamber is returned to the buffer reservoir via a length of Tygon tubing with a hypodermic needle inserted into its distal end. A needle with an internal diameter of 0.58 mm (20-gauge, 0.5-in. shaft) provides sufficient resistance to result in systolic and diastolic aortic pressures of approximately 145 and 75 mm Hg; use of a 23-gauge needle (inside diameter, 0.33 mm) produce aortic pressures of approximately 160/100 mm Hg (5). The oxygenator left atrial reservoir is adapted from apparatus that was described by Hems et al. (18) for liver perfusion and also used by Taeghtmeyer et al. (19) for heart perfusion. Perfusate enters the top of the oxygenator and spreads as a film over the entire inner surface of a series of glass bulbs. Cleaning of the oxygenator in a mixture of concentrated sulfuric acid and ammonium persulfate is required between each use to ensure spreading of an even film of buffer on the walls of the oxygenator. The lower end of the oxygenator terminates in a tapered (14/35) glass joint that is fitted with a Teflon stopper that contains a piece of stainless steel tubing (O.D., 0.132 in.). A short piece of Tygon tubing (I.D., one-fourth in.) connects this tubing to the atrial inflow cannula. A sidearm on the lower end of the oxygenator serves as an overflow that returns excess buffer to the reservoir. The height of the overflow above the level of the left atrium determines left atrial filling pressure (usually 14 mm Hg). A gas mixture (95 percent to 5 percent CO_2) that is saturated with water vapor enters the oxygenator via an upper sidearm and is carried into the buffer reservoir through the overflow sidearm. The cannula assembly with the heart attached to the aortic and atrial cannulae fits into the heart chamber, which is seated in the top of the buffer reservoir. In addition, the heart chamber has a Y-shaped sidearm that receives excess buffer from the oxygenator and outflow from the compliance chamber. The buffer reservoir is in Allihn condenser (20 cm in length, 29/42 standard taper joints) with a coarse sintered glass filter inserted in the lower end (3). The perfusate is recirculated with a peristaltic pump

(Cole-Parmer, Model 7545; pump head, No. 7016) whose output is maintained at 120 mL/min. Temperature of water circulating through the jacketed portions of the apparatus are maintained at 37°C. The minimum circulating volume is 40 mL in contrast to 65 mL in the earlier apparatus (3, 4); albumin-containing buffer can be oxygenated without formation of foam. In fact, a low concentration of albumin (0.2 percent) is required for even spreading of the perfusate on the walls of the oxygenator and optimal oxygenation. Modifications of the working heart method to allow for perfusion of rat hearts in a NMR spectrometer (5), to allow fetal and neonatal pig hearts to be perfused *in vitro* (20), and to allow for studies of myocardial ischemia (21) also have been described.

Heart work is begun by clamping the tube from the reservoir used for preliminary perfusion and unclamping the tubes supplying perfusate to the left atrial cannula and leading from the compliance chamber. Buffer entering the atrium passes into the ventricle, and ventricular contraction forces the fluid into the compliance chamber attached to the aortic cannula. This chamber is one-third filled with air (approximately 2 mL) to provide compliance to an otherwise rigid system. The volume of air is important in determining the size and shape of the aortic pressure curve and is adjusted to achieve systolic and diastolic pressures in the physiological range. When the ventricle contracts, pressure development in this chamber forces fluid out through a Tygon tube with a hypodermic needle in the distal end to offer resistance. Aortic output is measured by collecting flow from the needle. Coronary flow is measured by moving the heart chamber and buffer reservoir from below the heart and collecting the fluid dripping from the heart. If production of $^{14}CO_2$ from radioactivity substrates is to be measured, the apparatus can be made gas-tight as described earlier (22).

5. MECHANICAL PERFORMANCE AND ENERGY LEVELS OF WORKING HEARTS

Mechanical performance and content of high-energy phosphates are stable over 2 hr of perfusion of working rat hearts with a 20-gauge needle in the aortic outflow tract (Fig. 2). Stability is apparent in hearts supplied glucose, glucose-lactate-insulin, or glucose-palmitate-β-hydroxybutyrate. Systolic pressures are maintained at approximately 145 mm Hg for the first 90 min and are still at 90 percent of this value after 120 min of perfusion. Diastolic pressures average approximately 77 mm Hg and are well maintained throughout the 2-hr period. Hearts have an aortic output that averages 40–50 mL/min. Coronary flow averages 25–30 mL/min. The content of ATP is well maintained in hearts supplied any of the substrate mixtures. Creatine phosphate declines in hearts supplied only glucose as substrate but is stable in hearts supplied more physiological substrate mixtures. The ATP and creatine phosphate contents in these experiments are lower than observed in the later studies of Kira et al. (11) because the lyophilization of frozen hearts (5) resulted in some loss of

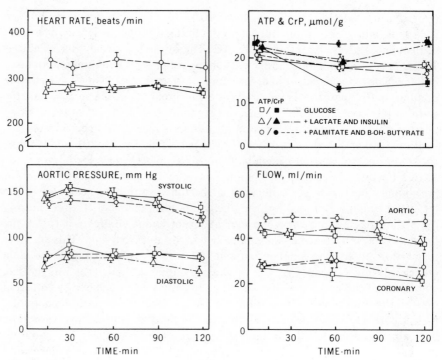

FIGURE 2. Stability of performance and energy levels in hearts with a 20-gauge needle in the aortic outflow tract. Substrate mixtures are denoted as follows: (*a*) glucose, 15 m*M*; bovine serum albumin, 0.2 percent; (*b*) lactate, 2 m*M*; glucose, 10 m*M*; insulin 400 μU/mL; bovine serum albumin, 4 percent; and (*c*) palmitate, 1.5 m*M*; DL-β-hydroxybutyrate, 10 m*M*; glucose, 8 m*M*; and bovine serum albumin, 4 percent. Creatine phosphate values are indicated by closed symbols. Contents of ATP and creatine phosphate are expressed per gram dry weight. Values are means ± SE of four to six hearts. Reproduced from Morgan et al. (5) with permission of the *American Journal of Physiology*.

high-energy phosphate content. When a 23-gauge needle supplies the outflow resistance (Fig. 3), mechanical performance is not as stable as with a 20-gauge needle. Systolic pressures average approximately 160 mm Hg for the first 60 min. During this period these hearts maintain a pressure about 10 percent higher than those having a 20-gauge needle as outflow resistance; by the end of 2 hr of perfusion, the systolic pressures are similar despite a different resistance in the aortic outflow tract (Figs. 2 and 3). Diastolic pressures are approximately 100 mm Hg when a 23-gauge needle is used. Higher resistance in the aortic outflow tract results in redistribution of cardiac output from aortic to coronary flow. Aortic flow averages approximately 10 mL/min and is stable during the 2-hr period; coronary flow falls from about 35 mL/min to about 25 mL/min over the 2-hr period. Content of ATP and creatine phosphate is well maintained with the exception of the content of creatine phosphate in hearts supplied glucose as substrate.

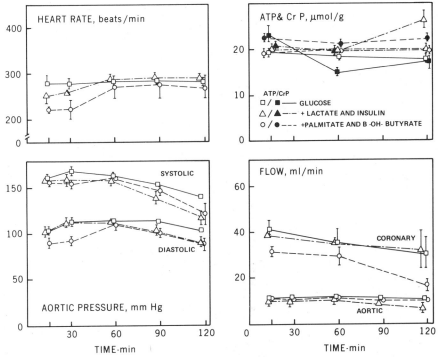

FIGURE 3. Stability of performance and energy levels in hearts with a 23-gauge needle in aortic outflow tract. Substrate mixtures are denoted as in Figure 2. Values are means ± SE of four to six hearts. Reproduced from Morgan et al. (5) with permission of the *American Journal of Physiology*.

Oxygen tension of buffer leaving the oxygenator is 623 ± 10 and 603 ± 21 mm Hg when 20- and 23-gauge needles are located in the aortic outflow tract, respectively. Oxygen tension of the coronary effluent that is obtained from the pulmonary artery averages 210 ± 9 and 284 ± 14 mm Hg in the presence of 20- and 23-gauge needles, respectively. These findings indicate that the working heart is well oxygenated.

The working rat heart is a preparation in which performance and energy levels generally are stable for periods of 1–2 hr. When a 20-gauge needle supplies the outflow resistance, systolic and diastolic pressures, heart rate, and total cardiac output are approximately the same as found in the intact rat.

6. PERFUSION OF HEARTS BY THE LANGENDORFF TECHNIQUE

The apparatus originally described in 1965 (3) is still used for many experiments. Recently, a new apparatus has been constructed that is based on the oxygenator used for the working heart (Fig. 4). This apparatus has a minimal circulating volume of approximately 8 mL, makes use of the more efficient oxygenator,

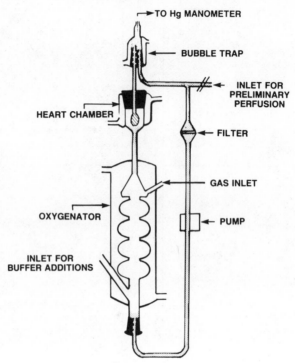

FIGURE 4. Apparatus for perfusion of Langendorff preparations with a small volume of perfusate. The oxygenator and pump is as described for the working heart. The coarse glass filter is 10 mm in diameter. The bubble trap and heart chamber are jacketed glass joints, 10/30 size for the bubble trap and 24/40 for the heart chamber. The tubing, other than that in the pump head (No. 7014) is made of Teflon (0.042 in. inside diameter).

and is adapted for addition and removal of radioactive substrates. The small circulating volume allows for economical use of high concentrations of radioactive substrates. The tissue content of ATP and creatine phosphate and heart rate are stable in these hearts for 6 hr when supplied 20 mM glucose, 400 μU insulin/mL, and 50 μg gentamicin/mL.

To use the apparatus, a measured volume of perfusion medium is placed in an oxygenator and is pumped from the oxygenator through the aortic cannula. After all air bubbles are removed from the tube connecting the bubble trap and aortic cannula, the pump is turned off. The rubber stopper containing the aortic cannula is then secured with a castaloy clamp alongside the heart chamber. The clamp on the tube leading from the reservoir for preliminary perfusion is removed and any air bubbles are dispelled. A fluid level is maintained in the bubble trap as indicated (Fig. 4). The heart is secured to the aortic cannula, as described above. At the end of the preliminary perfusion, the inlet from the preliminary perfusion reservoir is clamped, the heart is secured in its chamber, and the pump is started. The buffer used for preliminary perfusion has the same composition as that used in the subsequent period of recirculation. Pump speed is adjusted to maintain the desired aortic pressure as monitored by the mercury manometer. The stopper in the heart chamber must fit tightly to prevent formation of bubbles and foam in the tube leading to the oxygenator. An accurate estimate of the circulating volume can be obtained by isotope dilution using an extracellular marker such as [^{3}H]sorbitol.

7. CHOICES BETWEEN THE LANGENDORFF PREPARATION AND WORKING HEART FOR METABOLIC STUDIES

The advantages and disadvantages of these preparations are listed at the beginning of this chapter. The best preparation for a given experiment will depend upon the experimental objective. For example, oxygen consumption increases as a function of peak systolic pressure or pressure–time integral in both Langendorff preparations and working hearts, even though the working heart pumps fluid and does external work (Fig. 5). In fact, intraventricular pressure development is not needed to obtain the effects of increased aortic pressure on oxygen consumption or substrate utilization (Fig. 6). The rate of oxygen consumption is increased 70 percent by raising aortic pressure from 60 to 120 mm Hg and the rate is unaffected by draining the ventricle. When glucose uptake is measured at 60 mm Hg aortic pressure, rates are unaffected by insertion of a ventricular drain. An increase in aortic pressure to 120 mm Hg raises rates of glucose uptake by 50 percent in both control and drained hearts. Similarly, $^{14}CO_2$ production from 1-[^{14}C]pyruvate is increased by raising aortic pressure from

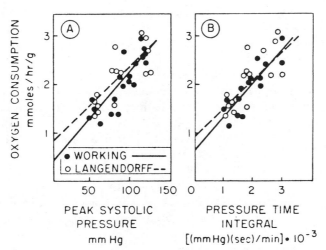

FIGURE 5. Correlation of oxygen consumption with peak systolic pressure and pressure–time integral of working and Langendorff preparations. The points represent individual hearts. Reproduced from Neely et al. (4) with permission of the *American Journal of Physiology*.

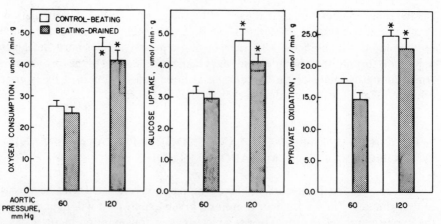

FIGURE 6. The effect of aortic pressure and drainage of the left ventricle on oxygen consumption, glucose uptake, and pyruvate oxidation in Langendorff preparations. Oxygen consumption is calculated from arteriovenous differences in oxygen tension (4). When glucose uptake is measured, production of ^3H_2O is determined using 2-[^3H]glucose after a 10-min exposure to allow ^3H_2O production to reach a steady state (23). After measurements at 60 mm Hg are completed, aortic pressure is raised to 120 mm Hg and the procedure repeated. Pyruvate oxidation is determined in a similar manner except that 1-[^{14}C]pyruvate is employed; 5 min are allowed for a steady state to be established; and coronary effluent is collected from the pulmonary artery without exposure to air for estimation of $^{14}CO_2$ (23). Intraventricular pressure development is prevented by cannulation of the left ventricular apex with a Teflon tube (18 gauge, 5 mm long). Values represent the mean ± S.E. of five to seven hearts.

60 to 120 mm Hg and is not reduced by insertion of a ventricular drain. These experiments indicate that an increase in ventricular pressure development is not required for the increase in oxygen consumption and substrate utilization in response to an elevation of aortic pressure. In regard to effects of aortic pressure on protein synthesis (14), the effect is obtained even though all beating is arrested with tetrodotoxin (Fig. 7). Protein synthesis is measured in Langendorff preparations supplied glucose during the second hour of perfusion at an aortic pressure of either 60 (open bars) or 120 mm Hg (shaded bars). When hearts are perfused at 60 mm Hg, there is no difference in the rates of protein synthesis under these conditions. When aortic pressure is raised to 120 mm Hg, the rate of protein synthesis is increased to the same extent in control-beating, drained-beating, and arrested-drained hearts. Oxygen consumption is increased by raising aortic pressure in the first two groups but not in the arrested-drained preparation. These results indicate that the mechanical effects on cardiac metabolism are observed in Langendorff preparations as well as in working hearts. Hormonal effects also are readily seen in the Langendorff preparation. What then are the indications for using the more technically demanding working preparation? These indications include a) a desire (often more emotionally than scientifically based) to most closely simulate the *in vivo* situation (5), b) the need to evaluate the mechanical function of the heart

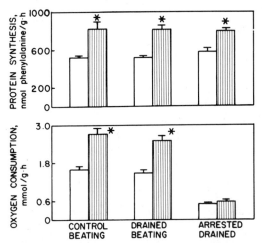

FIGURE 7. Effect of ventricular drainage and cardiac arrest on protein synthesis and oxygen consumption. Hearts are perfused initially for 10 min with an aortic pressure of 40 mm Hg with buffer that contains 15 mM glucose, 0.4 mM phenylalanine, and plasma levels of 19 other amino acids. This buffer is discarded after a single pass through the heart. Perfusion is continued by recirculating 30 mL of the same buffer containing glucose and 0.2 percent bovine serum albumin. [U-^{14}C]Phenylalanine is added after 70 min of perfusion to measure protein synthesis during the second hour. A ventricular drain is inserted as described in Figure 6. Hearts are arrested with tetrodotoxin (10–130 min; 9 μg/mL). Hearts perfused with an aortic pressure of 60 mm Hg during 10–130 min are indicated by open bars and those perfused at 120 mm Hg by shaded bars. Values represent the mean ± S.E. of 6–8 hearts. Data are from Kira et al. (11).

as affected by hormones or diabetes (8, 9), or c) the need to induce the highest possible rates of oxygen consumption (19, 23). In other experimental situations the Langendorff preparation, either control-beating, beating-drained, or arrested-drained preparations, is a suitable and in many instances a preferred experimental model.

REFERENCES

1. O. Langendorff, *Arch. Gesamte Physiol.* **61**, 291 (1895).

2. H. E. Morgan, M. J. Henderson, D. M. Regen, and C. R. Park, *J. Biol. Chem.* **236**, 253 (1961).

3. H. E. Morgan, J. R. Neely, R. E. Wood, C. Liebecq, H. Liebermeister, and C. R. Park, *Fed. Proc.* **24**, 1040 (1965).

4. J. R. Neely, H. Liebermeister, E. J. Battersby, and H. E. Morgan, *Am. J. Physiol.* **212**, 804 (1967).

5. H. E. Morgan, B. H. L. Chua, E. O. Fuller, and D. Siehl, *Am. J. Physiol.* **238**, E431 (1980).

6. E. T. Fossel, H. E. Morgan, and J. S. Ingwall, *Proc. Natl. Acad. Sci. USA* **77**, 3654 (1980).

7. J. Wikman-Coffelt and R. J. Coffelt, *IEEE Transactions on Biomedical Engineering* **29**, 448 (1982).

8. M. M. Bersohn and J. Scheuer, *Circ. Res.* **40**, 510 (1977).

9. T. F. Schaible, A. Malhotra, W. A. Bauman, and J. Scheuer, *J. Mol. Cell. Cardiol.* **15**, 445 (1983).

10. G. Arnold, F. Kosche, E. Miessner, A. Neitzert, and W. Lochner, *Pflügers Archiv.* **299**, 399 (1968).

11. Y. Kira, P. J. Kochel, E. E. Gordon, and H. E. Morgan, *Am. J. Physiol.*, in press.

12. H. E. Morgan, J. R. Neely, and Y. Kira, *Basic Res. Cardiol.*, in press.

13. T. Takala, *Basic Res. Cardiol.* **76**, 44 (1981).

14. H. A. Krebs and K. Henseleit, *Hoppe-Seyler's Z. Physiol. Chem.* **210**, 33 (1932).

15. J. M. Fisher and M. Rabinovitz, *Biochem. Biophys. Res. Commun.* **108**, 851 (1982).

16. A. Mohindru, J. M. Fisher, and M. Rabinovitz, *Nature* **303**, 64 (1983).

17. B. H. L. Chua, K. E. Giger, B. J. Paine, J. D. Robishaw, and H. E. Morgan, *Am. J. Physiol.*, unpublished.

18. R. Hems, B. D. Ross, M. N. Berry, and H. A. Krebs, *Biochem. J.* **101**, 284 (1966).

19. H. Taeghtmeyer, R. Hems, and H. A. Krebs, *Biochem. J.* **186**, 701 (1980).

20. J. C. Werner, V. Whitman, R. R. Fripp, H. G. Schuler, and H. E. Morgan, *Am. J. Physiol.* **241**, E364 (1981).

21. J. R. Neely, M. J. Rovetto, J. T. Whitmer, and H. E. Morgan, *Am. J. Physiol.* **225**, 651 (1973).

22. K. Ichihara, J. R. Neely, D. L. Siehl, and H. E. Morgan, *Am. J. Physiol.* **239**, E430, 1980.

23. K. Kobayashi and J. R. Neely, *Circ. Res.* **44**, 166 (1979).

B

AUTOMATED METHODS OF MASS ISLET ISOLATION

DAVID W. SCHARP, JULIE LONG, MARY FELDMEIER, BARBARA OLACK, SUSAN O'SHAUGHNESSY, AND CAROL SWANSON

Washington University School of Medicine, Department of Surgery, St. Louis, Missouri

1. INTRODUCTION

When Moskalewski (1) first developed the technique of islet isolation in 1965 using collagenase digestion of the pancreas, he opened the door to investigations which began to identify islet function, culture, and transplantation. Compared with previous techniques, his fine chopping of the pancreas, gentle digestion at 37°C for 30 min, and islet purification by sedimentation gave relatively large numbers of isolated islets compared with previous investigators. Up to this time all other techniques have essentially been modifications of his collagenase digestion. Lacy (2) in 1967 improved the yield of islets by cannulation of the pancreatic duct and an injection of balanced salt solution, which mechanically distended and disrupted the gland prior to the digestion. This technique was quite adequate for *in vitro* studies of islet function since one did not need excessively large amounts of islet tissue for study. The majority of islets isolated for many of the methodologies described in this book utilize this basic isolation technique. Attempts at improving the isolation procedure were directed next at the purification process. Lindall (3) was the first to use Ficoll to successfully isolate intact islets, but did not study its effect on insulin release. Our laboratory was unable to retrieve viable islets from Ficoll consistently until we dialyzed and lyophilyzed it, removing various impurities from the commercial material. (4) The use of Ficoll gradients has become the standard technique for islet purification for most transplantation studies and many other types of studies needing large numbers of viable islets.

When Ballinger and Lacy (5) in 1972 first demonstrated the feasibility of islet transplantation using an inbred strain of Lewis rats which had been made diabetic by streptozotocin, it became obvious that a rapid method of islet isolation and purification was required. In addition, attempts to apply this technique to other types of pancreas, including human, met with only partial success. Finding ourselves at this impasse, we began examining various components of the collagenase techniques. Through these studies we developed the digestion–filtration technique which permits complete digestion of pancreatic pieces while separating the islets from the enzymes when they are released (6, 7). This technique has also been confirmed by other investigators to increase significantly the yield of islets (8, 9). This method will be presented in detail in Section 2.

We also began examining different methods of distending the pancreas and have determined that venous distension gives a greater yield of islets than ductal distension, at least in the dog (10–12). We still were not able to achieve successful single-donor to single-recipient islet transplantation in dogs. Then Horaguchi and Merrell (13) described a method of perfusing the canine pancreas with collagenase prior to attempting islet isolation by mechanical passage through a 400-μm screen and additional collagenase digestion. We began to develop a more automated method that utilized an autoisolator for a more efficient method of isolation (14, 15). This method is far from being standardized, however, we will describe the general concepts and approach under Section 3.

2. RAT DIGESTION–FILTRATION TECHNIQUE

This technique is described for isolating islets under sterile conditions from three rat pancreata, which are all placed in one screen. Additional animals can be done by adding additional sets of screens, keeping the three pancreata per screen ratio. A single technique can handle two sets of rats with the surgery but will need the assistance of another technician during the isolation procedure.

2.1. Materials

2.1.1. SOLUTIONS AND REAGENTS

Hanks' with HEPES (1 L)	
$NaHPO_4$	0.0478 g
$NaHPO_4$	0.0478 g
NaCl	8.0 g
KCl	0.4 g
$CaCl_2$	0.14 g
$MgSO_4-7H_2O$	0.2 g
KH_2PO_4	0.06 g
HEPES	5.958 g
Dextrose	1.0 g

Using double-distilled, deionized water, each reagent must be completely dissolved before adding the next in order to avoid precipitation. Adjust the pH to 7.4 with HCl or NaOH. Filter sterile with 0.22-μm disposable filter units (Nalgene, S).

Ficoll. Dialyzed or lyophilized Ficoll is essential. Either purchase reagent grade and dialyze against 44 L of distilled water in 24 hr or purchase from Sigma (Model F-9378, type 400DL). Dissolve 25 g Ficoll in 75 mL of HEPES (without dextrose), pH 7.4. Test pH with strips and adjust with HCl or NaOH. Steam autoclave to sterilize. Carmellization can occur if sterilization is too vigorous, noted by golden color. Use this stock to make 23, 20, and 11 percent Ficoll layers. If producing separate concentrations prior to sterilization, different rates of evaporation from each stock will alter the gradients.

Collagenase. The type of collagenase needed is that made especially for islets. These include Sigma (type V), Worthingon (type IV), or Boehringer Manheim. Unfortunately each lot is different and must be tried for ability to give maximal yields of viable islets. Different concentrations of each prospective lot should also be tried to find its optimum. Many lots are not adequate for isolating viable islets. There are also strain, age, and size differences in the donor strains of rats utilized which affect the yield of islets. It should be stored in a freezer under dessication.

Tissue Culture Media. We utilize RPMI 1640 (Gibco) modified with 10 percent calf serum, 100 mg/dL glucose, 25 mM HEPES, 2 mM L-glutamine, 100 μg/ mL penicillin, and 100 mg/mL streptomycin.

2.1.2. SUPPLIES

Operating Setup. Sterile packs: Prepare three 4 × 4 gauzes with holes precut for the rat abdomen as laparotomy drapes; twenty additional sponges; three 23-gauge needles; two 19-gauge needles; one set of Petri plates (10 cm diameter); one evaporation dish (Corning 3180); one 250-mL Gibco bottle with lid; three Pasteur pipette bulbs; one tissue pipette (transfer pipette sawed off at bottom of neck); one 50-mL round bottom centrifuge tube with lid; two 12-mL conical centrifuge tubes; one 25-mL Erlenmeyer flask with stopper and 19-gauge needle; three 8-in. 4.0 Ethicon silk sutures; one 60-mesh rat digestion–filtration screen (16); One digestion–filtration chamber (50-mL syringe barrel cut off to accommodate the length of the digestion–filtration screen you've chosen to use); one #5 1/2 black rubber stopper (hollowed partially on the smaller end to hold the digestion–filtration screen, must have precise fit to retain preparation); one each of straight scissors, small curved scissors, small curved forceps, toothed forceps, straight forceps; two chopping scissors (medium sized curved); three small curved clamps; two 500-mL beakers. All of these items are placed into a sterilizing tray wrapped and sterilized.

Operating Area. Two nurses caps; two surgical masks; two pairs sterile gloves; one package wrapped sterile cannulae (six PE-50, bevelled on one end, 10 in.); one 1-cc syringe for Hanks'; two 4-way stop cocks; one Bardic intravenous extension tubing; one Bardic 3-way stopcock with tubing for Hanks'; two 50-cc syringes; seven 20-cc syringes (1 for Ficoll); five 10-cc syringes (3 for Ficoll); two 3-cc syringes; two additional 1-cc syringes; Betadine solution for skin preparation; one corning 1-ml pipette and bulbs; several siliconized and sterile Pasteur pipettes, 9 in.

2.1.3. EQUIPMENT

A thermostat-controlled, 37°C water bath large enough to permit adequate shaking using the Burrell wrist action shaker with clamps for digestion–filtration chamber mounted at 90° from rotating shaft. Refrigerated centrifuge. Dissecting microscope. Phillips–Drucker table-top centrifuge (Model L-708).

2.2. Operating Procedure

At the start of the day one should check the water bath temperature, at 37°C, and remove the collagenase from the freezer to warm up for weighing. Remove sterile 25 percent Ficoll and load into syringes with 19-gauge needle using 7 mL of 25 percent and 5 mL each of 23 percent, 20 percent and 11 percent. One liter of sterile Hanks' with 100 mg/dL glucose should be brought to pH 7.4 with sterile NaHCO$_3$ or HCl. Fill three 20-cc syringes with Hanks' and attach 23-gauge needles. Then attach cannulae and prime with Hanks'. Pour small amount of Hanks' into evaporation bowl and cover with Petri plate. Obtain rats for the day and inject with pentobarbital sodium (Abbott, 50 mg/mL) at 4 mg/100 g body weight intraperitoneally. Shave abdomen and place in groups of three on backs in operating area. Prepare abdomen with betadine. Drape with precut sponges and other sponges for sterile area. Make midline incision from xyphoid to bladder through skin. Locate linea alba and incise into peritoneal cavity. Lift up xyphoid with forceps and clip off at the base. Unfold gauze sponge and place over rib area. Push down and out exposing liver. Pull liver up and out over chest cavity holding in place with gauze. Pick up duodenal loop, identify junction of bile duct, and place curved clamp across loop. Locate bile duct and choose site for cannulation using small curved forceps. Place suture loosely around duct. Prepare cannula for insertion. Pick up with small curved forceps and make small transverse incision into the top of the duct with small curved scissors. Guide cannula into duct about 5 mm and distal toward pancreas. Secure with suture. Prepare all rats with cannulae before distending any. When all are ready, begin pancreatic distension. Slowly start distension with Hanks', being certain pancreas is distending. If duodenum begins to distend, reposition clamp on cannula. Too much pressure can rupture duct or pancreas prematurely. When all are distended, remove pancreas quickly. Neutral red added to distension Hanks' fluid helps to identify the pancreas, which stains red from surrounding fat. Pick up the spleen; remove it and surrounding fat. Tease pancreas from stomach, duodenum, and small intestine. Pick up pancreas and remove remaining fat and lymph nodes. Place in evaporator bowl with Hanks'.

2.3. Isolation Procedure

2.3.1. SET UP DIGESTION FILTRATION

Chopping the pancreas in the evaporation dish using the two curved scissors initiates the isolation procedure. Hold both curved scissors in one hand with the curves matching the side of the bowl. Stop at least three times and wash with Hanks'. Fatty tissue will float and should be decanted. After chopping is completed, pour into syringe barrel and record pancreatic volume, which determines the amount of collagenase needed. Use tissue pipette to recover all the pancreas. Usually the volume of three rat pancreata will fall between 4 and 6 mL, which will be used as shown in Table 1 to determine the digestion.

Load the chopped pancreas into the screen. Place the cork onto the top of the screen securely. Place the screen and cork into the barrel of the syringe and push it all the way to the bottom, centering it. Push a 19 gauge needle through the cork and into the center of the screen. Attach a stopcock at each end. Turn the stopcocks so fluid can only run through the chamber. Secure the chamber by running 1/2 in. adhesive tape around it longitudinally, including the stopcocks as well. Attach the Bardic extension tubing. While one person is loading the chamber, the other should be weighing the needed collagenase for the entire procedure. The amount needed depends upon the lot (10 mg/mL or greater) and the volume of pancreas to be digested (Table 1).

2.3.2. DIGESTION PROCESS

The process runs in interrupted steps. The digestion–filtration chamber is loaded with collagenase and placed in the shaker clamp in the 37°C water bath. It runs for 2 min. The chamber is removed and flushed with Hanks'. New collagenase is loaded and the digestion repeated for another 2 min. After this the digestions are each only 1 min in length. At the completion all the pancreatic tissue should be digested leaving only fibrous debris in the chambers.

1. *First Digestion Step (0–2 min).*   Looking at Table 1, assume one has 5.0 mL of chopped pancreas. Using a 3-mL syringe, draw up 2.5 mL of the collagenase solution. The collagenase concentration (e.g., 10, 20, or 30 mg/mL) has been determined by previous trials. One does not add any additional Hanks' on the first digestion step. Attach the syringe to the cork side of the chamber (detach the Bardic tubing). Open stopcocks to the chamber, inject the collagenase, close the stopcocks completely, and reattach the Bardic tubing to the cork end. The other end of the tubing should already be attached to the luer-lock end of the syringe barrel. Place chamber into clamps and tighten. Run shaker on setting 10 for 2 min with the chamber immersed in the water. During this 2-min period, draw up the next volumes needed for the chamber, referring to Table 1. Thus, with 5.0 mL of chopped pancreas one draws up 2.5 mL of collagenase, 5.0 mL of Hanks', and 35 mL of Hanks' in separate syringes. When the timer goes off, remove chamber from water bath and blot. Remove Bardic tube from cork end of chamber and hold the end over the waste beaker. Attach in the 50-mL syringe with 35 mL of Hanks'. Inject the Hanks' while gently shaking the chamber and discharge contents of chamber into waste beaker. Remove syringe, pull in 50 mL of air, reconnect and inject the air into the chamber holding luer end down. This clears out the digestate. Since we have never found significant islets in the first digestate, we discard it.

TABLE 1. Use of Digestion–Filtration Screens

| Digestion Time | Volume of Chopped Pancreas per Screen[a] | | | | | | | | | | | | | | |
| | 4.0 mL | | | 4.5 mL | | | 5.0 mL | | | 5.5 mL | | | 6.0 mL | | |
	C	H	T	C	H	T	C	H	T	C	H	T	C	H	T
0–2 min	2.00[b]	0	2.00	2.25	0	2.25	2.50	0	2.50	2.75	0	2.75	3.00	0	3.00
2–4 min	2.00	4.00	6.00	2.25	4.50	6.75	2.50	5.00	7.50	2.75	5.50	8.25	3.00	6.00	9.00
5 min	1.00	5.00	6.00	1.12	5.63	6.75	1.25	6.25	7.50	1.38	6.87	8.25	1.50	7.50	9.00
6 min	0.50	5.50	6.00	0.56	6.19	6.75	0.62	6.88	7.50	0.69	7.56	8.25	0.75	8.25	9.00
7 min	0.25	5.75	6.00	0.28	6.47	6.75	0.31	7.19	7.50	0.35	7.90	8.25	0.38	8.62	9.00
8 min	0.12	5.88	6.00	0.14	6.61	6.75	0.16	7.34	7.50	0.17	8.08	8.25	0.19	8.81	9.00

[a] C = Volume of collagenase; H = volume of Hanks'; T = total added volume.
[b] One leaves each of these volumes the same and changes the collagenase concentration, e.g., 10 mg/mL, 20 mg/mL, 30 mg/mL, depending upon the activity of any given lot.

231

2. *Second Digestion (2–4 min).* Inject into the chamber 2.5 mL of collagenase and close the stopcock. Attach the 10-mL syringe, open stopcock, and inject 5.0 mL of Hanks'. Close stopcock, remove syringe, and reattach the Bardic tubing. Place chamber back into shaker and start second 2-min digestion period. Again pull up all solutions for the third digestion period. In the example from Table 1 of 5.0 mL this would be 1.25 mL of collagenase, 6.25 mL of Hanks', and 35 mL Hanks' for flushing the chamber. At the end of the 2 min, remove chamber and hold the end of the Bardic tube over the 50 mL round-bottomed tube for the preparation, rinse with 35 mL of Hanks' and flush with air. Reload chamber with collagenase and Hanks' and place into the shaker for the next digestion period. While it is running, the preparation must be saved. Cap the 50 mL tube and spin in the centrifuge for 20 sec at 2000 rpm. (This is a table-top Drucker, which rapidly reaches rpm—adjust accordingly). Carefully decant supernatant and place on ice while waiting for the next preparation.

3. *Third Digestion (5 min).* Having loaded the 1.25 mL of collagenase and 6.25 mL of Hanks' into the chamber, it only runs from now on for 1-min digestion times. Pull up the solutions for the fourth digestion. Rinse with Hanks' and air while collecting the islet preparation again in the 50 mL round-bottomed tube. Spin and pour off supernatant.

4. *Fourth Digestion (6 min).* Inject 0.62 mL collagenase (1-mL syringe) and 6.88 mL of Hanks'. Shake for 1 min. Rinse and collect as before. Spin and save islet pellet.

5. *Fifth Digestion (7 min).* Inject 0.31 mL of collagenase and 7.19 mL of Hanks'. Shake for 1 min. Rinse as before and save islet pellet.

6. *Sixth Digestion (8 min).* Inject 0.16 mL of collagenase and 7.34 mL of Hanks'. Shake for 1 min. Rinse and collect pellet.

2.3.3. PURIFICATION PROCESS

Gently try to remove all the excess Hanks' from the last pellet. Now add 7 mL of the 25 percent Ficoll to the pellet and vortex to suspend the tissue evenly. Place tube in rack. Very carefully add the 23 percent Ficoll (5 mL) on top of the 25 percent layer by running the Ficoll gently down the side while rotating the tube. Add the 20 percent and 11 percent layers in an identical way resulting in a discontinuous gradient. Hanks' can be added on top of the 11 percent layer if desired. Balance the tubes and spin at 800g for 10 min. When complete, examination of the tube should reveal islets at the 11–20 percent interface and some at the 20–23 percent interface. Initially one should examine all layers and interfaces to document islet location. The islets from this point should only be handled by siliconized pipettes. Each pipette should be prewetted with solution to prevent sticking. Use the 1-mL Corning pipette to aspirate the islet tissue off the interface. Try to remove as little Ficoll in the process as possible. Place islet preparation into a 12-mL conical centrifuge tube. Then fill to 12 mL with Hanks'. Mix well and centrifuge at 2000 rpm on the Drucker for 20 sec. Aspirate supernatant and fill to 12 mL again with Hanks'. Resuspend pellet and centrifuge at 1500 rpm up to speed and off. Aspirate again, and resuspend the islets in Hanks'. Recentrifuge up and down again at 1500 rpm. Aspirate off supernatant, but this time fill to 12 mL with tissue culture media. Resuspend the pellet in the media and take up and down to 1000 rpm. Add media again and suspend. Now the islets are ready for examination, counting, perifusion studies, or other work. This series of light spins gives a cleaner islet preparation while eliminating the Ficoll. But, if one wants the maximal numbers of islets such as for transplantation, one should spin longer at each spin in order not to lose many of the smaller islets that are washed away with light spinning.

The chamber is disassembled by removing the Bardic tubing and tape and pulling the needle out of the stopper. To remove the screen, place an empty 50 mL syringe full of air to the stopcock. Invert the chamber so that the air pressure gradually blows the cork and the screen out of the syringe barrel. Examination of the screen should be done to be certain your collagenase concentration is sufficient to leave only fibrous debris. The stainless steel screens must be carefully cleaned with a brush in water. Do not use any kind of soap or detergent since it tends to increase protein and tissue sticking. Boil the screens in distilled water for 30 min between each use. New screens must be boiled for 30 min in 0.2 M KOH prior to their first use. Follow this with a 30 min boiling in distilled water.

Verification of the islets should be accomplished. The first method is by appearance. Normal islets are intact, smooth, and full with a whitish to opaque color and often tend to be sticky. Poor islets are transparent, tend to float, and are often quite fragmented. Histologic confirmation of the preparation is mandatory with hemotylin-eosin and aldehyde fuschin staining. The best *in vitro* demonstration of viable islets is their ability to release insulin in a perifusion system (17). The use of the dissecting microscope aids in picking the islets *in vitro*. With practice, one should be able to run the procedure from pancreatectomy to islets within 60 min. Greater than 90 min in preparation usually means a poor islet preparation.

3.   DOG AUTOISOLATOR PROCESS

The previous technique's primary difficulty is that it is a discontinuous process. Besides being perhaps less efficient than a continuous device, it also has numerous opportunities for contamination. While convenient for digesting small amounts of tissue, it is not manageable for handling the large quantity of tissue that is required for dog or human islet transplantation. We are therefore modifying this technique to eliminate these shortcomings and to develop a process suitable for human islet transplantation. This developmental process is far from complete. We will be therefore presenting concepts primarily, rather than actual finished methodology as we present this technique.

Figure 1 presents the general outline for this digestion process. After pancreatectomy, the pancreas is perfused with collagenase (0.2 percent), type I (Sigma), by cannulation of the pancreatic duct. The collagenase is pumped at 5 mL/min and is recycled (14, 15). The end point of digestion is difficult to determine but usually 1 min/g of pancreas gives a suitable predigestion. After this step the partially digested pancreas is removed and loaded into the auto-isolator device. Figure 2 gives the schematic diagram for this process. The collagenase (Sigma, type V) is contained in a reservoir at 37°C and connected through a pump and flow meter to the autoisolator. The released islets from the autoisolator are then collected in calf serum at 4°C. There are further washing steps required to clean up the preparation. Figure 3 presents the

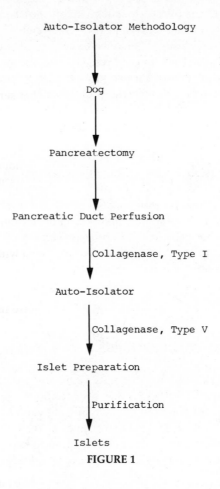

FIGURE 1

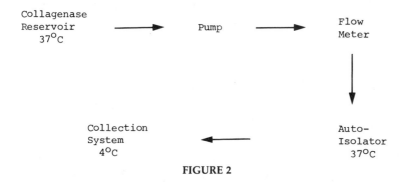

FIGURE 2

schematic representation of the autoisolator itself. The enzyme entering the device goes through a manifold to divide it into separate screen chambers. These chambers have been previously loaded with the chopped, partially digested pancreas. With the flow rate at 40 mL/min the digestion goes on within the screen such as it did with the rat process. But, now the enzyme flow carries any isolated islets out of the digestion screens. The islets are collected within the chamber and flow out of the device where they are cooled to 4°C and buffered with calf serum to retard the digestion process. This process gives a sufficient amount of isolated dog islets to permit successful islet autotransplants (14, 15).

The major problem with this islet preparation is that it is heavily contaminated with exocrine and duct cells. Thus, the purification step in Figure 1 is currently the most limiting problem. Ficoll gradients have not been very helpful in this regard. The autoisolator process has eliminated the major problems of the discontinuous process of digestion–filtration developed for the rat. Still, numerous modifications are underway to permit the ability to place the pancreas in on one side of such a device and obtain purified islets on the other side. This is the type of process required for large-scale islet isolation and the goal of our future efforts.

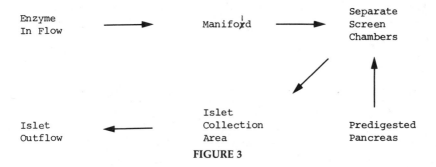

FIGURE 3

REFERENCES

1. S. Moskalewski, *Gen. Comp. Endocrinology* **5**, 342 (1965).

2. P. E. Lacy and M. Kostianovsky, *Diabetes* **16**, 35 (1967).

3. A. Lindall, M. Steffes, and R. Sorenson, *Endocrinology* **85**, 218 (1969).

4. D. W. Scharp, C. Kemp, M. Knight, W. F. Ballinger, and P. E. Lacy, *Transplantation* **16**, 686 (1973).

5. W. F. Ballinger and P. E. Lacy, *Surgery* **72**, 175 (1972).

6. D. W. Scharp, J. J. Murphy, W. T. Newton, W. F. Ballinger, and P. E. Lacy, *Surgery* **77**, 105 (1975).

7. D. W. Scharp, J. J. Murphy, W. T. Newton, W. F. Ballinger, and P. E. Lacy, *Transplantation Proceedings* **7**, 739 (1975).

8. A. Shibata, C. W. Ludvigsen, S. P. Naber, M. L. McDaniel, and P. E. Lacy, *Diabetes* **25**, 667 (1976).

9. A. Orsetti, A. M. Puech, M. Zouari, C. Guy, and F. Passebois, *J. Annu. Diabetology*, **66** (1977).

10. R. Downing, D. W. Scharp, and W. F. Ballinger, *Transplantation* **29**, 79 (1980).

11. D. W. Scharp, R. Downing, R. C. Merrell, and M. Greider, *Diabetes* **29**, 19 (1980).

12. D. W. Scharp, R. Downing, R. Merrell, S. Nunnelley, D. Kiske, and M. Greider, *Islet Isolation, Culture and Cryopreservation*, Thieme-St. Ratton, New York, 1981, p. 152.

13. A. Horoguchi and R. C. Merrell, *Diabetes* **30**, 455 (1981).

14. J. A. Long, L. Britt, B. J. Olack, and D. W. Scharp, *Transplantation Proceedings* **15**, 1332 (1983).

15. D. W. Scharp, J. A. Long, B. J. Olack, and L. Drummer, unpublished.

16. Custom Fabrications, P. O. Box 327, Glen Carbon, IL 62034.

17. P. E. Lacy, M. M. Walker, and C. J. Fink, *Diabetes* **21**, 987 (1972).

C

AUTOMATED METHODS FOR ISOLATING AND PURIFYING ISLET CELLS FROM THE PANCREAS

DAVID W. SCHARP, JULIE LONG, MARY FELDMEIER,
BARBARA OLACK, SUSAN O'SHAUGHNESSY,
AND CAROL SWANSON

*Washington University School of Medicine, Department of Surgery,
St. Louis, Missouri*

1. INTRODUCTION

One of the frustrating problems in attempting to isolate islets from the human pancreas is the inability to control the digestion process sufficiently to stop it at the right time to produce intact islets. Instead, we find the process tends to continue uncontrolled, resulting in few islets and many single cells. Because of our inability to understand the islet isolation process well enough to control it, we have been looking at alternative approaches. We have developed a process that purposely produces single cells from the pancreas and then attempts to purify the islet cells from this cellular preparation. Section 2 will detail the process as it was developed. This is the technique developed in dogs (1–3), used in neonatal pigs (4), and recently in humans (5, 6). The last section of this chapter describes the attempts to apply the autoisolator system described in Vol. 1C, Section IV B) to the problem of single-cell isolation (7, 8).

2. SINGLE-CELL PREPARATION

2.1. Reagents, Supplies, and Equipment

2.1.1. SOLUTIONS

Table 1 presents the solutions utilized for the isolation of the pancreatic single cells. They fit into the digestion process as described below. We also use as tissue culture media RPMI 1640 supplemented with 10 percent calf serum, 100 mg/dL glucose, 2 mM L-glutamine, 100 U/mL penicillin and 100 mg/mL streptomycin.

2.1.2. REAGENTS

Collagenase, type I (Sigma) is used for pancreatic ductal perfusion as a preliminary step to single-cell preparation when utilizing the cells for transplantation studies. Trypsin is the primary digesting enzyme but also varies in its potency by supplier and from lot to lot as has been noted for collagenase. We have used crude trypsin preparation (Gibco) 1:250 and Enzar T trypsin (Reheis, Armour). Each requires testing to find the optimal lot and concentration.

2.1.3. EQUIPMENT

Eberbach shaker water bath (6250), 37°C water bath, refrigerated centrifuge, and gyrotational bath (New Brunswick, G76) are needed in addition to the routine laboratory equipment.

2.1.4. SUPPLIES

10-mL and 25-mL Microfernbach culture flasks (Bellco). 12-mL conical centrifuge tubes with caps.

TABLE 1.

Solution A	
NaCL	136 mM
KCL	2.7 mM
HEPES	25 mM
Glucose	5.5 mM
Penicillin	100 U/mL
Streptomycin	100 μg/mL

Solution B	
Solution A	95 mL/100 mL
Calf Serum	5 mL/100 mL

Solution C	
Solution A	95 mL/100 mL
Calf Serum	5 mL/100 mL
EDTA	20 mg/100 mL
Trypsin	100–150 μg/100 mL

Solution D	
Solution A	90 mL/100 mL
Calf Serum	10 mL/100 mL

50 mL conical centrifuge tubes with caps.

250 mL conical centrifuge tubes with caps.

Siliconized transfer pipettes.

Siliconized Pasteur pipettes.

1, 3, 5, 10, 35, and 50 mL plastic syringes.

14-gauge 3-in. stainless steel reusable spinal needles

40 μm Nytex filter (Tetco).

Evaporation bowl (Pyrex 3180).

Medium-length curved scissors.

50 mL Erlenmeyer flask.

2.2. Single-Cell Suspensions

Mongrel dogs are anesthetized with sodium pentobarbital and a midline laparotomy performed. For initial studies the left lobe of the pancreas can be easily removed and used for isolation studies. A complete pancreatectomy is required for transplantation studies. While technically challenging, it is much easier in the dog than in humans to perform a complete pancreatectomy leaving the duodenum intact. Whichever method is chosen, the pancreas is removed and the pancreatic duct is cannulated with an intravenous catheter (Angio cath, 22 g–18 g) or PE-50 tubing. The catheter is sutured in place with 4.0 silk suture. One hundred milliliters of solution A (Table 1) is injected rapidly into the cannula, resulting in distension of the pancreas. The pancreas is chopped into 1-mm pieces and washed with solution B. Five milliliter aliquots of washed, chopped pancreas are distributed among 50 mL Erlenmeyer flasks. These contain 10 mL of solution C with trypsin. The digestion proceeds in a stepwise fashion. An initial 5-min digestion is done at 37°C in the Eberbach at slow speed. The remainder of the digestion times are each 2 min. Between each digestion period the tissue is triturated, further disrupting it mechanically. This is done by drawing it through the 3-in., 14-gauge needle attached to a 20 mL syringe and forcing the preparation back into the flask several times. This becomes easier with each step as the digestion progresses. The flask is then tipped to one side to permit the heavier pieces to settle. The single cells are aspirated from above the heavier particulate material and placed into solution D. Three milliliters of solution C is added to the digestion flask for the next digestion step. Multiple 2-min digestions are continued until only fibrous material remains in the digestion flask. The final digestate is centrifuged at 600g at 4°C for 10 min. It is then resuspended in solution D and filtered through the Nytex filter (40 μm mesh) to yield the pancreatic single-cell suspension. The cells are kept at 4°C until the digestion is complete to reduce aggregation and maintain viability. A total cell count using tryphan blue exclusion is done for determining the yield and viability.

2.3. Purification

Discontinuous Ficoll gradients are utilized to partially purify the islet cells from the remaining cell types. The gradient is made as described in Vol. 1C, Section IV B. Ficoll (25 percent) is made and sterilized; 23, 20, and 11 percent concentrations are layered on top in a 50 mL round-bottomed centrifuge tube. The final cell preparation is suspended in the 25 percent layer. The gradient is spun at 800g for 15 min. Islet cells scatter over the top three layers, which are combined and washed with solution B to remove the Ficoll. A final cell count and viability are recorded.

2.4. Rotational Tissue Culture

RPMI 1640 supplemented with 150 mg/dL glucose, 2 mM glutamine, 100 U/mL penicillin, 100 mg/mL streptomycin, 10 percent calf serum, and 25 mM HEPES is used for the culture. The Ficoll is washed from the cells by two rinses with solution B. Depending upon the cell yield, one uses either the 10 or 25 mL Microfernbach flasks. From 1 to 5 × 10^6 cells are placed in 4 mL of media in the 10 mL Microfernbach flasks. From 1 to 5 × 10^7 cells are placed in 10 mL of media in the 25 mL Microfernbach flask. Gyrotational culture is used to increase cellular reaggregation. The New Brunswick (G76) is used to provide the 37°C environment and 110 rpm. The conditions of gyrotational culture have been well described by Moscona (9). The important variables are types of tissue, species of origin, cell concentration, temperature, and speed of rotation. Optimal conditions must be developed for each tissue and species of origin. Islet cell aggregation begins in hours, but does not produce solid aggregates for 3–4 days. Therefore, one must centrifuge the preparation for the first media change. We have chosen to do the first media change at 24 hr. We routinely centrifuge the preparation at 600g for 10 min. Thereafter, media changes are performed every 2–3 days by aspiration of the supernatant from above the aggregates. Because the aggregates contain the major islet cell types, we have chosen to call them pseudoislets (1). Media samples are stored for radioimmunoassay of insulin, glucagon, somatostatin, and pancreatic polypeptide. Amylase, glucose, and total protein assays complete the evaluation. The pseudoislets are now ready for further *in vitro* study such as perifusion, morphologic evaluation, or transplantation studies. Moscona also described the phenomenon of "sorting out" as a function of culture duration in which the cells migrate within their aggregates to form their own domains of cell types. We have observed the same type of sorting out within the pseudoislets. This may have an effect on their function, but needs additional study to better document it with the islet cell types.

3.   AUTOMATED METHODS

There is a great deal of analogy between the basic and automated methods of pancreatic single-cell methods and those previously described for intact islet isolation. The process in Section 2 is a discontinuous method of single-cell production. While an effective method of producing pancreatic islet cells, it is not maximally efficient because of the discontinuous process of handling the cells. Our first attempts to automate the system were to use the single screens developed for rat islet isolation and simply pump trypsin through the pancreatic pieces entrapped within the screens (7). This method was effective in eliminating the discontinuous approach and resulted in the first semiautomated method of pancreatic cell preparation.

We have recently evaluated the autoisolator as a technology for single-cell preparation from the pancreas (8). The basic schematic is similar in setup to that described for the intact islet preparation. Modifications for the single-cell preparation are illustrated Figure 1. The trypsin enters the autoisolator after being pumped from the enzyme reservoir. It flows through a manifold which disperses it evenly into five streams for entry into the screen chambers. Chopped, predigested pancreatic pieces have been previously loaded into the screen chamber. We have found that predigestion of the pancreas with collagenase, type I (Sigma), which is pumped through a cannula in the pancreatic duct, increases the yield of single cells. This is a finding similar to that seen with intact islet preparations. The pore size of 140 μm permits release of the single

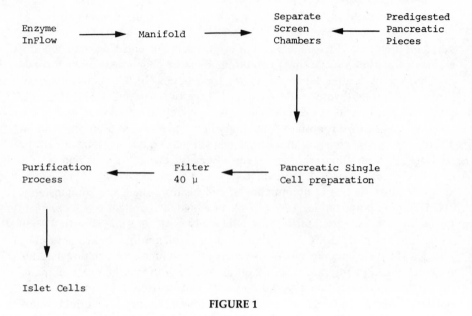

FIGURE 1

cells which can be removed from the chamber by the enzyme flow. Passage over a 40-μm (Nytex) filter entraps any particulate material, usually of ductal or vascular origin, that would cause aggregation of the isolated single cells. The pancreatic single-cell preparation is then ready for a purification step.

Since this process is still under development, we do not now have a finalized purification process to produce islet cells. Our first purification method uses Ficoll gradients as described in Section 2.3, however, this technique is only partially effective in purifying the islet cells. While the α cells seem to favor the lower layers, β cells preferentially migrate to the lighter densities of the Ficoll. Significant contamination with ductal and exocrine cells still exists even with the Ficoll. While selective aggregation from rotational tissue culture techniques are helpful, better methods of purification are being developed.

The Beckman elutriator (a JE-6B rotor used on a J6B centrifuge) shows significant promise for removing the larger exocrine cells (8). The apparatus consists of a special rotor which contains a chamber that permits inflow of media at the bottom and outflow from the top. After loading cells into the rotor, we balance the centrifugal force toward the bottom of the chamber, against the force of the fluid moving in a direction 180° opposite. Loading a population of mixed-cell size at low flow rates, a gradient is set up with the smaller cells on top. By increasing the flow rate, one can flush these cells out, separating them from the larger cells. We balance the flow rate versus the rpm of the rotor using a normogram for a selected cell size. This process is quite effective in removing the larger exocrine cells from the smaller islet, ductal, endothelial, white and red cells at a window setting of 12 μm. While the elutriator by itself is not as efficient, it can be connected in line with the outflow from the autoisolator and filter. This method is effective, but additional modifications and purification techniques are currently under development.

REFERENCES

1. D. W. Scharp, R. Downing, R. C. Merrell, and M. Greider, *Diabetes* **29** (suppl. 1), 19 (1980).
2. R. L. Gingerich, D. W. Scharp, M. H. Greider, E. S. Dye, and K. A. Mousel, *Regulatory Peptides* **5**, 13 (1982).
3. D. W. Scharp, R. C. Merrell, R. L. Gingerich, M. H. Britt, R. Downing, M. M. Feldmeier, and D. Kiske, unpublished.
4. L. D. Britt, P. C. Stojeba, C. R. Scharp, M. H. Greider, and D. W. Scharp, *Diabetes* **20**, 580 (1981).
5. D. W. Scharp, M. M. Feldmeier, R. V. Rajotte, K. DeSchryver, and M. Bell, *Diabetes* **29** (suppl. 2), 18A (1980).
6. D. W. Scharp, R. L., Gingerich, K. DeSchryver, N. White, J. Santiago, M. Bell, R. V. Rajotte, M. M. Feldmeier, D. Kiske, and S. Kristoff, unpublished.
7. D. W. Scharp, R. Downing, R. C. Merrell, S. Nunnelly, D. Kiske, and M. Greider, in *Islet Isolation, Culture, and Cryopreservation*, K. Federlin and R. G. Bretzel (eds.), Thieme-Stratton, New York, 1981.
8. D. W. Scharp, J. A. Long, M. M. Feldmeier, B. J. Olack, S. O'Shaughnessy, and C. Swanson, unpublished.
9. A. A. Moscona, "Recombination of Dissociated Cells and the Development Cell Aggregates," in *Cells and Tissues in Culture*, E. N. Willmer (ed.), Academic Press, New York, 1965, p. 489.

D

ISOLATION OF ISLETS FROM MICE AND RATS

J. BRUNSTEDT, J. H. NIELSEN, Å. LERNMARK, AND THE HAGEDORN STUDY GROUP

Hagedorn Research Laboratory and the Steno Memorial Hospital, Gentofte, Denmark

1.   INTRODUCTION

The endocrine pancreas in most adult mammals only comprises 1–2 percent of the pancreas. It was therefore a major advance for the study of islet physiology and biochemistry when Moskalewski in 1965 introduced the collagenase digestion technique for the isolation of islets of Langerhans (1). Since then numerous investigators have utilized this method with various modifications and improvements as reviewed recently (2). In this chapter we shall describe protocols for collagenase digestion of the pancreas from either rats or mice. Both protocols include gradient centrifugation to separate the islets from the pancreatic digest. The two procedures illustrate how the original technique (1) may be varied to increase the yield of isolated islets and to meet specific experimental purposes. It may, for example, be advisable to subject the isolated islets to a period of culture in order to allow the islet cells to regenerate from possible degradation of membrane components during the collagenase treatment (3). A brief culture period may also be useful to assist in selecting those islets which have suffered the least damage by the isolation procedure. The choice of the culture medium for a postisolation culture of islets has been discussed previously (4).

2.   ISOLATION OF MOUSE ISLETS

Although slight modifications in the collagenase concentration and digestion time may be necessary when different mouse strains are used for islet isolation, the following procedure has been successfully applied to several strains of mice (5–8). The application of a Percoll gradient centrifugation to isolate the islets from the digest has been described in detail (7).

2.1.   Reagents

2.1.1.   HANKS' BALANCED SALT SOLUTION (HBSS)

Hanks' balanced salt solution (available from, e.g., Flow Laboratories, Irvine, Scotland, U.K., or prepared according to Table 1) is supplemented by the

Members of the Hagedorn Study Group are K. Brunstedt, D. Jensen, R. Jørgensen, A. M. Olesen, T. Funder, T. Dyrberg, S. Bækkeskov,

TABLE 1. Preparation of Modified Hanks' Balanced Salt Solution (HBSS) for Isolation of Rat Islets

Hanks' 10× Stock Solution

NaCl	72 g
KCl	4 g
$Na_2HPO_47H_2O$	0.9 g
KH_2PO_4	0.6 g
$MgSO_47H_2O$	1.0 g
$MgCl_26H_2O$	1.0 g
Double-distilled H_2O to a final volume of 1 L	

Hanks' 1× Working Solution

Hanks' 10×	100 mL	150 mL	200 mL
1.4 percent (w/v $CaCl_2$	10 mL	15 mL	20 mL
7 percent (w/v) $NaHCO_3$	2.5 mL	3.75 mL	5 mL
D-glucose	1 g	1.5 g	2.0 g
Double distilled H_2O to final	1.0 L	1.5 L	2.0 L

Adjust pH to 7.4 with NaOH and keep the solutions tightly capped on ice. An islet isolation experiment with 8 rats usually requires 250–500 mL bovine serum albumin (BSA)-free and 1.0–1.5 L BSA-containing Hanks'. BSA, penicillin, streptomycin, or HEPES from stock solutions may also be added as required (see text).

addition of 25 mM N-2-hydroxyethylpiperazine-N'-2-ethane sulfonic acid (HEPES), 100,000 IU/L penicillin, and 100 mg/L streptomycin. Mix 500 mL HBSS with 12.6 mL 1 M HEPES buffer (pH 7.4) and 10 mL of a mixture of 5000 IU/mL penicillin and 5 mg/mL streptomycin (Flow Laboratories). Check pH and adjust if necessary to pH 7.4. Make the modified HBSS fresh and keep at 4°C.

2.1.2. COLLAGENASE SOLUTIONS

Crude collagenase from *CL. Histolyticum* (Type II, Worthington Biochemicals, Freehold, NJ) is dissolved to a final concentration of 1.5 mg/mL. A collagenase solution of half-strength, 0.75 mg/mL, in HBSS will also be used. Other types of collagenase from Worthington or different preparations from other manufacturers may be used after testing of each batch (2). The collagenase solutions are prepared the same day and kept at 4°C.

2.1.3. PERCOLL SOLUTIONS

Three Percoll (Pharmacia, Uppsala, Sweden) solutions are made:

1. *Percoll 90 percent.* Mix 88 mL Percoll with 10 mL of 10 times concentrated Hanks' balanced salt solution (10 × HBSS) (Flow Laboratories or

prepared according to Table 1), 2 mL of 1 M HEPES, pH 7.4, and 0.5 mL of 7.5 percent sodium bicarbonate solution.

2. *Percoll, Density 1.089.* Mix 6 mL 90 percent Percoll with 3 mL modified HBSS solution.

3. *Percoll, Density 1.062.* Mix 4 mL 90 percent Percoll with 5 mL modified HBSS solution. Prepare fresh and keep at 4°C.

2.1.4. CULTURE MEDIUM

RPMI 1640 (Flow Laboratories) is used after being supplemented with 20 mM HEPES, 300 mg/L L-glutamine, 0.35 g/L sodium bicarbonate, 100,000 IU/L penicillin, 100 mg/L streptomycin, and 10 percent newborn calf serum (available from several biochemical companies). Adjust pH to 7.2 and store at 4°C.

2.2. Preparation of Tissue

Mice weighing 20–30 g are fasted overnight and killed by cervical dislocation. The abdominal skin is rinsed with 70 percent ethanol and opened with sterile scissors and forceps without injuring the peritoneum. After changing to a new set of sterile instruments, the peritoneal cavity is cut open without touching the surrounding skin. The pancreas is most simply localized by finding the spleen and carefully lifting it up toward the midline with a pair of forceps. The pancreas is removed by cutting from the splenic lobe, following the attachment to the stomach and the duodenum as far down along the intestine as possible. The tissue is placed in a Petri dish and rinsed in cold modified HBSS. Attached fat and lymphnodes are removed by careful dissection. The dissected pancreas may be inspected in the stereomicroscope to assist in localizing lymph nodes.

2.3. Collagenase Treatment

The dissected pancreas is placed in a sterile 20 mL glass scintillation vial containing 4 mL of 1.5 mg/mL collagenase solution. Four to six glands may be added to each vial. The vials are placed in a solid thermostat at 37°C (Model BT3, Grant, Barrington, U.K.), placed on a shaking table (Model SM, Edmund Bühler, Thübingen, GFR) (Fig. 1). This shaker is run at a speed of 150 rpm. Any metabolic shaker with vigorous shaking speed should prove useful. The vials are incubated with shaking for 13–15 min and the supernatant fluids transferred to 10–15 ml siliconized (Prosil-28, PCR Research Chemicals, Inc., Gainesville, FL) conical polystyrene centrifuge tubes kept on ice. The undigested pancreas is allowed to remain in the vial and 4 mL of the 0.75 mg/mL collagenase solution is added. Each vial is again placed in the thermostat and shaken for another 5 min. Collect the supernatant fluids as above, leaving the remainder of the pancreas in the vial and adding another 4 mL of the 0.75 mg/mL col-

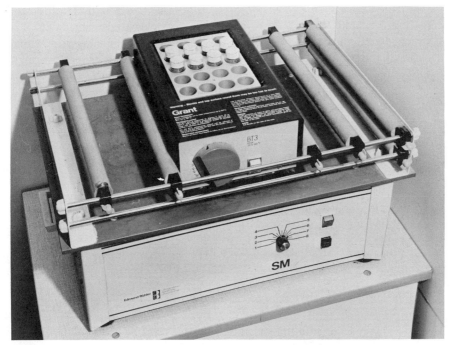

FIGURE 1. Metabolic shaker with solid thermostat used for the collagenase digestion of mouse pancreas.

lagenase solution. Shake once more for 5 min and repeat this collagenase treatment for one or more 5-min periods until the pancreas is completely digested. Often the largest number of islets are liberated from the pancreatic parenchyma after four to six incubations.

2.4. Islet Purification

The supernatants are allowed to sediment ($1g$ on ice) and are washed twice by sedimentation in ice-cold modified HBSS. It is advisable to carry out the washing procedure of the first collagenase digestions while the final 5-min collagenase digestions are being completed. This will minimize the exposure of the islets to collagenase. The last wash is by centrifugation at $200g$ for 1 min in a cooling centrifuge (Beckman model TJ-6, Fullerton, CA). Discard the supernatant fluid. Make sure that all HBSS is carefully removed. A Pasteur pipette connected to a water pump is useful for this purpose.

Resuspend the pellet in 3 mL *Percoll, density 1.089*. Use a vortex mixer with care and make sure that all clumps of tissue are broken up. Place the tube in a rack and layer carefully 3 mL of *Percoll, density 1.062*, on top. All tubes are centrifuged for 10 min at $800g$. The islets are located in the interphase and are removed by aspiration with a siliconized Pasteur pipette and placed in a bacteriological Petri dish (Nunc, Roskilde, Denmark).

The islets are collected under a dissecting microscope with a siliconized constriction pipette. The islets are now ready for the desired experiments. The yield of islets is normally 50–100/mouse pancreas, but as many as 400 may occasionally be obtained. In experiments with islets to be used after an overnight culture, 50–100 islets are placed in 50-mm bacteriological Petri dishes containing 5 mL of culture medium (RPMI 1640 with 10 percent newborn calf serum) for overnight culture. The appearence of isolated mouse islets viewed in a phase-contract microscope after tissue culture is shown in Figure 2.

3. ISOLATION OF RAT ISLETS

This method has been developed for the preparation of large quantities of rat islets (9). The details about the tissue chopper (Fig. 3), which was constructed for processing of human pancreas for transplantation, has been described previously (10).

3.1. Reagents

3.1.1. MODIFIED HANKS' BALANCED SALT SOLUTION (HBSS)

Hanks' balanced salt solution (available from several biochemical companies or prepared according to Table 1) is supplemented with 25 mM HEPES (pH

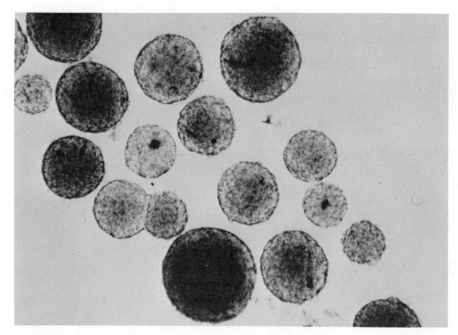

FIGURE 2.   Isolated mouse islets kept in culture overnight. Phase-contract microscopy.

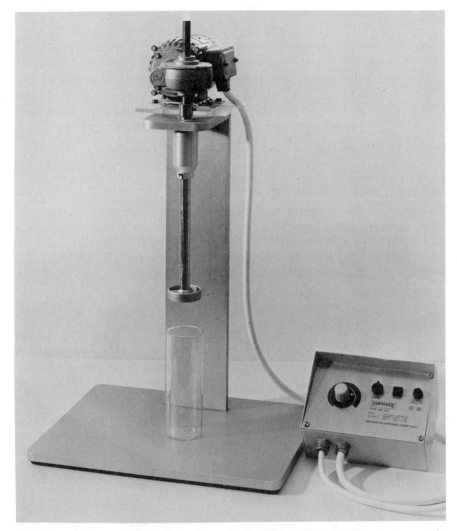

FIGURE 3. Tissue chopper with counterrotating knives used for preparing rat pancreata for collagenase digestion. The chopper is described in detail elsewhere (10).

7.4), 100,000 IU/L penicillin, and 100 mg/L streptomycin (see above). Make fresh and keep at 4°C.

3.1.2. HBSS with 1 percent Bovine Serum Albumin (BSA)

Bovine serum albumin of high quality (e.g., chromatographically purified fraction V from Miles, Elkhart, IN) is dissolved in HBSS. Check pH and adjust, if necessary, to 7.4 with NaOH and filter through a 0.22-μm filter (Millex-GS, Millipore, Bedford, MA). Keep at 4°C.

3.1.3. COLLAGENASE SOLUTIONS

Crude collagenase from *Cl. Histolyticum* [type IV Worthington, Freehold, NJ or other types from this or other manufacturers may be used after testing each batch (2)] is dissolved to a final concentration of 8 mg/mL in modified HBSS previously supplemented with 5 mg/mL D-glucose. Prepare the same day and keep at 4°C.

3.1.4. FICOLL SOLUTIONS

Stock Solution.   A Ficoll stock solution is prepared one day in advance by weighing 22.8 g Ficoll 400 (Pharmacia, Uppsala, Sweden) and then adding modified HBSS to a final weight of 100 g. All Ficoll solutions are conveniently prepared by weighing Table 2). Allow the Ficoll to dissolve slowly by leaving the sealed jar or beaker overnight in a refrigerator. Alternatively, Ficoll and modified HBSS are weighed into a jar with a tight screw cap and allowed to shake at 37°C for 30–60 min in a metabolic shaker.

Ficoll Solution 1.   18.5 g stock solution is weighed and modified HBSS added to a final weight of 20.0 g.

Ficoll Solution 2.   17.4 g stock solution is weighed and modified HBSS added to a final weight of 20.0 g.

Ficoll Solution 3.   9.3 g stock solution is weighed and modified HBSS added to a final weight of 20.0 g.

All Ficoll solutions are kept at room temperature (21–23°C) before use.

TABLE 2.   **Preparation of Ficoll Solutions for Separating Rat Pancreatic Islets from the Pancreatic Collagenase Digest**

Ficoll Solution[a]		1	2	3
Isolation of	x^b	18.5	17.4	9.3
islets from	y^c	20	20	20
8 rats				

[a] Ficoll stock solution: add Hanks' solution without bovine serum albumin (BSA) to 22.8 g Ficoll 400 to a final weight of 100 g.
[b] x is grams of Ficoll stock solution.
[c] y is final weight by adding Hanks' solution without BSA.

3.1.5. Culture Medium

RPMI 1640 is supplemented with 20 mM HEPES, 300 mg/L L-glutamine, 0.35 g/L sodium bicarbonate, 100,000 IU/mL penicillin, 100 mg/L streptomycin, and 10 percent newborn calf serum. Mix all ingredients, purchased or prepared, as sterile stock solutions adjusted to pH 7.2, and stored at 4°C.

3.2. Preparation of Tissue

Eight male rats weighing 100–150 g (e.g., Wistar or Sprague–Dawley) are fasted overnight. Alternatively, rats weighing 150–250 g may be treated with pilocarpine 1 hr before starting the islet isolation procedure (9, 11). The rats are decapitated and the abdominal skin is rinsed with 70 percent ethanol. Each rat is dissected with one set of sterile instruments to separate the skin from the peritoneum. The abdomen is opened with another set of sterile instruments and the pancreas localized. The pancreas is removed by carefully cutting with a pair of scissors either from the splenic part toward the duodenal part or vice versa. The glands are placed in a beaker with ice-cold modified HBSS. Remove fat and lymph nodes with scissors and forceps from one pancreas at a time kept in a Petri dish with fresh modified HBSS. All pancreata are thereafter placed in a 500-mL sterile glass beaker containing 100 mL cold modified HBSS, and minced in a tissue chopper with counterrotating knives (10) (Fig. 3) until pieces of about 1.5 × 1.5 mm are obtained.

3.3. Collagenase Treatment

The tissue suspension is divided into four 50 mL sterile plastic centrifuge tubes (Falcon, Oxnard, CA). The tissue is allowed to sediment and the supernatant fluid is discarded. Modified HBSS is added to each tube in a final volume of 5 mL, and the content of each tube poured into sterile 20 mL scintillation vials. Each centrifuge tube is thereafter rinsed with 5 mL of 8 mg/mL collagenase solution (final concentration 4 mg/mL) and also transferred to the scintillation vials. The vials are incubated horizontally for 15–20 min at 37°C in a metabolic shaker (Fig. 4). The shaking rate is vigorous, about 200–250 rpm. The incubation is terminated either by adding 10 mL modified HBSS with 1 percent BSA to each vial or by pouring the content of each vial into a 50 mL centrifuge tube containing modified HBSS with 1 percent BSA.

If a tissue chopper is not available, rinse pancreata once or twice and place in 20 mL glass scintillation vials and minced with a pair of scissors in a final volume of 6 mL of 4 mg/mL collagenase solution and incubated as mentioned above.

3.4. Islet Purification

Each centrifuge tube is filled with cold modified HBSS containing 1 percent BSA, and the content mixed by shaking for a few seconds before centrifugation

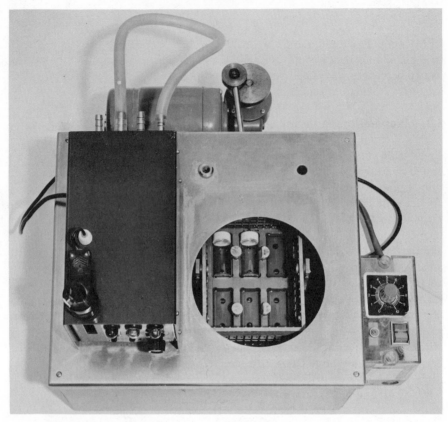

FIGURE 4.   Metabolic shaker used for the collagenase digestion of rat pancreas.

for 1 min at 200g. The supernatant fluid is discarded, and this washing step repeated twice. After the last wash, 10 mL Ficoll stock solution is added to the pellet and mixed vigorously by vortexing. It is imperative that all tissue clumps be broken up and dispersed within the Ficoll solution. A gradient is formed by careful addition of 4 mL of Ficoll solution 1, 4 mL of Ficoll solution 2, and finally 4 mL of Ficoll solution 3. Disposable plastic or glass 5 mL volumetric pipettes are useful to layer the gradients, which is most easily accomplished by having the test tube stabilized in a rack and very gently adding each Ficoll solution with the pipette kept at the tube wall just above the Ficoll solution already present in the test tube.

The gradients are centrifuged for 10 min at 800g in a centrifuge (such as Beckman model TJ-6, Fullerton, CA) run without cooling and brake. The islets are recovered at the interphase between layers two and three. Some islets may be found between layers one and two. The exocrine cells will be pelleted. The islets are transferred with a siliconized (Prosil-28, PCR Research Chemical Inc., Gainesville, FL) Pasteur pipette into a 50-mL centrifuge tube containing

10–15 mL cold HBSS, modified with 1 percent BSA. The tube is rotated slowly while the islets are gently picked up into the Pasteur pipette to avoid excess Ficoll being transferred with the islets. Note that lymph nodes and pieces of ducts and capillaries are also in the different Ficoll interphases. Many islets may not be seen with the naked eye but will be transferred along with visible islets and contaminating tissue. Our experiments with continuous gradients have met with little success to improve the separation of islets from contaminating tissues and yield of islets.

The islets are washed twice by centrifugation for 1–2 min at 200g in modified HBSS with 1 percent BSA or in any type of medium useful for the ensuing experiment. The islets are resuspended and placed in a bacteriological Petri dish (Nunc, Roskilde, Denmark). Islets are then individually selected with a siliconized constriction pipette in a dissecting microscope at 15 × magnification. In case there is an extensive amount of contaminating tissue, it is recommended that the final picking of islets is repeated. The islets are ready to use after this final step. In case an overnight culture period is preferred, 50–100 islets are picked into bacteriological Petri dishes containing culture medium (RPMI 1640 with 10 percent newborn calf serum) and cultured overnight at 37°C. The yield of islets is normally 100–200/rat pancreas. It should be noted that the average rat islet isolated by this procedure has a dry weight of 0.5–1 μg and that the recovery of islets from the entire pancreas is 2–10 percent only. Multiple factors involved are the production batch of collagenase, nutritional state and degree of starvation of the animal, age of the rats, and, in particular, the time allowed from removal of the pancreatic gland until the commencement of the collagenase digestion. A strict time schedule is recommended for the best result. About eight rats per person appears optimal, and it is better to repeat the isolation procedure rather than increasing the number of rats per islet preparation.

4. SUMMARY AND CONCLUSIONS

Mouse and rat islets are readily prepared by collagenase digestion of the pancreas and separation of the islets from the digest by gradient centrifugation. Still, the collagenase itself appears critical since it represents a crude mixture containing undefined amounts of various proteolytic enzyme activities (2). One batch of Worthington, Type IV collagenase was found to be composed of four major and some minor bands following sodium dodecyl sulfate (SDS) gel electrophoresis (unpublished observations). The day-to-day variation in the function of collagenase-isolated mouse demonstrate a highly variable pattern of insulin release into the culture medium (Fig. 5). The period with low insulin response to glucose could be traced to a certain batch of collagenase. Therefore, each new batch should be tested before use and a purchase of larger quantities.

Rodent islets are relatively easy to distinguish from the exocrine tissue by their different opacity in incident illumination. Contamination with lymph

ng / 10 ISLETS x 2 h

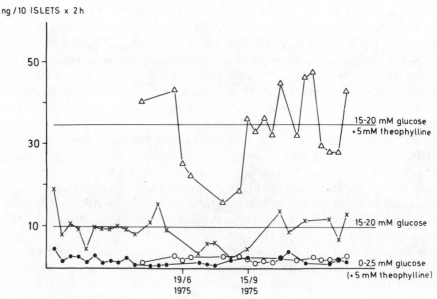

FIGURE 5. Effect of collagenase on insulin release in response to glucose and theophylline in mouse islets isolated on different days. In the interval indicated in the figure, one particular batch of collagenase was used to isolate the islets.

nodes may occur. Lymph nodes may be present also within the pancreatic parenchyma and hence are not easily seen during the preparation of the pancreas before collagenase digestion. Lymph nodes can be distinguished from the islets by illumination in green light (12). In order to get familiarized with the pancreatic lymph nodes, these can be stained by injecting 20–30 μL of 0.01 percent Evans blue solution in saline into the hind foot pads of the animals a few hours or even the day before decapitation. The blue color is taken up by the lymph node macrophages but not by islet cells.

The gradient centrifugation requires completely dispersed tissue, which is not always obtained. Clumping may be due to the presence of DNA leaking out from damaged cells. Clumping due to DNA may be avoided by the addition of DNase during or after the collagenase digestion (13).

Damage to membrane proteins may be circumvented by allowing the islets to recover under tissue culture conditions (3). The ability of mouse islets to release insulin in response to stimulation with glucose and theophylline after culture for up to 1 year is shown in Figure 6. The overnight culture period may be regarded as a pretreatment period to allow the islet cells to adapt to the *in vitro* conditions to be used in the subsequent experiments and thereby permit less variability between experiments.

Alternative isolation procedures than those described above may be employed such as microdissection (14) of the islets which, however, is time consuming. The collagenase digestion can also be carried out by hand shaking (15) or by

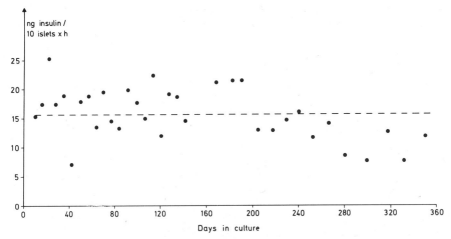

FIGURE 6.   Insulin release in response to 22 m*M* glucose and 5 m*M* theophylline from mouse islets maintained in tissue culture medium RPMI 1640 supplemented with 10 percent newborn calf serum for up to 1 year. Each symbol represents the amount of insulin released during a 1-hr stimulation period of the same group of islets tested repeatedly.

the use of a magnetic stirrer with a stirring bar having a pivot ring to prevent complete digestion of both the exocrine parenchyma and islets (16). Although we found the gradient centrifugation most useful, the islets may be collected directly from the digested tissue, following careful washings by centrifugation or sedimentation as described in the section on human islet isolation and culture (Vol. IB, IV H).

REFERENCES

1. S. Moskalewski, *Gen. Comp. Endocr.* **5**, 342 (1965).

2. J. H. Nielsen and Å. Lernmark, in *Cell Separation: Methods and Selected Applications*, Vol. 2, T. G. Pretlow and T. P. Pretlow (eds.) Academic Press, New York, 1983, p. 99.

3. L. Turcot-Lemay, A. Lemay, and P. E. Lacy, *Biochem. Biophys. Res. Comm.* **63**, 1130 (1975).

4. A. Andersson, *Diabetologia* **14**, 397 (1978).

5. M. W. Steffes, O. Nielsen, T. Dyrberg, S. Bækkeskov, J. Scott, and Å. Lernmark, *Transplantation* **31**, 476 (1981).

6. T. Dyrberg, S. Bækkeskov, and Å. Lernmark, *J. Cell Biol.* **94**, 472 (1982).

7. J. Brunstedt, *Diabete Metab. (Paris)* **6**, 87 (1980).

8. J. H. Nielsen, *Endocrinology* **110**, 600 (1982).

9. Å. Lernmark, A. Nathans, and D. F. Steiner, *J. Cell Biol.* **7**, 606 (1976).

10. A. J. Matas, D. E. R. Sutherland, M. W. Steffes, and J. S. Najarian, *Surgery* **80**, 183 (1976).

11. M. Kuo, D. S. Hodgins, and J. F. Kuo, *J. Biol. Chem.* **248**, 2705 (1973).

12. E. H. Finke, P. E. Lacy, and J. Ono, *Diabetes* **28**, 612 (1979).

13. A. Buitrago, E. Gylfe, C. Henriksson, and H. Pertoft, *Biochem. Biophys. Res. Comm.* **79**, 823 (1977).

14. C. Hellerström, *Acta Endocr. (Cph)* **45**, 122 (1964).

15. A. Andersson and C. Hellerström, *Diabetes* **21** (suppl. 2), 546 (1972).

16. H. S. Tager, A. H. Rubenstein, and D. F. Steiner, *Methods Enzymol.* **37**, 326 (1975).

E

PREPARATION OF
ISLET CELL SUSPENSIONS

**Å. LERNMARK, T. DYRBERG, J. H. NIELSEN,
AND THE HAGEDORN STUDY GROUP**
Hagedorn Research Laboratory, Gentofte, Denmark

1. INTRODUCTION

Pancreatic islets are composed of several cell types. It has been estimated that the endocrine cells in an isolated islet represent about 60 percent of the parenchyma (cf. 1). The remainder are endothelial cells, nerve cells, and connective tissue cells including fibroblast and macrophages. Among the endocrine cells the β cell predominates (65–80 percent of the endocrine cells) while the α and PP (pancreatic polypeptide) cells are present in roughly equal proportions depending on which part of the pancreas the islets have been isolated. The α cells are predominantly found in the splenic part, while PP cells dominate the islets in the duodenal part. δ cells, which comprise 5–10 percent of the endocrine cells are found in islets at all locations (2, 3). Cells producing other polypeptide hormones may also be found, and the presence of such cells, as well as the cellular composition and size of islet, may vary with the age of the animal (1–3). It is an important consideration that islets isolated by standard collagenase techniques often represent the medium-sized to large islets only (see chapters on islet isolation).

After disruption of the capillary system, the dense parenchyma of the isolated islet organ relies on simple diffusion from the extracellular medium into the center. This characteristic, as well as the cellular complexity of the islet organ, make preparations of single cells more useful in many experiments. The possibility that cell-to-cell interactions may still occur in preparations of isolated cells may make it necessary not only to prepare dispersed islet cells but also to separate and purify individual islet cell subtypes (see chapters on islet cell separation).

Several approaches to preparation of islet cell suspensions have been described (ref. 1). The two different techniques described in this chapter represent a chemical, nonenzymatic and an enzymatic approach to obtaining dispersed cells.

2. PREPARATION OF ISLETS CELLS

In certain experiments it is advisable to avoid the use of proteolytic enzymes since they are known to attack cell membrane components, while for other purposes a mild proteolytic treatment may be acceptable. Cells are prepared (Table 1) from isolated pancreatic islets as described in previous chapters (4, 5). Both freshly isolated and cultured islets may be used.

2.1. Reagents

2.1.1. RPMI-HEPES

RPMI 1640 (available from several biochemical companies) is supplemented with 20 mM N-2-hydroxyethylpiperazine N'-2-ethanesulfonic acid (HEPES),

Members of the Hagedorn Study Group are K. Brunstedt, D. Jensen, R. Jørgensen, A. M. Olesen, T. Funder, J. Brunstedt, T. Dyrberg, S. Bækkeskov, J. H. Nielsen, and Å. Lernmark. The support of the foundation Nordisk Insulinlaboratorium, the National Institutes of Health (Am 26190), and the Danish Medical Research Council is acknowledged.

Table 1.   Preparation of Dispersed Islet Cells.

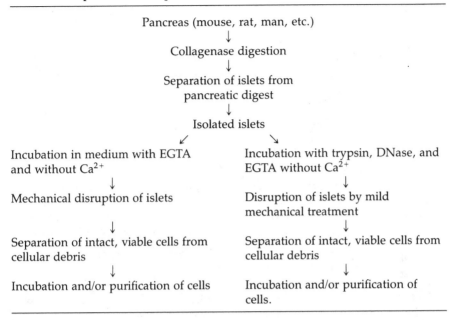

Pancreas (mouse, rat, man, etc.)
↓
Collagenase digestion
↓
Separation of islets from
pancreatic digest
↓
Isolated islets

Incubation in medium with EGTA and without Ca^{2+}	Incubation with trypsin, DNase, and EGTA without Ca^{2+}
↓	↓
Mechanical disruption of islets	Disruption of islets by mild mechanical treatment
↓	↓
Separation of intact, viable cells from cellular debris	Separation of intact, viable cells from cellular debris
↓	↓
Incubation and/or purification of cells	Incubation and/or purification of cells.

300 mg/L L-glutamine, 0.35 g/L sodium bicarbonate, 100,000 IU/L penicillin, and 100 mg/L streptomycin, pH 7.2. Store at 4°C.

2.1.2.   RPMI-EGTA-BSA

RPMI-HEPES is supplemented with 2 mM EGTA and 1 percent (w/v) bovine serum albumin (BSA) (Pentex bovine albumin, fraction V, reagent grade; Miles Laboratories Inc., Elkhart, IN). The pH is adjusted to 7.4 and the medium filtered through a 22-μm filter (Millipore, Bedford, MA). Store at 4°C. The bovine serum albumin is selected with care since individual batches may contain insulin-degrading activity.

2.1.3.   RPMI-EGTA-TRYPSIN-DNASE

RPMI-HEPES is supplemented with 2 mM EGTA, 100 μg/mL trypsin, and 2 μg/mL DNase. (All reagents used were from Sigma, St. Louis, MO. DNase may also be obtained from Worthington Biochemicals, Freehold, NJ.)

2.1.4.   RPMI–4 PERCENT BSA

RPMI-HEPES is supplemented with 4 percent (w/v) BSA and filtered through a 22-μm filter (Millipore). Adjust pH, if necessary.

2.2. Nonenzymatic Disruption of Islets

Pancreatic islets are prepared according to the protocols (4, 5). The islets are selected under a dissecting microscope after Percoll (mouse islets) or Ficoll (rat islets) gradient centrifugation directly into RPMI-EGTA-BSA medium. The islets are washed by centrifugation (50g for 5 min) with RPMI-EGTA-BSA in a 12 mL siliconized conical polystyrene centrifuge tube, resuspended in 10 mL RPMI-EGTA-BSA, and allowed to sediment at room temperature. Discard the top 9 mL of supernatant and transfer the remaining 1 mL with the islets to a 4 mL Minisorb centrifuge tube (Nunc, Roskilde, Denmark). Up to 1000 islets can be handled per Minisorb tube.

Allow the islets to sediment for 5 min and remove the supernatant. Repeat this procedure twice. After the last washing by sedimentation, leave approximately 1 mL RPMI-EGTA-BSA and aspirate the islet suspension gently five to seven times with a siliconized Pasteur pipette with a blunted end. Avoid formation of foam. At this stage it should be possible, by looking through the tube, to see the islets disrupted into a homogeneous cell suspension.

The Pasteur pipette with a blunt-ended tip is prepared as follows: Siliconize (Prost-28, PCR Research Chemicals, Inc., Gainesville, FL) a 145-mm disposable glass Pasteur pipette. Rotate the tip of the pipette nearly vertically in the flame of a Bunsen burner to allow the tip to melt and form a symmetrical hole of about 0.1–0.2 mm in diameter. Allow the pipette to cool and then test that RPMI-EGTA-BSA can be taken up into the pipette and ejected straight out of it. The islets should be compressed while passing the orifice, thereby forcing them to be broken up into single cells.

Transfer the cell suspension carefully to a 4 mL Minisorb tube containing 2.5 mL RPMI-4 percent BSA. If there still are intact islets left, these are allowed to sediment. Allow the islets to sediment for 2–3 min in RPMI-EGTA-BSA and repeat the aspiration. Transfer the cell suspension to RPMI-4 percent BSA. Centrifuge at 4°C for 10 min at 50g. Remove the supernatant and leave the cell pellet in a known volum (by comparing with another tube).

Resuspend the cells and examine a 10-μL sample in a hemocytometer. Determine cell number, number of single cells, and viability using a dye exclusion test. Light microscopy of freshly dispersed mouse islet cells often reveals a mixture of single cells in addition to clumps or clusters of various sizes (Fig. 1). Cell clumps appear to be due to a mixture of incompletely dispersed cells and single cells reaggregating after being pelleted by centrifugation. The contribution of the latter phenomenon may be diminished by centrifugation of the freshly prepared cell suspension through RPMI-4 percent BSA against a cushion of 30 percent (w/v) BSA in HEPES-RPMI (6). The cells are collected from the interface between the 4 percent and 30 percent BSA layers and resuspended in fresh medium.

In a number of studies (6–9) collagenase-isolated islets were mechanically disrupted using a micromixer (Fig. 2). The micromixer was a modified Beckman micromixer (Model 154, Beckman Instruments, Mountainside, NJ). In this

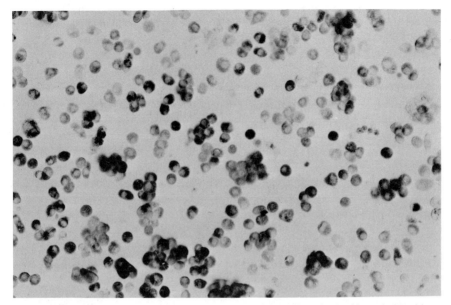

FIGURE 1. Light microscopy of freshly dispersed islet cells stained with methylene blue.

procedure the islets are washed by sedimentation in RPMI-EGTA-BSA and batches of 100 islets/200 μL medium transferred to 550-μL polypropylene microtest tubes (Milian Instruments, Geneva, Switzerland). The islets are disrupted by mechanical shaking for 10 sec. The longer the shaking time, the smaller the number of intact cells recovered. After shaking, intact islets and islet debris are allowed to sediment and the supernatant containing cells is transferred to a conical centrifugation tube containing RPMI-4 percent BSA. Fresh RPMI-EGTA-BSA medium is added to the microtest tube and the shaking–sedimentation procedure repeated until all islets are disrupted.

Preparations of dispersed cells from freshly isolated mouse islets resulted in a yield of 138,000 ± 13,000 (mean ± SEM, $n = 41$) cells per pancreas, corresponding to 1000–1500 cells per islet. The proportion of single cells was 85 ± 2 percent. Viability was > 90 percent. When applied to islets from newborn rats after 48 hr of culture, the yield of cells was 620 ± 75 per islet, and the viability was 65 ± 3 percent ($n = 13$).

2.3. Enzymatic Disruption of Islets

Freshly isolated or cultured islets are transferred at room temperature to siliconized, conical polystyrene 12-mL centrifuge tubes containing 10 mL RPMI-EGTA-BSA. The islets are allowed to sediment and the supernatant is discarded. The islets, kept in as small a volume as possible, are transferred to a 4 mL Minisorb tube containing 1 mL RPMI-EGTA-trypsin-DNase. Incubate the islets

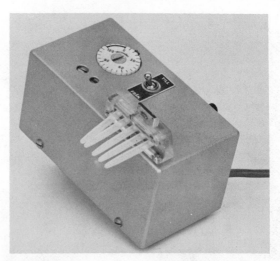

FIGURE 2.   Modified Beckman micromixer used for mechanical disruption of collagenase-isolated pancreatic islets.

for 30 min at room temperature. Remove the supernatant and wash the islets three times by 5-min sedimentation in 1 mL RPMI-EGTA-BSA. The islets are resuspended thereafter in 0.5 mL RPMI-EGTA-BSA and dispersed by aspiration three times with a siliconized Pasteur pipette with a blunt-ended tip (see above). Allow nondispersed islets to sediment for 1 min and layer the supernatant, which now contains dispersed cells, on top of 3–5 mL RPMI-4 percent BSA in a siliconized 12 mL centrifuge tube. Repeat the aspiration and sedimentation procedure until all islets are disrupted.

Centrifuge the cell suspension through the RPMI-4 percent BSA at 50g for 10 min at 4°C. Resuspend the cells and examine them under a microscope as mentioned above.

The yield and viability of cells from islets kept in tissue culture often appear higher with the enzymatic compared to the nonenzymatic procedure. In our experience cultured human islets are particularly resistant to the chemical procedure alone.

3.   SUMMARY AND CONCLUSION

Suspensions of dispersed islet cells are easily prepared by treatment with the Ca^{2+}-chelating agent EGTA alone (7, 10) or combined with a proteolytic enzyme like trypsin (11) or dispase (12). Since proteolytic enzymes are known to attack surface membrane components, it is advisable either to avoid enzymes or to reduce the concentration and exposure time as much as possible. However, in the interest of an increased yield of cells, enzymatically prepared cells may be subjected to a subsequent culture for 6 hr or longer to regain surface antigens (13). It must then be noted that the islet cells have a strong tendency to reaggregate during culture, often to form so-called pseudoislets (14).

Chelating agents may also affect membrane structure and function. The length of time of exposing the islets to EGTA should therefore be kept at a minimum. This may be achieved by the gentle mechanical treatment described above and by the immediate transfer of the cells to a complete medium with out EGTA. Cells prepared in this way release insulin in response to glucose (7, 9, 15) and react with various membrane-directed antibodies (6, 10, 15, 16).

REFERENCES

1. J. H. Neilsen and Å. Lernmark in *Cell Separation: Methods and Selected Applications*, Vol. 2, T. G. Pretlow and T. P. Pretlow (eds.), Academic Press, New York, 1983, p. 99.

2. D. Baetens, F. Malaisse-Lagae, A. Perrelet, and L. Orci, *Science* **206**, 1323 (1979).

3. F. Malaisse-Lagae, Y. Stefan, J. Cox, A. Perrelet, and L. Orci, *Diabetologia* **17**, 361 (1979).

4. J. Brunstedt, et al., "Isolation of rat and mouse islets," this volume.

5. J. H. Nielsen, et al., "Isolation of human islets," this volume.

6. Å. Lernmark, T. Kanatsuna, C. Patzelt, K. Diakoumis, R. Carroll, A. H. Rubenstein, and D. F. Steiner, *Diabetologia* **19**, 445 (1980).

7. Å. Lernmark, *Diabetologia* **10**, 431 (1974).

8. L. Å. Idahl, Å. Lernmark, M. Söderberg, and B. Winblad, *Medical Biol.* **58**, 101, (1980).

9. L. Å. Idahl, Å. Lernmark, J. Sehlin, and I. B. Täljedal, *Pflügers Arch.* **366**, 185 (1976).

10. T. Dyrberg, S. Bækkeskov, and Å. Lernmark, *J. Cell Biol.* **94**, 472 (1982).

11. D. G. Pipeleers and M. A. Pipeleers-Marichal, *Diabetologia* **20**, 654 (1981).

12. J. Ono, R. Takaki, and M. Fukuma, *Endocrin. Japan* **24**, 265 (1977).

13. D. Faustman, V. Hauptfeld, J. M. Davie, P. E. Lacy, and D. C. Schreffler, *J. Exp. Med.* **151**, 1563 (1980).

14. D. W. Sharp, R. Downing, R. C. Merrell, and M. Greider, *Diabetes* **29** (suppl. 1), 19 (1980).

15. T. Kanatsuna, Å. Lernmark, A. H. Rubenstein, and D. F. Steiner, *Diabetes* **30**, 231 (1981).

16. S. Bækkeskov, T. Kanatsuna, L. Klareskog, D. A. Nielsen, P. A. Peterson, A. H. Rubenstein, D. F. Steiner, and Å. Lernmark, *Proc. Nat. Acad. Sci. USA* **78**, 6456 (1981).

F

PERIFUSION OF SV 40 TRANSFORMED HAMSTER β CELLS TO STUDY INSULIN SECRETORY DYNAMICS

RONALD S. HILL AND A. E. BOYD III

Department of Medicine, Baylor College of Medicine, Houston, Texas

1. INTRODUCTION

Since Burr et al. (1) introduced a perifusion system to study insulin secretory dynamics from pancreatic pieces and Lacy et al. (2) from isolated islets, this technique has proven to be an extremely powerful method to evaluate the relative potencies of various secretagogues (3) and the role of Ca^{2+} fluxes (4, 5), other ions (6, 7), or cytoskeletal proteins (1, 8, 9) in the biphasic release of insulin. However, *in vitro* biochemical studies of perifused islets are limited by both the number of islets which can be prepared and the cellular and hormonal heterogenity of the islets. Recently, Santerre et al. (10) developed a hamster β cell line (HIT) by transforming Syrian hamster pancreatic islet cells with Simian virus 40 (SV 40). This line was cloned and shown to release insulin in response to glucose, glucagon, and 3-isobutyl-methylxanthine. We have developed a method to perifuse monolayers of the HIT cells grown on coverslips to probe the involvement of cytoskeletal proteins in the transport and release of insulin. New methods in cell biology, such as the low light level camera or microinjection of specific monoclonal or polyclonal antibodies or fluorescently labeled molecules into the HIT cells, can be applied to further study the secretory process. In addition, the transformed cells can be injected into hamsters pretreated with antilymphocyte serum, and the subsequent solid tumors can then serve as a source of large amounts of homogenous tissue for biochemical studies.

2. HIT CELL POPULATION

The derivation and preliminary studies characterizing the insulin product and the stimulus-secretion coupling of the transformed hamster cell line (HIT) has been published (10). In brief, islets were isolated from Syrian hamsters, further purified by centrifugation in a density gradient, and then dissociated into single-cell suspensions with trypsin and EDTA. After 4 days in culture, these cells were transformed by treatment with SV 40 virus. Colonies of the transformed cells were isolated in soft agar and cloned as monolayers. The original isolates were recloned several times before propogation as mass colonies and preparation of frozen stocks.

We received subclone HIT-T15 at passage 72 and used this line for our initial studies. There is a gradual decrease in the basal and insulin stimulated secretion with time in culture. However, earlier passages of the cells, which have been frozen back and then thawed and grown in culture, retain their secretory potential. It is important to obtain as early a passage as possible and to freeze back cells from each passage so that one always has a source of early-

This work was supported by the Diabetes and Endocrinology Research Center, Grant No. AMⱬ3033 awarded by the National Institute of Arthritis, Diabetes, Digestive and Kidney Diseases, Training Grant No. AM07348 (RSH) and NIH Grant No. AM23033 (AEB). Thanks to Susan Medved and Lucy Whitlock for their help with some of the technical aspect of these studies and to Donna Turnquist for preparation of the manuscript.

passage cells for future studies. In our laboratory the cells have a doubling time of 38 hr and a plating efficiency of 80 percent. When subcultured and grown at high density, the cells tend to self-associate and form clumps of cells rather than a true monolayer. When grown at low density on coverslips, the cells form monolayers. The cells contain approximately 2600 ng of insulin/mg of protein and are virtually 100 percent positive for the insulin antigen by immunofluorescence. Figure 1 shows indirect immunofluorescence of the cells grown on coverslips using the technique we have developed for insulin-secreting cells (11). The cultures are incubated at 37°C in 5 percent CO_2 and air and are routinely maintained in RPMI 1640 medium with 10 percent fetal calf serum, 10 μg/mL glutathione, 10^{-7} M selenous acid, 100 μg/mL streptomycin, and 100 U/mL penicillin.

We have subsequently grown the HIT cells as solid tumors in hamsters using the following protocol. On days −1, 0, 1, 4, 7, 11, 15, 18, and 25, fifty- to sixty-gram Syrian hamsters (Harland Sprague–Dawley, Indianapolis, IN) were injected subcutaneously with 0.25 mL of rabbit hamster antilymphocyte serum (M.A. Associates, Bethesda, MD). On day 0, the hamsters were injected subcutaneously with 6×10^6 cells suspended in 0.2 mL of RPMI 1640 plus 10 percent fetal bovine serum. Subcutaneous tumors first appeared in approximately 4 weeks and can then be transplanted to hamsters which have not been primed with antilymphocyte serum.

3. PERIFUSION SYSTEM

The perifusion system consists of a pump to move media from the pump chamber over the cells, which are housed in the 25-mm Swinnex chamber and

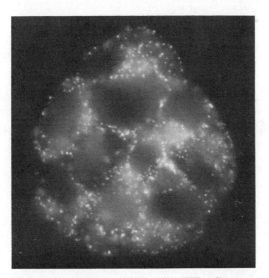

FIGURE 1.   Insulin immunofluorescence of HIT cells. HIT cells were stained with affinity-purified guinea pig anti-insulin serum and rabbit FITC-labeled anti-guinea pig IgG. Note that all cells are positive for insulin and that the insulin occurs in discrete granules.

a means to collect effluent fractions. We use and eight-chamber Gilson Minipuls 2 pump to perifuse up to four chambers simultaneously. A Harvard Apparatus peristaltic pump may also be used. The Gilson Blue-Yellow (⅛-in. outside diameter, 1/16-in. inside diameter) pump chambers are used at a flow rate of 1 mL/min. Tygon tubing (⅛-in. outside diameter, 1/16-in. inside diameter OD, 1/16" ID) is used to connect the pump chamber to the reservoir of media and to the cell chamber (Fig. 2). Connections are made using ¼ in. outside diameter × ⅛-in. diameter tygon tubing cyclohexanone to seal the connections. The end of the tubing, which is submersed into a beaker of perifusion media, is attached to an 8-cm length (3-mm diameter) of glass tubing to ensure the tubing remains firmly in the bottom of the media container. Media are switched by physically moving the tubing to the new media container while the pump is momentarily (< 5 sec) switched off. The tubing is connected to the cell chambers using a male leur-lock connector. A section of effluent tubing is connected to the other side of the chamber using a female leur-lock connector.

In constructing these perifusion chambers, the following points must be kept in mind. First, all chambers must be of exactly the same dimensions to ensure uniform flow in each chamber. Second, tubing lengths must be chosen

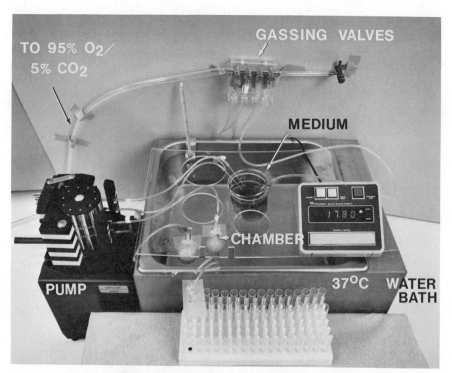

FIGURE 2. The perifusion system. The perifusion system consists of a peristaltic pump to deliver media, a 37°C water bath, a Plexiglass holder for media and chambers, a device to collect fractions, a cylinder of 95 percent O_2/5 percent CO_2 and valves, and the perifusion chambers.

to ensure easy, rapid movement from one media to another and that all chambers can be submerged in the water bath and fractions can be easily collected. Third, dead space should be kept to a minimum to prevent slow mixing of experimental medium and basal medium during changeover. If for a particular set of experiments less dead space is needed, smaller diameter tubing (except for the pump chamber) may be used and silicone rubber added to the Swinnex chambers to reduce their dead space. Fourth, all perifusion chambers should be clearly labeled, using a color-coding system to ensure that samples are not confused during collection.

The fractions are collected using a simple device. A piece of stiff plastic (approx. 3 × 6 cm) is drilled with four holes centered over the spacings of the collection tubes. The effluent from the perifusion chamber is connected to a vacutainer needle, which has had the sharp ends cut off and filed down. The tubing can then be quickly screwed into the collection plate device. Fractions are changed by manually moving all four perifusion effluent tubings simultaneously. Fractions are collected in 12 × 75-mm test tubes or 15-mL conical centrifuge tubes. The cell chambers and media containers are maintained at 37°C in the same water bath. A Plexiglass template is used to hold the media container and perifusion chambers in the water bath (Fig. 2).

3.1. Media

Standard perifusion media consists of Krebs–Ringer bicarbonate of the following composition (in mM): NaCl, 118.5; KCl, 5.94; $CaCl_2$, 2.54; $MgSO_4$ 1.19; KH_2PO_4, 1.19; $NaHCO_3$ 25.00. Media is prepared as four stock solutions: (I) 474.0 mM NaCl; (II) 10.16 mM $CaCl_2 \cdot 2H_2O$; (III) 4.76 mM KH_2PO_4; (IV) 21.76 mM KCl, 100 mM $NaHCO_3$, 4.76 mM $MgSO_4$. These are stored at 4°C and should be made fresh every 4 weeks.

Media is prepared on the day of the experiment by mixing equal volumes of solutions I–IV. Approximately 25 percent extra media is made for each experiment to ensure no shortage of media during perifusion. Media is supplemented with 1 mg/mL bovine serum albumin (fraction V) and glucose as needed. Media is equilibrated to pH 7.40 by gassing with 95 percent O_2 and 5 percent CO_2. Brass aquarium gang valves (from a local pet store) are used to control gas flow between several different media (Fig. 2). HEPES (N-2-hydroxyethylpiperazine-N'-2 ethanesulfonic acid) may be added to further stabilize the pH. Other components of the media are then added as needed for each experiment. Variations of this basic media may be made depending on experimental needs. We have tested two additional media: Hanks' balanced salt solution and Schubart's PO_4-free media (12). Both of these media also gave good stimulation to depolarization with high potassium. In selecting alternative media, it is important to check to see if the media holds pH satisfactorily and if the secretory response parallels that of the Krebs–Ringer bicarbonate media.

3.2. Cells for Perifusion

Cells cultured as above are subcultured 3 days before an experiment with 500,000 cells/well in a 12-well plate. Each well has one 18-mm circular #1 cover glass (Bellco, Vineland, NJ). On the day of the experiment each coverslip containing about 300,000 cells is transferred to a 25-mm Swinnex chamber (Millipore) without a filter which is filled with basal media. Remove any air bubbles which were allowed in the chamber. The pump tubing is prefilled with basal media, then connected to the chamber—again being careful not to allow air into the chambers.

Perifusion consists of simply pumping basal media over the cells for a given period of time, switching the media of the test chambers to experimental medium, and collecting timed fractions. Fractions are assayed using a standard insulin RIA. Insulin levels of serially diluted perifusate samples should parallel the insulin RIA standard curve. Secretion rates are calculated using the flow rate, the time of collection, and concentration of insulin in the fractions. Secretory rates may then be expressed on a per cell basis by counting the cells on the coverslips after perifusion using standard techniques.

4. VALIDATION

4.1. Flow Rate

The flow rate is determined before, during, and after the perifusion. Prior to and after perifusion, 10-min fractions are collected into 15 mL conical centrifuge tubes, the volumes recorded and flow rates calculated. Periodic tubes (12 × 75 mm) are preweighed and then reweighed after collection of perifusion media. From the weight, the volume of the media can be determined and flow rate during perifusion calculated. If graduated conical centrifuge tubes are used, flow rates can be determined from the volumes and collection times. The Gilson pump is extremely reliable in providing a constant flow rate during perifusion.

4.2. Turnover

Turnover time in the system is measured in three ways. First, a small amount of [^{125}I] labeled compound ($\sim$ 2000 cpm/mL) is added to a beaker of perifusion media. The perifusion system is started and five 1-min basal fractions are collected. Then the media is switched to the media with the label and timed fractions are collected to calibrate the system. For example, a 5 min. period of 15-sec fractions followed by 10 min of 1 min fractions are collected and the medium is then switched to nonradioactive medium. Approximately 10 more 1 min fractions are collected. Figure 3 demonstrates the turnover profile of this system. Second, concentrations of a test agent like glucose are measured

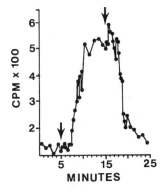

FIGURE 3. Turnover profile of the perifusion system. Media was switched to [^{125}I]-containing media at 5 min. The dead space of the system is 2.5 mL and the flow rate 1 mL/min, so that the increase in radioactivity should begin 2.5 min after the media change. The arrowheads indicate when the media was changed. Counts decrease after media was switched back to basal.

in the fractions collected furing perifusion. The levels of glucose or other secretagogues in the perifusate should follow the pattern predicted by the radioactive turnover data. This ensures that within the limits of the system a brisk changeover to stimulation media occurs with minimal mixing of secretagogues. Third, the total volume of the perifusion system (tubing, pump chamber) is measured. From the known flow rate and the measured dead space, a turnover time can be calculated. The three values should be in close agreement. In our system the dead space is 2.5 mL, the flow rate 1 mL/min. Therefore, media is physically switched 2.5 min before the desired media is collected. If stimulation is to begin at 60.0 min, the media switch is made at 57.5 min and stimulation media is first collected from minute 60 to 61.

4.3. Secretory Profile

During initial experiments it is essential that a complete secretory profile including a postexperimental period in basal medium be determined (Fig. 4). Four significant points must be kept in mind. First, the secretory profile of cells during the basal period must reach a stable baseline before stimulating the cells. This is important since artificially high secretory rates are observed initially. Second, by simultaneously perifusing paired chambers with basal or the experimental media, it is possible to obtain a minute-to-minute comparison of stimulated versus basal secretion. Third, insulin stimulated secretion should parallel the change in secretagogues levels and that predicted by the turnover studies. Fourth, when the secretagogue is removed from the media, secretion rates should return to basal levels. These points support a physiologically significant secretory process.

4.4. Other Controls

Media pH should be carefully monitored throughout the perifusion to ensure that no change in pH occurs, particularly between the basal and experimental media. Since insulin secretion is known to be dependent on extracellular Ca^{2+}

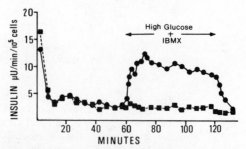

FIGURE 4. Perifusion secretory profile of the HIT cells. Two chambers containing HIT cells were perifused, one from minute 0 to 60 and 120 to 135 in basal media (0.3 ng/mL glucose) and from 60–120 min in high glucose (3.5 mg/mL) plus 0.1 mM 3-isobutyl-methylxanthine (●, HG/IBMX), the other chamber (■) was perifused with basal throughout. The HIT cells initially released large amounts of insulin, which then established a stable basal rate. HG/IBMX induced a brisk, highly significant response which remained elevated during the entire experimental period. Upon switching back to basal medium, secretion returned to control levels.

(13, 14), omitting Ca^{2+} and adding EGTA should eliminate the secretory response. Figure 5 demonstrates the secretory response to 40 mM K^+ by the HIT cells. When Ca^{2+}-free media with 1 mM EGTA is present, basal (before 60 min) secretion is decreased and the stimulated response is eliminated. When Ca^{2+} is returned at 75 min, the secretory response then occurs. To ensure that changes of pressure within the chambers do not correlate with changes in

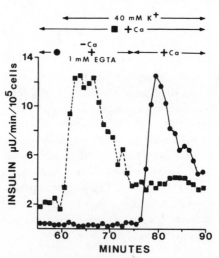

FIGURE 5. Calcium dependency of K^+-induced secretion. One set of chambers ($n = 4$) received basal medium (0.3 mg/mL glucose) with 2.54 mM Ca^{2+} and one set received basal medium without Ca^{2+} plus 1 mM EGTA ($n = 4$). Both were stimulated at 60 min with 40 mM K^+. Both basal and stimulated release were significantly inhibited in the Ca^{2+}-free chambers compared to controls. At 75 min the Ca^{2+}-free chambers continued in 40 mM K^+ media, now with 2.54 mM Ca^{2+}. Upon replacement of the calcium a brisk stimulatory response was detected in these chambers.

secretory rate and that pressure does not build during perifusion, pressure profiles can be determined using a pressure transducer.

Cell viability after perifusion is determined by (i) vital stains such as acridine orange/ethidium bromide, (ii) returning the coverslip to the growth media overnight and remeasuring the basal and stimulated secretory rates the next day, (iii) determining the plating efficiency of the postperifused cells, and (iv) structural evaluation at both the light and EM level. The cells should meet all the criteria of viablity after perifusion. Finally, insulin extraction by acid–alcohol (15) is performed postperifusion and the percentage of insulin released during stimulation determined. Physiological secretory rates are characterized by release of a small percentage of the total insulin content. Having performed these controls, one can be sure that the secretory patterns observed represent a physiological response of the HIT cell to the experimental substances.

5. SUMMARY

The HIT cell perifusion system described provides several unique advantages to other model insulin secretory systems. The HIT cells can be easily grown and maintained in tissue culture obviating the need to isolate islets. These cells provide a uniform population which form tumors in hamsters pretreated with antilymphocyte serum and provide large quantitites of tissue for biochemical studies. The combination of the perifusion system and HIT cell culture line enables the application of powerful new technologies in cell biology to the problem of insulin secretion.

By using perifusion the dynamic nature of the secretory profile can be characterized. The rapidity of the response, the peak secretory rate, the ability or inability to sustain a secretory response, as well as simply giving the total insulin released can be measured. In addition, the perifusion system can be used to discriminate between first- and second-phase effects as well as delayed responses induced by test agents. Thus, the perifusion system provides a more complete understanding of the secretory profile than a static system. In deciding whether to use a perifusion system for a given problem, these advantages must be weighed against the greater time and effort required to develop à perifusion system and the large number of samples generated by each experiment.

REFERENCES

1. I. M. Burr, W. Stauffacher, L. Balant, A. E. Renold, and G. M. Grodsky, *Acta Diabet. Lat.* **6**, 580 (1969).
2. P. E. Lacy, M. M. Walker, and C. J. Fink, *Diabetes* **21**, 987 (1972).
3. J. C. Henquin, *Diabetologia* **18**, 151 (1980).
4. P. R. Flatt, P. O. Berggren, E. Gylfe, and B. Hellman, *Endocrinology* **107**, 1007, (1980).

5. M. Kikuchi, C. B. Wollheim, E. G. Siegel, A. E. Renold, and G. W. G. Sharp, *Endocrinology* **105**, 1013 (1979).

6. W. J. Malaisse, A. C. Boschero, S. Kawazu, and J. C. Hutton, *Pflugers Archiv.* **373**, 237 (1978).

7. J. Sehlin, *Am. J. Physiol.* **235**, E501 (1978).

8. P. E. Lacy, N. J. Klein, and C. J. Fink, *Endocrinology* **92**, 1458 (1973).

9. W. B. Rhoten, *Comp. Biochem. Physiol.* **47A**, 959 (1974).

10. R. F. Santerre, R. A. Cook, R. M. D. Crisel, J. D. Sharp, R. J. Schmidt, D. C. Williams, and C. P. Wilson, *Proc. Natl. Acad. Sci. USA* **78**, 4339 (1981).

11. A. E. Boyd III, W. E. Bolton, and B. R. Brinkley, *J. Cell Biol.* **92**, 425 (1982).

12. U. K. Schubart, S. Shapiro, N. Fleischer, and O. M. Rosen, *J. Biol. Chem.* **252**, 92 (1977).

13. G. M. Grodsky and L. L. Bennett, *Diabetes* **15**, 910 (1966).

14. R. D. G. Milner and C. N. Hales, *Diabetologia* **3**, 47 (1967).

15. I. A. Mirsky, *Methods in Investigative and Diagnostic Endocrinology, Vol. 2B, Peptide Hormones*, American Elsevier, New York, 1973, p. 823.

G

MEASUREMENT OF ACTIN AND IDENTIFICATION OF ACTIN- AND CALMODULIN-BINDING PROTEINS IN INSULIN-SECRETING CELLS SECRETING CELLS

T. YAP NELSON, M. C. SNABES, AND A. E. BOYD III
Department of Medicine, Baylor College of Medicine, Houston, Texas

1. INTRODUCTION

An understanding of the transport and secretion of insulin requires methods to identify and then quantitate the cellular proteins that facilitate the movement of insulin and its precursors from the site of synthesis to the plasma membrane. Many of the molecular events involved in the secretory process are undoubtedly regulated by "cytoskeletal" proteins, an array of structural and regulatory elements suspended in a lattice network of the cytoplasm. This report describes methods which are useful for studying the role of two cytoskeletal proteins, actin and calmodulin, in insulin secretion.

2. ACTIN

Understanding the role of actin in cellular processes requires a means of quantitating changes in the number and assembly state of actin molecules. In pancreatic islets or insulinoma cells actin exists in several forms; G-actin, a polypeptide of 42,000 daltons which in the presence of ATP and magnesium polymerizes to form filamentous F-actin. Early methods to measure actin used densitometry of stained electrophoretic gels to study changes in actin content (1). Blikstad et al. exploited the unique property of soluble or G-actin to bind to DNase I with high affinity and inhibit the enzymatic hydrolysis of DNA (2). Although the inhibition assay measures both soluble (G) and filamentous (F) actin, the procedure requires lengthy spectrophotometric determinations of DNA hydrolysis and is relatively insensitive, measuring actin in the microgram per milliliter range.

In our attempts to develop an actin radioimmunoassay, we, like Morgan et al. (3) found that small differences in the primary structure of actin from various species or even from different tissues in the same species resulted in marked differences in the binding of actin to actin antibodies. It was difficult to quantitate absolute amounts of nonmuscle actin in pancreatic islets using antiactin antibodies we had raised against highly purified rabbit skeletal muscle actin and the same actin as the label and standard. However, we had measured actin in pancreatic islets by the DNase I inhibition assay of Blikstad and knew that the enzyme would bind to actin in the islet. We then set out to develop an actin assay which used the DNase I enzyme as the ligand and utilized the competition between unlabeled rabbit skeletal muscle actin and [^{125}I] labeled actin for the DNase I. Bound and free actin are separated by a two-step immunoprecipitation of the actin–DNase I complex (4).

2.1. Purification of Actin

Rabbit skeletal muscle actin is purified by the method of Spudich and Watt (5). This method has recently been outlined in detail by Pardee and Spudich (6) who point out possible technical problems. The actin is stored as G-actin at 4°C with 0.05 percent sodium azide as a preservative or for more prolonged storage at −70°C, the actin is divided into small aliquots. Thawing and refreezing causes a partial loss in activity.

2.2. Preparation of Antisera

Electrophoretically pure DNase I (Sigma grade EP) is dissolved in 0.9 percent NaCl, emulsified in an equal volume of Freund's complete adjuvant, and injected intradermally and subcutaneously into 2-month-old New Zealand white rabbits. Four hundred micrograms of DNase I is injected initially and at 6-week intervals, and 200 μg is injected subcutaneously in incomplete Freund's adjuvant. The DNase is quite antigenic and antibody suitable for use in the assay is obtained after the second injection. Anti-rabbit IgG is obtained by injecting a sheep or goat using a similar injection schedule with 2.0 mg of rabbit IgG as the antigen. Test bleeds are obtained at 2-week intervals following each booster injection, and upon removal the blood is allowed to clot, and the serum obtained by centrifugation at 6000g for 20 minutes at 4°C. The serum is aliquoted in small fractions and stored at −20°C.

2.3. Radioiodination of Actin

Approximately 5–10 μg of G-actin is radioiodinated by the method of Bolton and Hunter (7). [^{125}I]actin is separated from free [^{125}I] Bolton and Hunter reagent by chromatography at 4°C on a Sephadex G-75 column (1.5 × 40 cm) previously equilibrated with the assay buffer (5 mM phosphate, 50 mM NaCl (pH 7.5), 0.1 percent (w/v) gelatin, 0.2 mM ATP, 1 mM Mg acetate, 0.2 mM CaCl$_2$, 0.05 percent NaN$_3$). Thirty drop fractions are collected and actin determined by the DNase I inhibition assay (2). We usually use only the three peak tubes and refer to this material as [^{125}I]actin.

The elution profile of the actin iodination mixture shows two peaks (Fig. 1). The first peak contains iodinated actin which retains biologic activity. It inhibits DNase I and will polymerize under the appropriate conditions. The specific activity of the actin in this peak expressed as the ratio of the cpm/ng of actin averages 1.0 ± 0.3 × 10^3 Ci/mmol or about 0.5 molecules of iodine per molecule of actin. There is no detectable DNase I inhibitory activity in

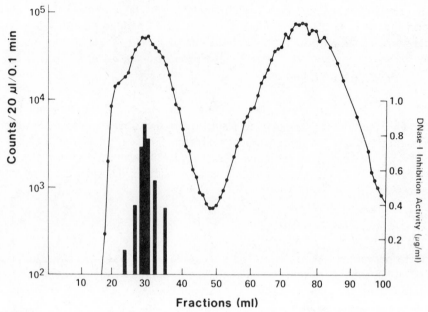

FIGURE 1. The elution profile of an actin iodination mixture applied to a Sephadex G-75 column. Actin was iodinated as described and applied to to a 1.5 × 40-cm Sephadex G-75 column and eluted in 30-drop fractions. Actin in the column fractions was determined by the DNase I inhibition assay, and [^{125}I]iodine was assayed in a γ counter. The micrograms of actin are depicted by the bars from the individual column fractions assayed. The second [^{125}I]iodine peak contain no DNase I inhibition activity.

the second peak. The [^{125}I]actin is diluted to 50,000 cpm/μL with assay buffer and stored at 4°C. This is used for up to 4–6 weeks after iodination.

2.4. Preparation of Cell and Tissue Extracts for Actin Measurements

Cells and tissues for actin measurements are collected on ice and placed in cold lysis buffer containing 0.1 percent Triton X-100 in 90 mM KCl, 2 mM Mg acetate, 0.2 mM ATP, 0.2 mM DTE, 0.1 mM ethylene glycol *bis*(β-aminoethylether)-$N,N,N',N,'$-tetraacetic acid (EGTA), 1.0 mM NaN$_3$, and 10 mM PIPES (pH 6.9). The suspension is then vortexed or homogenized. The lysate is centrifuged at 15,000g for 5 min in an Eppendorf microfuge and the supernatant is collected for meaurement of soluble actin. For measurement of F-actin, the pellet is resuspended in lysis bufer plus an equal volume of the depolymerization buffer, 1.5 M guanidine hydrochloride (Gdn-HCl), 1.0 M Na-acetate, 1.0 mM CaCl$_2$, 1.0 mM ATP, and 20 mM Tris-HCl pH 7.5 (2). After incubation on ice for 10 min to depolymerize actin filaments, the sample is centrifuged at 15,000g for 5 min and the supernatant is used for analysis of actin.

2.5. Actin Assay

The sensitivity of the immunoprecipitation assay can be altered by varying the amount of the ligand, DNase I. We have employed either 2.0 or 17.5 ng of DNase I per assay tube. Actin standards or experimental samples are aliquotted into disposable glass tubes (12 × 75 mm) and brought to a volume of 500 μL with the assay buffer. For the less sensitive assay 17.5 ng of DNase I in 100 μL of assay buffer is added followed by 500 pg of [^{125}I]actin in 100 μL. This mixture is then incubated at 4°C for 2 hr before addition of 100 μL of a 1:10 dilution of anti-DNase I rabbit serum. After 4 hr at 4°C, 100 μL of a 1:2 dilution of sheep anti-rabbit IgG serum is added. After another 4 hr at 4°C, 3.0 mL of phosphate-buffered saline is added. The tubes are centrifuged at 1000g for 30 min, the supernatants are decanted, and the pellets are counted in a γ counter. The more sensitive assay uses 2 ng of DNase I incubated for 4 hr, 100 μL of 1:200 dilution of the anti-DNase I serum for 12 hr, and 100 μL of 1:8 dilution of the second step serum incubated for 8 hr.

It is possible to define nonspecific binding in two ways. In the first, nonspecific binding is considered to be the radioactivity which is not displaced by a 10,000-fold excess of unlabeled actin (5 μg/tube). For practical purposes, to conserve the amount of purified actin used in the assay, nonspecific binding can also be considered to be the radioactivity which is immunoprecipitated in the absence of DNase I. These two values are quite similar. Specific binding in the absence of competitor, defined as B_0, is equal to the difference between the total bound counts and the nonspecific counts divided by the total [^{125}I]actin counts in the assay tube. Specific binding in the presence of competitor, defined as B, is equal to the difference between the counts bound and the nonspecific counts divided by the total [^{125}I]actin counts originally in the assay tube. The statistical analysis and estimates of the unknown actin concentrations are peformed using the computer program of Duddleson et al. (8). This program does a logit transformation, tests for linearity and for parallelism of standards, and unknowns by an analysis of covariance.

All actins tested to date, purified rabbit skeletal muscle, sea urchin, and human platelet actin and cell homogenates from a variety of cell lines and tissue sources dilute in parallel in the assay. The average coefficient of variation of the assay at the 50 percent displacement point is 9 percent. The 17.5 ng assay has 50 percent displacement at 23.7 ± 3.4 ng of actin (± SE, $N = 8$); the assay with greater sensitivity, 2 ng of DNase I, has 50 percent displacement at 2.9 ± 0.3 ng of actin (± SE, $N = 5$). The average assay sensitivity for the 17.5 ng assay defined from the assay median variance ratio (9) is 4.9 ± 1.5 ng (± SE, $N = 5$) while the limit of detection, defined as 1 SE from the buffer control tube, is 1.73 ± 0.33 ng (± SE, $N = 5$). The 2 ng DNase I assay has a sensitivity of 0.24 ng and a limit of detection of 61 pg.

In order to use the binding–immunoprecipitation assay to measure both G- and F-actin, it is necessary to separate these forms before assay and to depolymerize the filamentous actin. The strategy employed is to rapidly and gently lyse the cells with a nonionic detergent and then separate a cytoskeletal fraction by centrifugation at 15,000g for 5 min. The supernatant is either diluted directly for assay or is diluted after incubation with the Gdn-HCl buffer; the F-actin in the cytoskeletal fraction is depolymerized in Gdn-HCl before dilution for assay. This strategy is not unique but does attempt to minimize the potential effects of the redistribution of actin during the initial fractionation. During the assay the concentrations of actin are routinely in the nanogram per milligram range, at least 100 times below the critical concentration for assembly; therefore, the actin remains in a nonfilamentous form available to DNase I. We have tested the low-speed extracts for the presence of additional F-actin by recentrifugation at 100,000g for 120 min. In hamster islets or insulinoma cells, Chinese hamster ovary cells, and sea urchin coelomocytes, we find no difference. Thus, under the lysis conditions employed, the bulk of the filamentous actin in these cells is present in a "cytoskeleton" which is sedimentable at relatively low-gravity forces. It should be noted that the criterion for discriminating G- and F-actin is substantially different from that used by Blikstad et al. (2). The inhibition assay relies upon the substantially higher rate of enzyme binding to G-actin to measure soluble actin in the presence of F-actin.

2.6. Summary

This assay provides a simple rapid method for quantitation of F- and G-actin. The sensitivity is over 1000-fold that of the DNase I inhibition assay and hundreds of samples can be assayed in 2 days. The data analysis is amenable to statistics used in radioimmunoassays and it is unnecessary to purify individual actins from the tissue or species of interest since all α-, β-, or γactins tested to date displace in parallel. DNase I is available in relatively pure form commercially, is highly antigenic, and the use of the DNase I and anti-DNase I obviate the need to characterize individual actin antibodies.

3.   IDENTIFICATION OF ACTIN- OR CALMODULIN-BINDING PROTEINS

A number of proteins which associate with actin have been identified in muscle and nonmuscle cells. Many appear to either regulate the assembly state of actin by binding to either end of actin filaments and altering actin polymerization or by linking actin filaments to cellular organelles like the plasma membrane or secretory granule. Previously, actin-binding proteins have been identified by solution chemical methodology. We developed a simple method to identify actin-binding proteins in cells or tissues (10) by gel-overlay, a technique first used to localize calmodulin-binding proteins (11). Both of these techniques are useful for the study of cytoskeletal proteins in islets or insulinoma cells and are described here. These techniques involve the specific interaction of radiolabeled actin or calmodulin with proteins separated on polyacrylamide gels and derive from a large body of work on the renaturation of proteins after solubilization in SDS.

Calmodulin is a major Ca^{2+}-binding protein found in all eukaryotic cells and appears to be involved in many Ca^{2+}-mediated processes including exocytosis. Since the level of calmodulin in the islet or β cell remains constant when insulin secretion is stimulated (12), identifying the β cell proteins which interact with calmodulin will be of major importance in understanding the role of this ubiquitous protein in secretion. The gel overlay system provides a simple method to identify calmodulin-binding proteins.

3.1. Isolation and Radioiodination of Rabbit Skeletal Muscle Actin

The isolation and radioiodination of the actin used for the label in the overlay procedure is performed as described in the previous section on the actin assay. The molecular weight markers obtained from Pharmacia are labeled using [^{125}I]iodine and the chloramine-T reaction (13). Thus, the molecular weight markers can be seen on both the stained gels and the autoradiographs.

3.2. Purification and Radioiodination of Calmodulin

The bovine testis calmodulin and [^{125}I]calmodulin we use is kindly supplied by J. Chafouleas who prepares the materials as described (14). Furthermore, [^{125}I]calmodulin prepared using these methods is now commercially available (Amersham) either as part of an RIA kit or in 10 or 50-μCi amounts. We have also purchased calmodulin from Calbiochem and iodinated it by the Bolton Hunter procedure (7) as described by Chafouleas et al. (14) and found it also to be satisfactory in the overlay procedure. The [^{125}I]calmodulin is diluted to 150,000 cpm/μL with 50 mM Na phosphate, 1 mg/mL gelatin, 100 mM NaCl, 0.05 percent NaN$_3$, pH 7.5, and stored at 4°C. We have obtained adequate results with 2-month-old tracer.

3.3. Cell Harvest, Homogenization, and Protein Assay

Monolayer cultures of 50–100 million hamster (15) or rat insulinoma cells (16) per flask are rinsed twice with cold phosphate-buffered saline to remove traces of the fetal calf serum supplement in the medium and harvested using a 5-min 37°C incubation with 5 mM EDTA in phosphate-buffered saline, pH 7.4, containing 0.1 mM DIFP and 0.1 mM PMSF as protease inhibitors. Extreme care should be exercised in the handling of solutions containing DIFP and PMSF. Gloves are worn routinely and the 0.1 M stock solutions are pipetted and stored in a fume hood.

Sometimes it is necessary to agitate the flask to release the cells from the surface. The cells are centrifuged at 1000g for 5 min, resuspended in a known volume of isotonic cell extraction buffer (10 mM MES, 5 mM Tris, pH 7.0, containing 0.25 M sucrose, 5 mM MgCl$_2$, 1 mM CaCl$_2$, 0.1 mM PMSF, and 0.1 mM DIFP) and counted. The suspension is recentrifuged and the pellet is resuspended in the same buffer at approximately 50 $\times$ 10^6 cells/mL. The cells are lysed in a Parr nitrogen cavitation bomb (225 psi, 5 min) for subsequent fractionation or sonicated (3 $\times$ 10-sec pulses) on ice for whole extracts. Protein concentrations are measured by the method of Bradford (17) using BSA as standard.

3.4. Gel Electrophoresis

Five to 50 μg protein from cell extracts or fractins are electrophoresed on 0.75- or 1.5-mm thick slab gels prepared using the Laemmli buffer system (18). When analysis on two-dimensional gels is desired, 100–200 μg protein is prepared using the SDS solubilization method of Anderson (19). Equal volumes of sample and solubilization buffer (0.05 M CHES (cyclohexylaminoethanesulfonic acid from Calbiochem), 2 percent (w/v) SDS, 10 percent (v/v) glycerol, 2 percent (v/v) β-mercaptoethanol, pH 9.5) are mixed and heated at 100°C for 5 min. The sample is focused and run in the second dimension as described by O'Farrell (20). When the actin- or calmodulin-binding activity of a relatively pure protein is evaluated, the protein can be either electrophoresed on SDS-containing Laemmli gels or in a Davis non-denaturing gel system (21).

3.5. Gel Overlay

This procedure is essentially that described by Glenney and Weber (11) and Carlin et al. (22). Immediately after electrophoresis, the proteins in the gel are fixed with 40 percent methanol and 10 percent acetic acid for 30 min at room temperature, with gentle shaking. The residual SDS and methanol–acetic acid is removed by washing with 10 percent ethanol. Four 30-min washes using 100 mL/wash or an overnight wash (250 mL) followed by a 30 min wash (250 mL) is sufficient for a 10 mL slab gel. The gel may be held in the 10 percent ethanol for up to 3 days without any adverse effects. The gel is then washed with 0.1 M imidazole, pH 7.0, for 10 min followed by another 10-min incubation in either calmodulin overlay buffer [1 mg/mL BSA fraction V (Sigma) in 20 mM imidazole, pH 7.0, 0.2 M KCl, 0.02 percent NaN$_3$ with 10 μM or 1 mM CaCl$_2$, or 1 mM EGTA] or actin overlay buffer [1 mg/mL BSA fraction V (Sigma) in 20 mM imidazole, pH 7.4, 0.2 M NaCl, 0.2 mM ATP, 1 mM MgCl$_2$, 0.05 percent NaN$_3$ with 0.2 mM or 1 mM CaCl$_2$ or 1 mM EGTA]. The gel is sealed in a polyethylene bag with a minimum volume of overlay buffer (20 mL for a 10 mL slab gel) containing approximately 0.6 μCi [^{125}I]calmodulin/mL or 1.0 μCi of [^{125}I]actin/mL. After 12–16 hr at 4°C with gentle agitation (Nutator), unbound radioactivity is removed by washing the gel for 2–3 days with overlay buffer (250 mL/10 mL gel) at 4°C until the radioactivity in the buffer decreases to background. Five sequential washes of 1-hr, 2 × 2-hr, overnight (12–16-hr), and a final 1-hr duration work well for a 10-mL slab gel. Larger gels take longer and it is important to reduce the radioactivity in the wash buffer to minimize gray background areas on the X-ray film. We have not tested if excessive washing results in the loss of specifically bound tracer from the gel. The gel is briefly rinsed with H_2O to remove the BSA, stained using 0.25 mg/mL Coomassie brilliant blue R250 in fixing solution and destained using the same solution without the dye. The gels are dried under vacuum and exposed for 12–24 hr at −70°C to Kodak X'Omat XAR-5 X-ray film using a DuPont Cronex Lightning Plus intensifying screen.

Gelatin was used in the original [125I]G-actin and [125I]calmodulin gel overlays with admirable results (10, 11). However, the same concentration of BSA (1 mg/mL) used in place of gelatin in the overlay buffers provides even sharper autoradiograms. Carlin et al. (22) showed that the addition of BSA to overlay preincubation buffers resulted in a tenfold increase in [125I]calmodulin binding by specific bands. They postulate that the possible neutralization of static charges, removal of residual denaturants, and blocking of nonspecific sites on the gel by BSA could explain this enhanced binding. However, the reason why BSA is better than gelatin in our hands is unclear. We have not tested the effect of combining gelatin and BSA in the overlay buffers.

We have tested three types of BSA fraction V preparations available from Sigma (A4503, A9647, and A8022) and do find differences in [125I]calmodulin binding using the different preparations. When optimal binding is desired, it is advisable to check the BSA in the overlay buffers using rabbit muscle phosphorylase B as a "standard" calmodulin-binding protein. Phosphorylase B is commercially available as a pure protein (Sigma) or as the 94,000-dalton marker in a molecular weight kit for SDS gels (Pharmacia). Phosphorylase B binds [125I]calmodulin in the overlay procedure and different BSA preparations give a range of 158–438 dpm [125I]calmodulin bound per microgram of protein. The amount of [125I]calmodulin bound is determined by cutting the phosphorylase band out of the dried gel (less background which is determined from an equivalent piece of dried gel with no protein) or by scanning the autoradiograms as described below.

DNase I does not bind in the overlay procedure and we have not found a commercially available standard actin-binding protein. Twenty micrograms of human platelet sonicate (10) shows binding activities predominantly at 90,000 and 40,000 daltons.

3.6. Quantitation of Binding

A standard curve is constructed by electrophoresis of increasing amounts (250–10,000 dpm) of the [125I]calmodulin or [125I]G-actin used in the overlays in a Laemmli slab gel. Unlabeled calmodulin or actin (5–10 μg) is added to each lane to coelectrophorese with the tracer. At the end of the run the gel is stained, destained, dried, and autoradiography is performed as described above. Exposure times are varied (2–20 hr, −70°C) to give multiple determinations of total disintegrations. (For example, 60,00 disintegrations = 250 dpm × 240 min = 500 dpm × 120 min.) Alternatively, replicate gels are prepared for autoradiography. When all the desired autoradiograms are obtained, the bands are excised from the dried gels and counted in a γ counter to determine the actual amounts of radioactivity (dpm) in the bands.

The autoradiograms are scanned on a Kontes Fiber Optic Scanner interfaced with a Hewlett Packard integrator. A standard curve is generated by plotting peak areas (arbitrary units) versus total disintegrations. All peak areas which registered "off scale" on the scanner are discarded. As seen in Figure 2, the linear range of the curve encompasses 0.2 to 1.0×10^6 disintegrations (0.5–4.0 area units). When quantitation of binding is desired, exposure times of autoradiograms from gel overlays are chosen to give peak areas in the linear range of the standard curve.

3.7. Specificity Studies

When an actin- or calmodulin-binding protein is identified, the specificity of binding should be tested using fresh [^{125}I]actin or [^{125}I]calmodulin. Three general criteria should be met: (i) Binding of the tracer should increase when increasing amounts of the binding protein are electrophoresed. (ii) Binding of the tracer should be displaced by preincubation or simultaneous incubation of the gel with the unlabeled protein. In addition, increasing the concentration of the nonradioactive actin or calmodulin in the overlay buffer should result in a corresponding decrease in binding of the iodinated actin or calmodulin

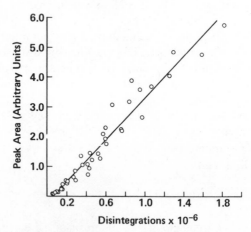

FIGURE 2.   The relationship between the autoradiographic image absorbance and total disintegrations occurring. Exposure from 2–20 hr at −70°C of samples containing from 250–10,000 dpm [^{125}I]calmodulin are represented. Conditions of electrophoresis, autoradiography, and scanning are described in the text. Linear regression analysis of all the points yields a y intercept of −0.18, a slope of 3.39×10^{-6}, and a correlation coefficient r of 0.943.

(Figs. 3 and 4). (iii) Binding of the tracer should be stable to high salt concentrations, 2 M KCl or NaCl instead of the 0.2 M in the overlay buffers. Since actin is thermolabile, heating the [^{125}I]G-actin tracer to 90°C for 3 min totally eliminates binding. In contrast, calmodulin is fairly stable and heating [^{125}I]calmodulin to 100°C for 15 min results in a reduction of binding.

Some actin-binding proteins are Ca^{2+} dependent and show decreased binding with 1 mM EGTA in the overlay buffer. All the "biologically significant" calmodulin-binding proteins should be Ca^{2+} dependent and show slightly less binding with 10 μM instead of 1 mM $CaCl_2$ in the overlay solutions and no binding in the presence of 1 mM EGTA.

In the case of both proteins it is advisable to further establish the relevance of binding by using other independent techniques. For actin we often start with a DNase I–Sepharose affinity column (23) and for calmodulin a calmodulin-Sepharose column (24).

The major advantage in the use of these overlay procedures is that individual binding proteins in complex mixtures can be identified by their relative molecular weights using microgram amounts of cell or tissue extracts. Side-by-side comparisons of binding proteins in different tissues are easily performed (25). Gel overlays are useful in the isolation of a binding protein since fractions from various purification steps can be rapidly screened and binding easily quantitated.

The gel overlay technique is limited to the detection of monomeric proteins which can renature under the conditions used. We do not see binding of [^{125}I]G-

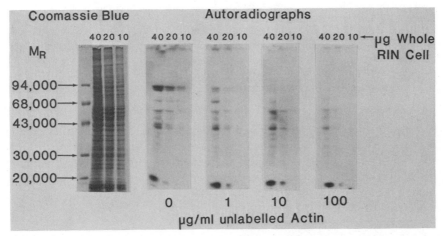

FIGURE 3. The effect of increasing concentrations of unlabeled actin or [^{125}I]actin binding. The first panel shows a Coomassie blue-stained 10 percent polyacrylamide gel with molecular weight markers on the left and 40, 20, and 10 μg whole RIN cell extract. Panels 2–5 are autoradiographs which document the displacement of [^{125}I]actin binding by unlabeled actin. The gels for panels 2–5 were preincubated with 0, 1, 10, or 100 μg/mL unlabeled actin for 8 hr before the addition of 0.1 μg/mL [^{125}I]actin. Similar results are obtained when the unlabeled actin and [^{125}I]actin are added to the gel overlay solution simultaneously.

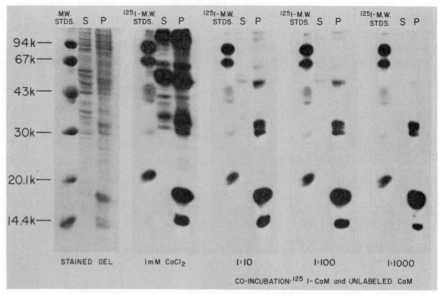

FIGURE 4. The effect of increasing concentrations of unlabeled calmodulin on $[^{125}I]$calmodulin binding. The left panel shows a Coomassie-stained 12.5 percent polyacrylamide gel with 20 μg each of a 1500g supernatant (S) and pellet (P); the second panel shows a control autoradiograph with no unlabeled calmodulin in the overlay solution. All overlay solutions contain 1.7 nM of $[^{125}I]$calmodulin (10^6 cpm/mL) and 1 mM $CaCl_2$. The next three panels show the autoradiographs with a 10-fold (17 nM), 100-fold (170 nM), and 1000-fold (1700 nM) excess of unlabeled calmodulin in the overlay solutions. The molecular weight markers electrophoresed in the first lane in each panel have been iodinated and are seen in both the Coomassie-stained gel and the autoradiographs. Note that a 10-fold excess of unlabeled calmodulin displaces almost all the $[^{125}I]$calmodulin binding activities in the supernatant. The putative histone bands in the pellet fraction account for the only remaining bands of binding activity observed at a 1000-fold excess of unlabeled calmodulin. The intensity of the bands corresponding to the molecular weight standards in constant for all four autoradiograms. This documents that the exposure time for all overlays was equivalent.

actin to purified DNase I or the high-molecular-weight actin-binding protein and myosin (26) found in human platelet extracts. Carlin (22) reports that troponin-I, which binds calmodulin in other assays, does not show binding in the gel overlay. When screening for binding activities, it is advisable to employ binding protein standards such as platelet extract for actin overlays and phosphorylase B for calmodulin overlays.

3.8. Summary

The actin and calmodulin overlay procedures provide a relatively simple means of identifying actin- or calmodulin-binding proteins for study of the role of these proteins from tissues or cells.

REFERENCES

1. R. T. Tregear and J. M. Squire, *J. Mol. Biol.* **77**, 279 (1973).

2. I. Blikstad, F. Markey, L. Carlsson, T. Persson, and U. Lindberg, *Cell* **15**, 935 (1978).

3. J. L. Morgan, C. R. Holladay, and B. S. Spooner, *Proc. Natl. Acad. Sci. USA* **77**, 2069 (1980).

4. M. C. Snabes, A. E. Boyd III, R. L. Pardue, and J. Bryan, *J. Biol. Chem.* **256**, 6291 (1981).

5. J. A. Spudich and S. Watt, *J. Biol. Chem.* **246**, 4866 (1971).

6. J. D. Pardee and J. A. Spudich, in *Methods in Enzymology*, Vol. 85, D. W. Frederiksen and L. W. Cunningham (eds.), Academic Press, New York, 1982, p. 164.

7. A. E. Bolton and W. M. Hunter, *Biochem. J.* **133**, 529 (1973).

8. W. G. Duddleson, A. R. Midgley, Jr., and G. D. Niswender, *Comput. Biomed. Res.* **5**, 205 (1972).

9. E. Wang and A. Goldberg, *J. Histochem. Cytochem.* **26**, 745 (1978).

10. M. C. Snabes, A. E. Boyd III, and J. Bryan, *J. Cell Biol.* **90**, 809 (1981).

11. J. R. Glenney and K. Weber, *J. Biol. Chem.* **255**, 10551 (1980).

12. T. Y. Nelson, J. Oberwetter, J. Chafouleas, and A. E. Boyd III, *Diabetes* **32**, 1126 (1983).

13. A. E. Boyd III, W. E. Bolton, and B. R. Brinkley, *J. Cell Biol.* **92**, 425 (1982).

14. J. G. Chafouleas, J. R. Dedman, and A. R. Means in *Methods in Enzymology*, Vol. 84, J. L. Langone and H. van Vunakis (eds.), Academic Press, New York, 1982, p. 138.

15. R. F. Santerre, R. A. Cook, R. M. D. Crisel, J. D. Sharp, R. J. Schmidt, D. C. Williams, and C. P. Wilson, *Proc. Natl. Acad. Sci. USA* **78**, 4339 (1981).

16. A. F. Gazdar, W. L. Chick, H. K. Oie, H. L. Sims, D. L. King, G. C. Weir, and V. Lauris, *Proc. Natl. Acad. Sci. USA* **77**, 3519 (1980).

17. M. M. Bradford, *Anal. Biochem.* **72**, 248 (1976).

18. U. K. Laemmli, *Nature (London)* **227**, 680 (1970).

19. N. G. Anderson, N. L. Anderson, and S. L. Tollaksen, Argonne Nat'l Lab Publication 79-2.

20. P. H. O'Farrell, *J. Biol. Chem.* **250**, 4007 (1975).

21. B. J. Davis, *Ann. N.Y. Acad. Sci.* **121**, 404 (1964).

22. R. K. Carlin, D. J. Grab, and P. Siekevitz, *J. Cell Biol.* **89**, 449 (1981).

23. F. Markey, T. Persson, and U. Lindberg, *Cell* **23**, 145 (1981).

24. J. R. Dedman, M. J. Welsh, and A. R. Means, *J. Biol. Chem.* **253**, 7515 (1978).

25. M. C. Snabes, A. E. Boyd III, and J. Bryan, *Exp. Cell Res.* **146**, 63 (1983).

26. K. Wang, J. F. Ash, and S. J. Singer, *Proc. Natl. Acad. Sci. USA* **12**, 83 (1975).

H

INTRAINSULAR REGULATION OF ISLET FUNCTION

H. SCHATZ AND G. SCHAFER

Center of Internal Medicine, University of Giessen, Giessen, Federal Republic of Germany

1. INTRODUCTION

The islets of Langerhans can be regarded as a disseminated endocrine organ composed of various cell types producing several hormonal peptides. One of them, insulin, has been studied most extensively. It is stored within the granules of the β cells. However, the maintenance of the steady state—that is, the interrelations between biosynthesis, release, and intracellular degradation of insulin within the islets—is not fully understood. On the other hand, the neighborhood of α, β, and δ cells (and PP cells) might result in direct local (paracrine) interactions between these cells. Although evidence has been accumulated that islet hormones may influence the function of islet cells producing other hormones, these experiments were mostly performed with *in vivo* administration or *in vitro* addition of exogenous hormones, leaving open the question of a physiological (paracrine) role of endogenously produced islet hormones for their neighboring cells.

2. GENERAL METHODS FOR STUDY OF ISLET FUNCTION WITH ISOLATED ISLETS

For studying intrainsular regulation of islet function with isolated islets, the following methods were used by us: static incubation, static culture, perifusion, and perifusion culture. Independent of the method applied, the procedure of islet isolation was always the same and will be briefly described first.

Two hours prior to decapitation, rats (150–200 g) are injected intraperitoneally with 0.5 mL of a solution of pilocarpine (2 percent). Before being removed, the pancreas is filled via the pancreatic duct with 2–5 mL of ice-cold Krebs–Ringer bicarbonate buffer (KRB buffer) containing aprotinine (Trasylol 800 kallikrein-inactivator units/mL) and 2.7 mmol/L glucose. The pancreas is minced by scissors or tissue chopper, and the mince is incubated in a collagenase–albumin solution with magnetic stirring at 37°C (for each pancreas, 20 mg collagenase and 10 mg bovine serum albumin are dissolved in 1 mL KRB buffer). During the 15–30-min digestion (depending on the type of collagenase) we check aliquots of the tissue to determine the time when most of the islets are free of acinar tissue, and then stop the digestion by adding ice-cold KRB buffer to the incubation mixture. After three washings with buffer the islets are collected under a dissecting (stereo-) microscope with Pasteur pipettes, or micropipettes. Petri dishes with bottoms painted black facilitate the recognition of islets.

2.1. Static Incubation of Islets

To carry out static incubations, isolated islets are transferred by pipetting to glass test tubes (total volume, 12 mL) containing usually 1 mL of buffer used for islet isolation (see above). When the same number of islets is present in all tubes, buffer is carefully removed using Eppendorf pipettes, and 1 mL of incubation buffer is added, consisting of KRB buffer containing 10 mg albumin/mL. To obtain the desired glucose concentration a 10 percent glucose solution is used. Studies of islet function are usually carried out at certain specific concentrations of D-glucose: 2.7 mmol/L (50 mg/dL), a low, substimulatory concentration; 5.6 or 8.3 mmol/L ($\triangleq$ 100 or 150 mg/dL), concentrations in the physiological range; and 11.1 or 16.7 mmol/L ($\triangleq$ 200 or 300 mg/dL), strongly stimulating concentrations.

For the study of insulin biosynthesis, the incubation buffer is further supplemented with 20 μg/mL of each of the following amino acids: Ala, Arg, Asp, Cys, Gln, Gly, His, Ile, Leu, Lys, Met, Pro, Ser, Thr, Tyr, Val. When estimating hormone synthesis by measuring the rate of incorporation of tritiated amino acids into islet proteins, the respective unlabeled amino acid is omitted. In our laboratory, we use two tracers: [^{3}H]leucine (20 μCi/mL) and [^{3}H]phenylalanine (50 μCi/mL). We usually take 5–10 islets per test tube containing 1 mL of buffer for studying insulin release. For studies of somatostatin release or insulin biosynthesis batches of 20–30 islets in 1 mL give reliable results.

When studying the influence of a wide variety of agents (Table 1) control tubes contain islets in buffer containing only the specified concentration of glucose. Whereas the incubation buffer of the experimental tubes is supplemented with the substances to be tested. In static incubations we have studied insulin release and/or biosynthesis under the influence of the agents listed in Table 1. Table 2 lists our studies on islet function under a variety of special conditions affecting the islets.

Prior to starting incubations, aliquots were taken for various analyses, tubes were gassed for 15 sec with O_2/CO_2 = 95:5 percent v/v (Carbogen), and then stoppered. Incubations were carried out in a metabolic shaking water bath (37°C) at 50 strokes/minute. Usually, incubation periods of 2 or 3 hr were chosen and samples taken hourly. Whenever tubes were unstoppered to remove samples, gassing with Carbogen was repeated.

Static incubations were performed not only with freshly isolated islets but also with islets maintained in static organ culture (precultivated islets). Concerning static with freshly isolated islets used in static incubations a prior period of preincubation (e.g., for 30 min) at a low or a medium glucose concentration may be useful to allow islets to recover from the isolation procedure.

2.2. Static Culture of Islets

For longer term culture experiments, we carry out the islet isolation under aseptic conditions: that is, isolation buffer is sterile-filtered and glassware and instruments are autoclaved. After separately incising the skin and peritoneum of the rat, the incision is covered with a sterile piece of cloth, open in the center to allow removal of the pancreas. Cultivated islets demonstrate well-

TABLE 1. Agents Tested in Our Laboratory on Isolated Pancreatic Islets Regarding Biosynthesis, Release, and Degradation of (pro-) Insulin and Release of Other Islet Hormones

Substance	Tested Concentrations	References
Glucose	0.5, 1, 1.5, 2, 3 mg/mL	1, 2
Mannoheptulose	3 mg/mL	3
2-Desoxyglucose	3 mg/L	3
Arginine	1–10 mmol/L	4, 5, 6
Leucine	1–10 mmol/L	4, 7
Lysine	1–10 mmol/L	5, 6
Amino acid mixture		8
Insulin	200 μU/mL; 2.5, 5, 25 mU/mL	3, 9–11
Anti-insulin serum	5, 10 μL/mL, binding capacity 5 mU (200 ng) insulin/mL	11, 12
Glucagon	5, 10 μg/mL	2, 8, 13, 14
Anti-glucagon serum	3.5 μL/mL binding capacity 2.5 ng glucagon/mL	12
Somatostatin	1, 10, 100, 1000 ng/mL	14, 15
Anti-somatostatin serum	5 μL/mL, binding capacity 10 ng somatostatin/mL	12
TRH	10^{-13}–10^{-5} g/mL	16
Anti-TRH serum	10 μg/mL, binding capacity 45 ng TRH/mL	16
Growth hormone	50 μg/mL	17
Human placental lactogen	50 μg/mL	17
ACTH	50 mU/mL	17
GIP	5 μg/mL	8
Secretin	0.2 U/mL	13
Pancreocymin	0.75 Ivy-U/mL	13
Gastrin	1 μg/mL	13
cAMP (db)	1, 10 mM	2, 15
Theophylline	1, 2.5, 10 mM	2, 15
Met-enkephalin	$2 \times 10^{-6}\ M$	18
DAMME	2×10^{-6}, $10^{-5}\ M$	18
β-Endorphin	$10^{-8}\ M$	18
β-Casomorphin-5	10^{-7}, $10^{-6}\ M$	18
Naloxon	$10^{-5}\ M$	18
Calcium omission	—	3, 5, 19, 20
Calcium increase	5 mmol/L	5, 20
Verapamil	8 μM	5, 20
Diazoxide	100 μg/mL	3, 5, 9, 20
Chlorprotixen	40–100 mmol/L	21
Lithium	15 mmol/L	22
Puromycin	10 μg/mL	3

TABLE 1. (*cont.*)

Substance	Tested Concentrations	References
Streptozotocin	200 µg/mL	23
α-Neuraminidase		24
β-Galactosidase		24
Hexosaminidase		24
Concanavalin A	0.4, 0.8, 2, 4 mg/mL	25
Tolbutamide	100, 250, 500 µg/mL	1, 6, 26, 27
Glibenclamide	2.5, 5, 10 µg/mL	1, 6, 19, 26, 27
HB 699	10, 50, 100 µg/mL	19, 22
Metformin	0.1–10 000 µg/mL	28
Phenformin	0.1–10 000 µg/mL	28

preserved function if kept free-floating during culture (39, 40). Plastic dishes from NUNC (Roskilde, Denmark) prevent attachment of islets and are therefore used. Each dish (diameter, 5 cm) is filled with 5 mL of medium RPMI 1640 and 1 mL heat-inactivated (56°C) newborn calf serum, yielding a final serum concentration of 16.7 percent. Medium is supplemented with 100 IU penicillin and 100 µg streptomycin/mL. Medium RPMI 1640 usually contains 11.1 mmol glucose/L (200 mg/dL).

For studying islet function also at lower glucose concentrations, we purchase a glucose-free medium RPMI 1640 (from GIBCO, Glasgow) and add appropriate amounts of a 10 percent glucose solution to obtain the desired glucose concentration. The respective test substances are added last. After transfer of islets to the Petri dishes containing medium, they are placed in an incubator with a humidified atmosphere of 5 percent CO_2 to 95 percent air at 37°C. Islets are cultivated usually for 2–3 days, however long-term culture studies have

TABLE 2.   Studies on Islet Function under Special Conditions Performed in Our Laboratory

Experimental Model	References
Fetal and newborn rats	16, 29
Sucrose fed rats	30, 31
Sulfonylurea treated rats	32
Growth hormone and ACTH treated normal rats	33
Hypophysectomized rats	17, 34, 35
Thyroidectomized rats	36
Genetically "diabetic" mice (gg diab)	30
Streptozotocin diabetic rats	37
Cryopreserved islets	38

been successfully performed in our laboratory for up to 6 weeks (5). Culture also improves β cell function after cryopreservation of islets (38).

2.3. Perifusion of Islets

Unlike static incubations, perifusion of isolated islets allows monitoring of dynamic aspects of islet function. This method is based on the principle of a continuous stream of medium surrounding the islets placed in an appropriate chamber. Medium leaving the islets (effluent) is collected in equal fractions for determination of the desired measurement (e.g., insulin, glucagon, or somatostatin). Islets are placed in sterile filter units (diameter, 13 mm; Millipore), the original filter of which is replaced by nylon gauze (pore size, 1 μm). Medium is transported from the reservoir flasks to the chambers through silicone tubing (inside diameter, 0.5 mm) and medium flow is kept constant by a six-channel peristaltic pump. For studies of insulin release, we employ a flow rate of 0.5 mL/min; for somatostatin flow rate is adjusted to 0.25 mL/min. Each chamber has two inlet tubes, one containing control medium, the other test medium. By means of three-way stopcocks either control or test medium reaches the chamber and is collected as effluent, the other medium being allowed to recirculate to its reservoir flask. Flasks, chambers, and as much tubing as possible are immersed in a water bath at 37°C. Media are continuously gassed with Carbogen to maintain physiologic pH. Care must be taken to insure that no air bubbles enter the chamber, since islets might then be removed from the system.

2.4. Perifusion Culture of Islets

The perifusion system described above has also been used by us to maintain islets during culture. For this purpose all parts of the system coming in contact with incubation and culture media are sterilized. Gassing of media is done directly as described whereas in the perifusion culture system of Gingerich et al. (41) CO_2 exchange in a gas chamber occurs through the tubing.

2.5. Extraction of Islets for Determination of Total Insulin

Insulin extraction from islets was performed according to the method of Davoren (42). Insulin was determined mainly after culture of islets in order to estimate the effect of long-term exposure to a stimulator or an inhibitor of insulin release and/or biosynthesis. After culture, islets were transferred to test tubes, washed with KRB buffer which was then totally removed. Four hundred microliters of acidic ethanol [1 mL HCl concentration in 50 mL ethanol (95 percent)] and 200 μL distilled H_2O were added and tubes were kept at 4°C overnight. On the next day, after sonication, aliquots were frozen after appropriate dilution with albumin-containing KRB buffer for radioimmunological insulin determination.

2.6.   Methods for Studying Insulin Biosynthesis in Isolated Islets

Measurement of the rate of incorporation of radioactively labeled amino acids into islet proteins is the technique most commonly employed to study insulin biosynthesis. Preferably, tritiated L-leucine or tritiated L-phenylalanine are used as tracers. Proinsulin of most mammals contains a high number of leucine-residues, but phenylalanine, in contrast to leucine, is barely oxidized in islet tissue (43). It should always be kept in mind that changes in the specific radioactivity of the intracellular free amino acid pool might be responsible for, or contribute to the measured data for amino acid incorporation. No such changes, however, were found for glucose, glucagon, and tolbutamide (13). After incubation of islets in the presence of the test substance and tracer amino acid, (pro-) insulin is separated from other islet proteins. Several separation techniques have been employed by us: column separation and two methods employing immunoprecipitation.

2.6.1.   SEPARATION BY COLUMN CHROMATOGRAPHY

The method is based on separating islet proteins according to their molecular weights. In the elution diagram three peaks appear. The first represents noninsulin proteins (high molecular weight, MW), the second proinsulin (MW~9000), and the third insulin (MW~6000). Sephadex G-50 fine or Biogel P-30 can be used as the stationary phase together with an acidic liquid phase. To prepare islet samples for column chromatography, we submit them to sonication (15 sec, 100W, at + 4°C), add 1 mg of pork insulin and 0.5 mL trichloroacetic acid (TCA, 30 percent), and maintain for 15 min at 4°C for precipitation. After centrifugation at 3600 rpm for 10 min, the supernatant is discarded and the precipitate dissolved in 1 mL of 1 M acetic acid. Samples are then applied on Sephadex G-50 fine columns (55–60 cm length, 1.2 cm inside diameter) and eluted with 1 M acetic acid. Samples (of 1 mL each) are collected with fraction collectors and 100 μL aliquots mixed with 5 mL of scintillator gel and radioactivity counted in a liquid scintillation spectrometer. Between separations, columns are eluted with 0.5 mL of a 2.5 percent (w/v) albumin–acetic acid solution for displacement of any radioactivity attached to the surfaces and the gel.

2.6.2.   ESTIMATION OF INSULIN BIOSYNTHESIS BY THE SEPHAROSE 4B TECHNIQUE

This method, first described by Berne (44), separates proinsulin and insulin from other islet proteins by binding to insulin antibodies (AIS) coupled to cyanogen-bromide-activated Sepharose 4B (AIS-Sepharose). For estimation of nonspecific binding, Sepharose 4B treated with normal guinea pig serum (GPS) is used (GPS-Sepharose). To prepare samples, the labeled media are withdrawn from the islets after incubation. Islets are then washed twice with a buffer (0.1 M NaCl, 0.04 M NaH$_2$PO$_4$·H$_2$O, = "buffer B") containing an excess of nonlabeled amino acid (the same as used for tracer) and frozen in 200 μL of that buffer. After thawing and sonication (see above), 100 μL of homogenate is diluted 1:7 with buffer B containing 0.5 percent (w/v) bovine serum albumin. Then 100 μL of the diluted sample is incubated with AIS- or GPS-treated Sepharose 4B in plastic tubes with rotation. After centrifugation and three washings with albumin–buffer B, the sediment is dissolved in 800 μL of a tissue solubilizer and transferred to liquid scintillation tubes.

For estimation of newly synthesized islet total protein, 1 mL of 5 percent TCA is added to 100 μL of the diluted sample. The mixture is allowed to precipitate for 1 hr at 4°C. After centrifugation, the sediment is treated further as described above.

For each new preparation of AIS-Sepharose, the respective binding capacity is determined using islet homogenates containing a tracer dose of [^{125}I]insulin. The amount of AIS-Sepharose yielding a more than 90 percent binding of immunoreactive material is then used for the following sample measurements.

2.6.3. PROTEIN A–SEPHAROSE C1-4B TECHNIQUE

This method is also based on immunoprecipitation of hormone, but in contrast with the Sepharose 4B method, formation of antigen–antibody complexes occurs first, followed by binding of the complexes to the Sepharose beads. Since this method gives lower nonspecific binding, we prefer it to the Sepharose 4B technique previously described. Islet samples are prepared in the same way. For incubation and washing, a glycine-albumin buffer is used: 1.5 g glycine, 0.26 g bovine serum albumin, 500 μL of the detergent Nonidet NP 40 per 100 mL, pH 9.00 (= "GA-buffer"). After sonication, 20 μL aliquots are pipetted into plastic tubes, together with 20 μL anti-insulin serum (AIS) or normal guinea pig serum (GPS, both diluted 1:7 with GA buffer) and 200 μL GA buffer (see above). After vortexing, the mixture is incubated for 1 hr at room temperature. Thereafter, 200 μL GA buffer containing 10 mg protein A–Sepharose are added. Tubes are stoppered and kept rotating for 15 min. After adding 1 mL GA buffer, tubes are centrifuged for 5 min at 3000 rpm and 21°C. The supernatant is discarded and this washing procedure repeated twice.

The sediment is suspended in 300 μL of 1 M acetic acid (0.5 percent bovine serum albumin) and transferred to a liquid scintillation vial. The tubes are rinsed with another 300 μL of the albumin–acetic acid. After adding 10 mL of Bioflour, radioactivity of the sample is counted in a liquid scintillation spectrometer. To estimate the incorporation rate of the tracer amino acid into total islet protein, 1 mL of TCA (5 percent) is added to 20 μL of the islet homogenate. The precipitates (1 hr at 4°C) are centrifuged and transferred with 600 μL of 1 M acetic acid into scintillation vials.

2.7. Methods for Studying Insulin Release from Isolated Islets

There are two different techniques for the study of insulin release which have already been mentioned above:

1. Static incubation of islets. Only relatively few aliquots of the media are taken at certain time intervals for determination of hormone content.
2. Perifusion of islets. This allows one to follow the dynamic pattern of insulin release continuously.

Both methods can be applied to freshly isolated as well as to cultured islets. By keeping islets in a perifusion system under culture conditions the dynamics of hormone release before and after a culture period can be compared without further manipulation of the islets.

2.8. Methods for Studying Intrainsular Insulin Degradation

For the study of intrainsular insulin degradation, islets prelabeled radioactively during culture can be used. In our experiments the procedure described by Halban et al. (45–49) was applied with some modification. Batches of 50 islets are cultivated for 3 days in 8.3 mM (150 mg/dL) glucose in the presence of 100 μCi [^{3}H]leucine (or 150 μCi [^{3}H]phenylalanine). Thereafter, all islets are washed three times in KRB buffer and a representative portion of islets is frozen in "buffer B" (see above). Remaining islets are divided between two or three new dishes containing control or test medium (e.g., test medium— 2.7 mM glucose and 100 μg diazoxide/mL; control medium—without diazoxide) and cultivated for another 24 hr in "cold" medium without radioactive amino acids. Content of labeled (pro-)insulin is then determined in the islets frozen after the prelabeling period, in islets further kept in cold medium, and in aliquots (50 μL) of medium. The amount of labeled hormone measured in islets after prelabeling is taken as an "initial value" (expressed as cpm per islet). The difference between this value and the sum of (pro-) insulin-bound radioactivity detected in islets and in media after the chase period (also calculated as cpm per islet) represents a measure of the amount of hormone degraded during the chase period. The greater the difference, the greater the degree of insulin degradation within the islets (degradation of insulin in media can be regarded as negligible).

2.9. Methods for Studying Paracrine Regulatory Mechanisms

Two approaches to study paracrine mechanisms within pancreatic islets have been used: addition of exogenous islet hormones to the incubation media containing isolated islets or addition of specific hormone antisera in vitro (see also Table 1). These experiments were performed in static (short-term and long-term) as well as in dynamic systems (see Sections 2.1–2.3). Short-term static incubations were done for 1–3 hr in 2.7 or 16.7 mM glucose. In studies on somatostatin release, a glucose concentration of 8.3 mM was also used. For perifusion experiments, 8.3 mM was the only glucose concentration employed. Here, flow rate was 0.25 mL/min and 2-min fractions were collected. Before the test agent (rat insulin or insulin antiserum) was introduced into the system, islets were preperifused with control medium for 30 min to achieve a constant level of hormone release. Perifusion with the test agent was then performed for an additional 30 min. According to our experience, hormone antisera should always be tested for specificity before use. For example, in a commercially available somatostatin antiserum we found cross-reactivity with glucagon (12).

3. SPECIAL STUDIES ON INTERRELATIONS BETWEEN BIOSYNTHESIS, RELEASE, AND DEGRADATION OF INSULIN

Using static incubation of islets for several hours, it can be seen that unlike, for example, glucose or leucine (1, 2, 4) several agents do not stimulate insulin biosynthesis although they do enhance release. With sulfonylureas, especially tolbutamide, an inhibition of [^{3}H]leucine and arginine uptake into proinsulin and insulin can be observed at a lower glucose concentration (1, 10), which appears not to be due to changes in the intracellular free leucine pool within the islets (13). Such changes must always be considered in incorporation studies. Similar findings as with tolbutamide were observed with the amino acid arginine (6) and with the insulin secretagogue HB 699 (19, 22). On the other hand, inhibition of insulin release by calcium omission (3, 20) or by the addition of diazoxide or verapamil (20) did not reduce insulin biosynthesis during 3 hr.

From a teleologic point of view the question arises whether a depleted— or overfilled—storage pool (e.g., after sulfonylureas and calcium omission, respectively) signals an increase or reduction of insulin biosynthesis later on, in order to maintain a steady rate in the insulin storage pool. A reduced—or enhanced—intrainsular insulin degradation might be an additional regulatory mechanism. To answer this question the technique of islet culture can be used. Substances which stimulate or inhibit insulin release were added during several days of islet culture and insulin biosynthesis or degradation was determined. Some agents apparently do not disturb islet function during short-term incubations. However, they might strongly depress islet function during longer culture periods. This has been observed with arginine and tolbutamide (4, 26). This can, at least in part, be overcome by shortening the culture period or by interposing a culture period without these agents in order to wash out inhibitory substances and/or to restore islet function (26).

Islets can be monitored during culture by simple counting under a stereomicroscope. In the presence of 10 mmol arginine, the number of islets does not decrease during 40 hr of culture. Sudden increases in insulin content of culture media during culture indicates leakage from deteriorated islets. A markedly decreased incorporation of labeled tracer amino acids into proinsulin/insulin or into the nonhormonal islet proteins (reflecting general protein synthesis) is a sign of nonspecific alteration of islets (6).

Such studies have produced evidence that the reduction of insulin release (by the omission of Ca^{2+} or by the addition of diazoxide and verapamil over

2 days) results in a feedback inhibition of (pro-) insulin biosynthesis (20). That is, studies on islets cultured in the presence of insulin secretagogues (e.g., sulfonylureas or arginine) which do not augment insulin biosynthesis (4, 26) have not provided evidence for such a feedback regulation: no compensatory increase in (pro-) insulin biosynthesis was observed after 2 days. It may be that other concentrations of these agents and/or glucose or other times should be used to detect this type of regulation.

Another approach is to administer such substances *in vivo* for longer periods [e.g., sulfonylureas have been administered to rodents for over several months (32)] and to study insulin content and islet function thereafter. Interestingly, reduced islet insulin content found *in vivo* after tolbutamide administration for several months corresponded to the reduced rate of insulin biosynthesis in *in vitro* experiments with tolbutamide present for several hours or days (27).

Intraislet insulin degradation should also be considered as one regulatory mechanism for maintaining a steady state of insulin storage pools. Prelabeled islets prepared, for example, by culturing islets with radioactive amino acids for 72 hr, can be used for studies of secretion. Following a second culture period, the remaining intact labeled hormone within the islets and the culture media can be estimated by appropriate immune binding techniques (see above). Using such techniques, it has been shown that insulin degradation is prevented by glucose-stimulated insulin release (45–47). From experiments with diazoxide to block insulin release, it appears that it is rather the concentration of glucose (and leucine) *per se*, and not the secretory process as such, that prevents intrainsular insulin from degradation within the islets (7).

Another approach to the study of insulin degradation is morphological examination. Ultrastructural changes in the β cell indicating an intracellular digestion of insulin granules have been observed in studies with diazoxide administered *in vivo* (48). Similarly, intracellular insulin degradation was correlated with ultrastructural alteration of islet lysosomes (49). Findings obtained by functional and morphological techniques, however, are not always in full agreement (7, 46, 49). Enzymes catalyzing insulin catabolism have been demonstrated in pancreatic islets (50, 51), including the thiol-protein disulfide oxidoreductase. If it is possible to prove its direct implication in the regulation of insulin content in pancreatic islets, measurement of its activity under various conditions might be an additional way to study insulin degradation within the β cell.

4. SPECIAL STUDIES ON PARACRINE REGULATION OF ISLET FUNCTION AND ON DIRECT FEEDBACK MECHANISMS

Administration of islet hormones both *in vivo* and *in vitro* has shown that the function of one type of islet cells can be influenced by hormonal products of the other islet cell types. In isolated islets an enhancing effect of glucagon on insulin and biosynthesis release was found (2; cf. 52, 53) as well as an inhibiting effect of insulin on α cell function (cf. 54) and an inhibition by somatostatin of insulin and of glucagon release (14, 15, 55–57, 87; cf. 58). However, the effect of insulin on pancreatic δ cell function has remained a matter for discussion.

Pancreas perifusion with exogenous insulin resulted in either unaltered (59–61) or inhibited (62, 63) release of somatostatin. Using isolated islets, Schauder et al. (64) did not observe a direct effect of insulin on δ cell function. In short-term incubation or perifusion studies with isolated islets, we were unable to detect any change in somatostatin release at low (2.7 mM), medium (8.3 mM), or high (16.7 mM) glucose concentration (11). Decreased somatostatin content in the medium from islets in culture in the presence of insulin gave rise to the suggestion that the culture conditions restored δ cell insulin receptors which had probably been altered by the collagenase treatment. When freshly isolated islets were precultured for 2 days and then tested in static or in dynamic incubations, a small inhibiting effect of exogenous insulin on somatostatin release became apparent (9).

Experiments with exogenous hormones, however, do not definitely answer the question concerning a local physiological effect of endogenously released islet hormones. Therefore, the action of immune-binding antisera on the content of endogenous islet hormones provides another way to study intraislet paracrine mechanisms. *In vivo* administration of somatostatin antiserum failed to affect insulin levels (65), a finding which can be interpreted as supporting the assumption of local actions of somatostatin within the pancreatic islets. In isolated islets the presence of somatostatin antiserum resulted in an enhancement of glucose- or leucine-induced insulin release. This occurred not only when the antiserum was added during a preincubation period before the test period (66, 67), but also when it was present during the test incubation (12). It should be noted, however, that differences were found depending on the glucose concentration. For example, after preincubation with somatostatin antiserum, insulin release was increased at low and medium but not at high glucose concentrations. When antiserum was present during the test, an increased insulin content in the medium was observed only at high (16.7 mM) but not at low (2.7 mM)(12) or medium (5.6 mM) glucose concentration (68). After addition of somatostatin antiserum to isolated islets, a stimulation of glucagon release was also observed (68).

In the presence of glucagon antiserum, the release of both insulin and somatostatin was greatly diminished (12). With statically incubated islets, somatostatin release was unchanged by insulin antiserum present at different glucose concentrations (12, 69). In perifusion experiments the administration of insulin antiserum caused a decreased somatostatin content of the effluant (9). The observation of Khokher et al. (70) that commercial γ-globulin and human immunoglobulin G preparations caused an insulinlike stimulation of lipogenesis in isolated adipocytes might provide an explanation for this— unexpected—result. Likewise, antiidiotypic antibodies, which might also exert insulinlike actions, could have been present in the insulin antiserum used in our experiments. Therefore, results obtained with hormone antisera should always be interpreted with caution regarding paracrine mechanisms.

In addition to the use of hormones or hormone antisera, destruction of β cells by certain agents can be useful in the study of intraislet paracrine mechanisms. For example, Patel and Weir (71) reported increased somatostatin content in islets of streptozotocin-diabetic rats, and Schusdziarra et al. (72) observed higher plasma levels of somatostatin in alloxan-diabetic dogs compared to normal dogs, suggesting a suppressive effect of insulin on the δ cell in the healthy state. However, it cannot be fully excluded that other islet cell types are also altered to some extent by these agents.

In conclusion, the results of the types of studies described above suggest multiple paracrine interactions of islet cells and their hormonal products: stimulation of α and δ cell function by glucagon, inhibition of α and β cell function by somatostatin and inhibition of α (and probably δ) cell function by insulin.

In the past several other (hormonal) peptides have been reported to be present within pancreatic islets, but their existence has not been definitely proven, apart from pancreatic polypeptide. However, immunoreactivity for thyrotropin-releasing hormone (TRH) has been found by several authors including ourselves (16) in quite large amounts within fetal and newborn islets, decreasing later in life. Studies of the effects of addition of TRH or TRH antiserum to isolated islets (cf. Table 1), on the other hand, have yielded negative or only small (of borderline significance) effects on insulin release; that is, somewhat higher in the presence of TRH and lower following the addition of TRH antiserum (16). An increase in arginine-stimulated glucagon release was also observed (73) as well as a decreased release of TRH from cultivated rat islets in the presence of somatostatin (74). Although it is attractive to speculate that local TRH might counteract local somatostatin action in paracrine regulation of islet cell function, there is as yet insufficient experimental evidence to support such a hypothesis.

A special problem in the field of intraislet paracrine interactions is the question of a direct feedback inhibition of insulin (also proinsulin and C-peptide) on β cell function. This is still unsettled, as is the question of possible analogous local effects of the other islet hormones on their own cellular sites of production. Addition of insulin or insulin antiserum to isolated islets did not result in a change in insulin release (10, 75; for a review, see 76) or in an altered rate of (pro-) insulin biosynthesis (3, 12). On the other hand, a reduction in the presence of exogenous insulin of glucose-stimulated insulin secretion *in vitro* has been reported (77–79). Ziegler et al. (79) have observed an enhancement of insulin output in the presence of insulin antibodies. However, it should be noted that different methods of insulin determination were used in these studies. Malaisse et al. (75) measured the quantity of unneutralized insulin antibodies, while Ziegler et al. (79) separated insulin from its antibody and determined free insulin by radioimmunoassay. Decreased insulin secretion was also reported to occur in *in vitro* experiments after administration of proinsulin (80) or homologous C-peptide (81).

Using morphological parameters, different results were obtained on the effect of insulin antibodies administered *in vivo* or *in vitro*. Complete degranulation of β cells was observed after infusion of insulin antiserum to rats (48, 82). On the other hand, islet ultrastructure was reported to be similar in control and antiserum-treated islets after 14 days of islet culture (57), with no difference in insulin release.

Another approach to study the problem is measurement of C-peptide release— for example, during insulin infusion in vivo, since C-peptide and insulin are released from β cells in equimolar amounts. In humans serum C-peptide concentrations did not decrease when plasma levels of insulin were elevated and blood glucose was kept at normoglycemic values, according to Shima et al. (83) and Zilker et al. (84). On the other hand, Beischer et al. (85) reported a decrease in C-peptide release in volunteers during insulin infusion using the glucose-clamp technique. In a more recent *in vitro* study of Beischer et al. (86), determination of immunoreactive rat C-peptide (and also insulin) after incubation of isolated rat islets under various conditions (varying glucose concentration, exogenous insulin, and insulin antibodies) brought about no evidence for a direct feedback inhibition of insulin on its own secretion.

In summary, after about two decades of research on this field, there is still no general agreement concerning the question of a direct feedback inhibition of insulin release.

REFERENCES

1. H. Schatz, V. Maier, M. Hinz, C. Nierle, and E. F. Pfeiffer, *FEBS Lett.* **26**, 237 (1972).
2. H. Schatz, V. Maier, M. Hinz, C. Nierle, and E. F. Pfeiffer, *Diabetes* **22**, 433 (1973).
3. M. Hinz, H. Schatz, V. Maier, C. Nierle, and E. F. Pfeiffer, in *VII. Karlsburger Symposium über Diabetesfragen*, H. Bibergeil, H. Fiedler, U. Poser (eds.), Karlsburg 1971, p. 100.
4. G. Schäfer and H. Schatz, *J. Endocrinol.* **91**, 255 (1981).
5. H. Schatz, B. Gonnermann, G. Schäfer, K. Leinweber, D. Gustson, and K. Federlin, *Horm. Metab. Res., Suppl.* **12**, 59 (1982).
6. H. Schatz, C. Nierle, and E. F. Pfeiffer, *Europ. J. Clin. Invest.* **5**, 477 (1975).
7. G. Schäfer, H. Daum, and H. Schatz, *Mol. Cell. Endocrin.* **31**, 141 (1983).
8. R. Schäfer and H. Schatz, *Acta Endocrin.* **91**, 493 (1979).
9. G. Schäfer, A. E. Heyer, and H. Schatz, *Diabetologia* **25**, 192 (1983).
10. H. Schatz and E. F. Pfeiffer, *J. Endocrin.* **74**, 243 (977).
11. G. Schnellbacher-Daum, G. Schäfer, and H. Schatz, *Diabetologia* **23**, 199 (1982).
12. H. Schatz and U. Kullek, *FEBS Lett.* **122**, 207 (1980).
13. H. Schatz, J. Otto, M. Hinz, V. Maier, C. Nierle, and E. F. Pfeiffer, *Endocrinology* **94**, 248 (1974).
14. J. Sieradzki, H. Schatz, C. Nierle, and E. F. Pfeiffer, *Horm. Metab. Res.* **7**, 284 (1975).
15. Y. Sako, H. Schatz, V. Maier, and E. F. Pfeiffer, *Horm. Metab. Res.* **9**, 347 (1977).

16. H. Schatz, A. Ferdussian, G. Schäfer, and S. Ahuja, *Akt. Endokr. Stoffw.* **2**, 94 (1982).

17. H. Schatz, V. Maier, M. Hinz, M. Schleyer, C. Nierle, and E. F. Pfeiffer, *Horm. Metab. Res.* **5**, 29 (1973).

18. M. Nieter, H. J. Teschemacher, and H. Schatz, *Diabetologia* **21**, 309 (1981).

19. M. Glatt and H. Schatz, *Diabete Metab.* **7**, 105 (1981).

20. K. P. Leinweber and H. Schatz, *Acta Endocrin.* **99**, 94 (1982).

21. B. Gonnermann and H. Schatz, unpublished results.

22. M. Glatt, Inaugural-Dissertation, University of Giessen, Giessen, 1983.

23. M. Hinz, N. Katsilambros, V. Maier, H. Schatz, and E. F. Pfeiffer, *FEBS Lett.* **30**, 225 (1973).

24. V. Maier, H. Schatz, M. Hinz, E. F. Pfeiffer, and J. Blessing, *Endokrinologie* **62**, 269 (1973).

25. V. Maier, C. Schneider, H. Schatz, and E. F. Pfeiffer, *Hoppe-Seyler's Z. Physiol. Chem.* **356**, 887 (1975).

26. B. Gonnermann, D. Gustson, and H. Schatz, *Horm. Metab. Res.* **13**, 411 (1981).

27. H. Schatz, D. Steinle, and E. F. Pfeiffer, *Horm. Metab. Res.* **9**, 457 (1977).

28. H. Schatz, N. Katsilambros, C. Nierle, and E. F. Pfeiffer, *Diabetologia* **8**, 402 (1972).

29. E. Heinze, H. Schatz, C. Nierle, and E. F. Pfeiffer, *Diabetes* **24**, 373 (1975).

30. B. Gonnermann, R. Schäfer-Spiegel, H. Laube, and H. Schatz, *Internat. J. Obesity* **6** (suppl. 1), 41 (1982).

31. H. Laube, H. Schatz, C. Nierle, R. Fussgänger, and E. F. Pfeiffer, *Diabetologia* **12**, 441 (1976).

32. H. Schatz, H. Laube, J. Sieradzki, W. Kamenisch, and E. F. Pfeiffer, *Horm. Metab. Res.* **10**, 23 (1978).

33. J. Sieradzki, H. Schatz, and E. F. Pfeiffer, *Acta Endocrin.* **86**, 813 (1977).

34. H. Schatz, Y. Abdel Rahman, M. Hinz, H. L. Fehm, C. Nierle, and E. F. Pfeiffer, *Diabetologia* **9**, 135 (1973).

35. H. Schatz, N. Katsilambros, M. Hinz, K. H. Voigt, C. Nierle, and E. F. Pfeiffer, *Diabetologia* **9**, 140 (1973).

36. N. Katsilambros, R. Ziegler, H. Schatz, M. Hinz, V. Maier, and E. F. Pfeiffer, *Horm. Metab. Res.* **4**, 377 (1972).

37. M. Hinz, N. Katsilambros, Y. Abdel Rahman, H. Schatz, V. Maier, E. Schröder, and E. F. Pfeiffer, *Diabetologia* **7**, 484 (1971).

38. B. Gonnermann, H. Schatz, R. Schäfer-Spiegel, R. G. Bretzel, J. Schneider, and K. Federlin, in *Islet Isolation, Culture and Cryopreservation*, Internat. Workshop Giessen 1980, K. Federlin and R. G. Bretzel (eds.), Thieme, Stuttgart-New York, 1981, p. 161.

39. A. Andersson, *Diabetologia* **14**, 397 (1978).

40. A. Andersson, R. Gunnarsson, and C. Hellerström, *Acta Endocr.* **82**, 318 (1976).

41. R. L. Gingerich, S. L. Aronoff, D. M. Kipnis, and P. E. Lacy, *Diabetes* **28**, 276 (1979).

42. P. R. Davoren, *Biochim. Biophys. Acta* **63**, 150 (1962).

43. T. O. Tijoe, G. H. J. Wolters, W. Konijnendijk, and P. R. Bouman, *Horm. Metab. Res.* **12**, 220 (1980).

44. C. Berne, *Endocrinology* **97**, 1241 (1975).

45. P. A. Halban, *Endocrinology* **110**, 1183 (1982).

46. P. A. Halban and C. B. Wollheim, *J. Biol. Chem.* **255**, 6003 (1980).

47. P. A. Halban, C. B. Wollheim, B. Blondel, and A. E. Renold, *Biochem. Pharmacol.* **29**, 2625 (1980).

48. W. Creutzfeldt, C. Creutzfeldt, H. Frerichs, E. Perings, and K. Sickinger, *Horm. Metab. Res.* **1**, 53 (1969).

49. L. A. H. Borg and A. H. Schnell, *Diabetologia* **21**, 252 (1981).

50. K. D. Kohnert, H. Jahr, S. Schmidt, H. J. Hahn, and H. Zühlke, *Biochim. Biophys. Acta* **422**, 254 (1976).

51. H. Zühlke, K. D. Kohnert, H. Jahr, S. Schmidt, K. Kirschke, and D. F. Steiner, *Acta Biol. Med. Germ.* **36**, 1695 (1977).

52. E. Samols and J. Harrison, *Metabolism* **25**, 1495 (1976).

53. E. Samols, G. Marri, and V. Marks, *Lancet* **II**, 415 (1965).

54. W. A. Müller, G. R. Faloona, and R. H. Unger, *J. Clin. Invest.* **50**, 1992 (1971).

55. S. Efendic, V. Grill, and R. Luft. *FEBS Lett.* **55**, 131 (1975).

56. H. J. Hahn and M. Ziegler, *Acta Biol. Med. Germ.* **35**, 439 (1976).

57. L. Turcot-Lemay and P. E. Lacy, *Diabetes* **24**, 658 (1975).

58. W. Norfleet, A. S. Pagliara, M. W. Haymond, and F. Matschinsky, *Diabetes* **24**, 961 (1975).

59. S. Kadowaki, T. Taminato, T. Chiba, K. Mori, M. Abe, Y. Goto, Y. Seino, S. Matsukura, M. Nozawa, and T. Fujita, *Diabetes* **28**, 600 (1979).

60. G. S. Patton, E. Ipp, R. Dobbs, L. Orci, W. Yale, and R. H. Unger, *Proc. Natl. Acad. Sci. USA* **74**, 2140 (1977).

61. G. C. Weir, E. Samols, S. Loo, Y. C. Patel, and K. H. Gabbay, *Diabetes* **28**, 35 (1979).

62. P. D. G. Gerber, E. R. Trimble, L. Herberg, and A. E. Renold, *Diabetologia* **19**, 275 (1980).

63. P. Schauder, J. Arends, H. Koop, and W. Creutzfeldt, 2nd Internat. Symposium on Somatostatin, Athens 1981, Abstract.

64. P. Schauder, C. McIntosh, U. Panten, J. Arends, R. Arnold, H. Frerichs, and W. Creutzfeldt, *Metabolism* **27** (suppl. 1), 1211 (1978).

65. G. S. Tannenbaum, J. Epelbaum, E. Colle, P. Brazeau, and J. B. Martin, *Metabolism* **27**, 1263 (1978).

66. H. Taniguchi, M. Hasegawa, T. Kobayashi, Y. Watanabe, K. Murakami, M. Seki, A. Tsutou, M. Utsumi, H. Makimura, M. Sakoda, and S. Baba, *Horm. Metab. Res.* **11**, 23 (1979).

67. H. Taniguchi, M. Utsumi, M. Hasegawa, T. Kobayashi, Y. Watanabe, K. Murakami, M. Seki, A. Tsutou, H. Makimura, M. Sakoda, and S. Baba, *Diabetes* **26**, 700 (1977).

68. N. Barden, M. Lavoie, A. Dupont, J. Côté, and J. P. Côté, *Endocrinology* **101**, 635 (1977).

69. K. Ejiri, H. Taniguchi, K. Murakami, M. Tamagawa, K. Ishihara, M. Utsumi, and S. Baba, 2nd Internat. Symposium on Somatostatin, Athens 1981, Abstract.

70. M. A. Khokher, S. Janah, and P. Dandona, *Diabetologia* **25**, 264 (1983).

71. Y. C. Patel and G. C. Weir, *Clin. Endocrin.* **5**, 191 (1975).

72. V. Schusdziarra, R. E. Dobbs, V. Harris, and R. H. Unger, *FEBS Lett.* **81**, 69 (1977).

73. J. E. Morley, S. R. Levin, M. Pehlevanian, R. Adachi, A. E. Pekary, and J. M. Hershman, *Endocrinology* **104**, 137 (1979).

74. L. O. Dolva, J. H. Nielsen, and K. F. Hanssen, *Diabetologia* **25**, 151 (1983).

75. W. J. Malaisse, F. Malaisse-Lagae, P. E. Lacy, and P. H. Wright, *Proc. Soc. Exp. Biol. Med.* **124**, 497 (1967).

76. H. Schatz, *Insulin: Biosynthese und Sekretion.* Thieme, Stuttgart, 1976.

77. H. Frerichs, U. Reich, and W. Creutzfeldt, *Klin. Wschr.* **43**, 136 (1965).

78. J. C. Sodoyez, F. Sodoyez-Goffaux, and P. P. Foa, *Proc. Soc. Exp. Biol.* **130**, 568 (1969).

79. M. Ziegler, H. J. Hahn, and D. Klatt, *Diabetologia* **4**, 148 (1972).

80. J. Dunbar, W. J. McLaughlin, M. F. Walsh, P. P. Foa, *Horm. Metab. Res.* **8**, 1 (1976).

81. T. Toyota, K. Abe, M. Kudo, K. Kimura, and Y. Goto, *Tohoku J. Exp. Med.* **117**, 79 (1976).

82. J. Logothetopoulos, J. K. Davidson, R. E. Haist, and C. H. Best, *Diabetes* **14**, (1965).

83. K. Shima, S. Morishita, N. Sawazaki, R. Tanaka, and S. Taru, *Horm. Metab. Res.* **9**, 441 (1977).

84. Th. Zilker, K. Paterek, R. Ermler, and P. Bottermann, *Klin. Wschr.* **55**, 475 (1977).

85. W. Beischer, M. Schmid, W. Kerner, L. Keller, and E. F. Pfeiffer, *Horm. Metab. Res.* **10**, 168 (1978).

86. W. Beischer, A. Michael, B. Maier, M. Maas, and L. Keller, *Diabetologia* **25**, 139 (1983).

87. L. Turcot-Lemay, A. Lemay, and P. E. Lacy, *Biochim. Biophys. Res. Comm.* **63**, 1130 (1975).

I

PANCREATIC MONOLAYER CULTURES

Preparation of Purified Islet Cell Cultures and Assessment of β Cell Replication

ALEXANDER RABINOVITCH

Department of Medicine, University of Miami School of Medicine, Miami, Florida

1. INTRODUCTION

Growth and differentiation of the insulin-producing β cells in pancreatic islets is considered to be controlled, in part, by interaction of nutrients, hormones, and growth-promoting factors, as has been demonstrated for most mammalian tissues (1). The islet β cell mass can be affected by food intake and diet composition (2–5), pregnancy (6–9), hormones such as cortisone (10–13) and growth hormone (14–16), and to a lesser extent glucagon (17) and hypoglycemic sulfonylureas (18–21). It is not completely clear, however, to what extent these effects observed *in vivo* reflect direct actions of the various factors on the islet β cells. Tissue culture provides a method of controlling the environment of the β cell and, thereby, allows one to quantitate the effect of a putative growth factor, to study its mechanism of action, and to dissect possible complex interactions between different factors.

Various techniques for isolation and long-term incubation of islets and islet cells *in vitro* have been developed since the original descriptions of Hellerstrom (22), Moskalewski (23), and Lacy and Kostianovsky (24). These methods include monolayer cell cultures of neonatal (25–28) and adult (29) rodent pancreas, organ cultures of the pancreas from fetal mice (30), fetal (31–33) and adult (34) rats and the human fetus (35, 36), and cultures of islolated islets from adult mice (37, 38), fetal (39) and adult (37, 40, 41) rats, and fetal (42) and adult (43, 44) humans. Islets have also been cultured on synthetic capillaries (45).

This chapter describes a method to prepare neonatal rat pancreatic islet cell monolayer cultures for study of islet β cell replication (46–48). The method is based on the procedure described by Lambert et al. (27) and modified by Chick et al. (28) and Punter et al. (49).

2. PREPARATION OF ISLET CELL MONOLAYER CULTURES

1. Three- to five-day old neonatal rats are used. Any rat strain can be used; we have used inbred Lewis (LEW/Crl BR) and outbred Sprague–Dawley

The author thanks Carol Quigley for expert and devoted technical assistance. This work was supported by a grant (AM25832) from the U.S. Public Health Service, National Institutes of Arthritis, Diabetes, Digestive and Kidney Diseases (NIADDK), by a Research Career Development Award (AM00552) of the NIADDK to the author, and by the Diabetes Research Institute Foundation.

[Crl:CD(SD)BR] rats (Charles River Breeding Laboratories, Inc., Wilmington, MA). A total of 60–120 rats is used per culture preparation.

2.   Sacrifice the rats, by decapitation, in groups of 12–20. Place the animals on their sides and attach them to a styrofoam board by pinning the legs to the board.

3.   After swabbing the animal's flank with 70 percent ethanol and entering the abdominal cavity through a small incision over the spleen, remove the pancreata aseptically in a laminar flow hood.

4.   Collect the pancreata in a Ca^{2+}- and Mg^{2+}-free phosphate-buffered saline (PBS) solution in a 50-mL screw cap Erlenmeyer flask.

5.   Wash the pancreata collected from all the rats in Ca^{2+}- and Mg^{2+}-free PBS by stirring gently on a magnetic stirrer for 10 min at room temperature.

6.   Remove the medium from the pancreata by decantation. Then, wash once with, and add, a prewarmed (37°C) solution of Ca^{2+}- and Mg^{2+}-free PBS (pH 7.6) containing 5.6 mM glucose, 1 mg/mL trypsin (1:250; Difco Laboratories, Detroit, MI), and 0.2 mg/mL collagenase (CLS IV, Worthington, Biochemical Corp., Freehold, NJ). The trypsin–glucose solution is prepared first and sterilized by filtration through a membrane (0.45 μ; Millipore Corp., Bedford, MA). Collagenase is weighed and dissolved in Ca^{2+}- and Mg^{2+}-free PBS, filtered, and added to the trypsin–glucose solution just before use. The trypsin–collagenase solution is kept at 4°C until added to the pancreata.

7.   Dissociate the pancreata by stirring the glands gently in the trypsin–collagenase solution (20 mL/100 pancreata) for 5–6 min at 37°C in a heating chamber with magnetic stirrer (Amicon Corp., Scientific Systems Division, Danvers, MA). Allow the tissue to settle for 2 min at room temperature. Collect the remaining cell suspension with a 14-gauge steel cannula and 20-mL plastic syringe and store at 4°C in 50-mL plastic centrifuge tubes (Corning Glass Works, Corning, NY) each containing 3 mL heat-inactivated fetal calf serum (Gibco Laboratories, Grand Island, NY).

8.   Add fresh trypsin–collagenase solution (15 mL per original 100 pancreata) to the undissociated tissue and repeat step 7 four to five times, pooling the cell suspensions. Dissociate any undigested tissue by aspirating several times gently through a 14-gauge steel cannula and 20 mL plastic syringe and add this to the pooled cell suspensions. Microscopic examination of the dissociated tissue reveals mostly single cells and small clusters (less than ~50 cells) and also some larger clusters (~50–500 cells).

9.   Wash the cells by centrifugation at 250 g for 10 min at room temperature. Remove the supernatants and resuspend the cells in tissue culture medium 199 with modified Earle's salts, L-glutamine, and phenol red (Gibco Laboratories), buffered with 25 mM sodium bicarbonate and supplemented with 100 U/mL penicillin, 100 μg/mL streptomycin, 0.25 μg/mL fungizone, 10 percent (v/v) heat-inactivated fetal calf serum, and 16.7 mM glucose (standard culture medium for islet monolayers). The cells are suspended in the standard culture medium to a volume of 1 mL per original pancreas dissociated.

10.   Plate out the cells in 100-mm plastic culture dishes (Falcon Labware, Division Becton, Dickinson & Co., Oxnard, CA), 10 mL/dish, and incubate overnight (16–20 hr) at 37°C in a water-saturated 95 percent air/5 percent CO_2 atmosphere. Since fibroblasts attach to the bottom of the dishes faster than do islet cells, this incubation serves to enrich the floating cells in islet cells.

11.   Decant the cell suspensions, shaking the 100-mm dishes before decanting to dislodge clusters of loosely attached cells. Fibroblasts are more firmly attached to the bottoms of the dishes. Pool the decanted cells and dilute in fresh standard culture medium to a volume of 4 mL per original pancreas dissociated.

12.   Plate the cells in 35-mm culture dishes (2 mL/dish) and incubate at 37°C in the 95 percent air/5 percent CO_2 incubator for 3 days. By this time, pancreatic acinar cells have died, and the attached cells are mainly islet cells and fibroblasts (Fig. 1A).

13.   Aspirate and remove the culture medium and unattached cells and cellular debris. Add fresh standard culture medium containing 2.5 µg/mL iodoacetic acid (Matheson Coleman and Bell, Cincinnati, OH). Punter et al. (49) were the first to demonstrate that iodoacetate (or iodoacetic acid) is a

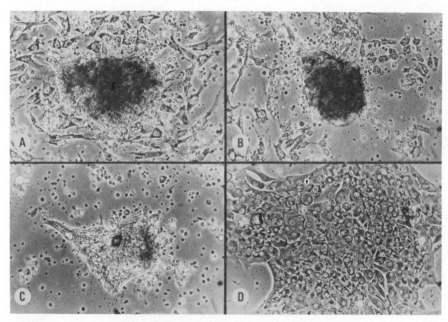

FIGURE 1.   Sequential phase-contrast photomicrographs (×400) of a newborn rat pancreatic monolayer culture. (A) Three days after dissociating the pancreata and plating the cells, a large cluster of islet cells is surrounded by fibroblasts. (B) Five hours after adding iodoacetic acid (2 µg/mL), many fibroblasts show retraction of their cytoplasmic processes and early necrosis. (C) One day after the iodoacetic acid treatment (for 5 hrs) no viable fibroblasts remain, only cellular debris, and islet cells are beginning to spread out. (D) Three days later (7 days after initial plating) the islet cells have spread out in a monolayer.

very effective agent to eliminate fibroblasts from pancreatic monolayer cultures without impairing islet β cell function (insulin release and biosynthesis) or ultrastructure. Iodoacetate was found to be superior to other SH reagents such as thiomerosal (50) or other methods used in attempts to selectively eliminate fibroblasts from pancreatic islet cultures, including omission of essential compounds from the medium, for example, L-cystine, (51) substitution of D-valine for L-valine (52) or differential trypsination (53).

14.   Examine the cultures, by phase-contrast microscopy 3 hr after addition of iodoacetic acid and each 30 min thereafter. At the first visible evidence of damage to fibroblasts (retraction of cytoplasmic processes and cellular necrosis), usually observed 3–5 hr after addition of iodoacetic acid (Fig. 1B), aspirate and remove the medium, and replace with fresh standard culture medium (rinse not necessary). Most, if not all fibroblasts rapidly die and detach over the next 24 hr (Fig. 1C), whereas the islet cell clusters spread out in monolayers over the next 2–3 days (Fig. 1D). If fibroblast removal is incomplete, a second treatment with iodoacetic acid can be used. This is applied 2–3 days after the first treatment to allow islet cells to spread out and attach more firmly to the bottom of the dishes.

15.   Replace the medium with fresh standard culture medium each 2–3 days. At 7–10 days after first plating the dissociated pancreatic tissue, the cultures are comprised of clusters (~10–200 cells) of islet cells well spread out in monolayers attached to the bottom of the dishes. Electron microscopic examination of the cells indicates that approximately 80 percent are β cells, 10 percent α cells, and 10 percent δ cells (54). Contamination with fibroblastic, endothelial, or acinar cells is negligible or absent, and experimental studies can be started on these purified islet cell monolayer cultures.

3.   ASSESSMENT OF β CELL REPLICATION

Replication of β cells in the islet monolayer cultures is assessed by determining the incorporation of [^{3}H]thymidine in nuclei of islet β cells in aldehyde-thionin-stained autoradiographs (29, 46–48).

1.   Add 10 μCi/mL [methyl-^{3}H]thymidine (40–60 Ci/mmol; Amersham Corp., Arlington Heights, IL) to the islet cell monolayer cultures during the last 16–20 hr of incubation in test or control media.

2.   Remove the culture media, wash the cultures three times in PBS, and fix the cells in Bouin's solution for 30 min in the dark at room temperature. Bouin's solution is made up of formaldehyde (75 mL) and picric acid (25 mL). This is kept in the dark at room temperature, and glacial acetic acid (2 mL) is added just before use.

3.   Wash the fixed cells by removing the Bouin's solution from the dishes and immersing the dishes in a large beaker filled with warm tap water running slowly for 3–4 hr, until microscopic examination (of wet cells) shows no trace

of yellow-brown residue from the Bouin's fixation. Allow the fixed cells to dry by inverting the dishes overnight at room temperature.

4. Stain the fixed cells with aldehyde-thionin, according to the method of Paget (55). The dishes can be stored in the dark for several weeks or directly processed for autoradiography.

5. The autoradiographic method of Caro et al. (56) is used. Work in a dark room, using a lamp with a red safelight filter No. 2 (Kodak, Rochester, NY). Add Ilford L-4 photographic emulsion (Polysciences, Inc., Warrington, PA) to the dishes. Pour 2 mL of the liquefied (45°C in a water bath) emulsion onto the first dish and rapidly decant into the next dish, inclining the first dish at a 45° angle to drain away from the cells (attached mainly at the center of the dish). Approximately 10 dishes can be processed over 1 min, then fresh liquefied emulsion is added in a similar fashion to the next 10 dishes.

6. Store the dishes in a light-proof box at 4°c for 3 days to expose the emulsion.

7. Process the autoradiographs in the dark with Kodak D-19 developer (1 mL/dish) for 3 min. Stop with one rinse of distilled water. Fix with Kodak rapid fixer (1 mL/dish) for 3 min. Rinse once with distilled water, and again after 5 min. Drain the dishes and allow to dry.

8. Determine the [^{3}H]thymidine-labeling index for β cells by counting approximately 500 aldehyde-thionin-stained cells (β cells) in each culture dish and scoring how many of these contain labeled nuclei (blackened overlying emulsion).

9. To confirm that the [^{3}H]thymidine-labeling index represents β cell replication, estimate the β cell mitotic index by adding 1 μg/mL N-desacetyl-N-methylcolchicine (Colcemid; Gibco Laboratories) to the cultures for 18 hr, in place of [^{3}H]thymidine, to arrest dividing cells in metaphase. Remove the medium carefully so as not to detach any cells in mitosis and carefully add a hypotonic solution (0.075 M KCL) for 15–30 min to swell the cells and improve identification of mitotic figures (57). Fix in Bouin's solution by adding the fixative slowly to dilute the hypotonic solution 1:1. Place the dishes in the dark for 10 min, remove the fixative, add fresh fixative for 10 min and repeat once. Rinse the cells with warm tap water, and stain with aldehyde-thionin. Determine the β cell mitotic index by counting approximately 500 aldehyde-thionin-stained cells in each culture dish and scoring how many of these contain nuclei with mitotic figures. In general, the effect of a substance on the [^{3}H]thymidine-labeling index of β cells is accompanied by a proportional effect on the β cell mitotic index; however, the absolute value for the β cell mitotic index may be lower than that for β cell labeling with [^{3}H]thymidine (46–48, 58).

REFERENCES

1. H. A. Armelin, K. Nishikawa, and H. G. Sato, in *Control of Proliferation in Animal Cells*, B. Clarkson and R. Baserga (eds.), Cold Spring Harbor, New York, 1974, p. 97.

2. S. Tejning, *Acta Med. Scand.* (suppl. 198) *128*:1 (1947).
3. R. N. Wissler, J. W. Findley, and L. E. Frazier, *Proc. Soc. Exp. Biol. Med.* **71**, 308 (1949).
4. M. A. Ashworth, N. C. Kerbel, and R. E. Haist, *J. Physiol. (London)* **171**, 25 (1952).
5. B. Petersson and B. Hellman, *Metabolism* **11**, 342 (1962).
6. T. Akehi, *Jap. J. Obstet. Gynecol.* **13**, 427 (1930).
7. B. Hellman, *Acta Obstet. Gynecol. Scand.* **39**, 331 (1959).
8. C. Hellerstrom, *Acta Soc. Med. Upsal.* **68**, 17 (1963).
9. L. Aerts and F. A. van Assche, *Diabetologia* **11**, 285 (1975).
10. F. X. Hausberger and A. J. Ramsay, *Endocrinology* **53**, 423 (1953).
11. C. Hellerstrom, *Acta Soc. Med. Upsal.* **68**, 1 (1963).
12. H. Kern and J. Logothetopoulos, *Diabetes* **19**, 145 (1970).
13. A. A. Like and W. L. Chick, *Am. J. Path.* **75**, 329 (1974).
14. K. C. Richardson and F. G. Young, *Lancet* **116**, 1098 (1938).
15. B. W. Volk and S. S. Lazarus, *Diabetes* **11**, 426 (1962).
16. S. A. Bencosme, V. Tsutsumi, J. M. Martin, and H. K. Akerblom, *Diabetes* **20**, 15 (1971).
17. B. Petersson and B. Hellman, *Acta Endocrinol.* **44**, 139 (1963).
18. M. A. Ashworth and R. E. Haist, *Can. Med. Assoc. J.* **74**, 975 (1956).
19. W. Gepts, J. Christophe, and J. Mayer, *Diabetes* **9**, 63 (1960).
20. J. M. B. Bloodworth, Jr., *Metabolism* **12**, 287 (1963).
21. S. C. Bunnag, N. E. Warner, and S. Bunnag, *Diabetes* **15**, 597 (1966).
22. C. Hellerstrom, *Acta Endocr.* **45**, 122 (1964).
23. S. Moskalewski, *Gen. Comp. Endocrinol.* **5**, 342 (1965).
24. P. E. Lacy and M. Kostianovsky, *Diabetes* **16**, 35 (1967).
25. I. Hilwig, S. Schuster, W. Heptner, and E. V. Wasilewski, *Z. Zellforsch. Mikrosk. Anat.* **90**, 333 (1968).
26. I. A. Macchi and E. H. Blaustein, *Endocrinol.* **84**, 208 (1969).
27. E. A. Lambert, B. Blondel, Y. Kanazawa, L. Orci, and A. E. Renold, *Endocrinol.* **90**, 239 (1972).
28. W. L. Chick, V. Lauris, J. H. Felwelling, K. A. Andrews, and J. M. Woodruff, *Endocrinol.* **92**, 212 (1973).
29. M. Kostianovsky, M. L. McDaniel, M. F. Still, R. C. Codilla, and R. E. Lacy, *Diabetologia* **10**, 337 (1974).
30. T. E. Mandel, S. Collier, W. Carter, L. Higginbotham, and F. I. R. Martin, *Transplantation* **30**, 231 (1980).
31. L. R. Murrell, *Exp. Cell Res.* **41**, 350 (1966).
32. O. D. Hegre, R. C. McEvoy, V. Bachelder, and A. Lazarow, *Diabetes* **22**, 577 (1973).
33. R. C. McEvoy, O. D. Hegre, and A. Lazarow, *Differentiation* **6**, 17 (1976).
34. L. E. Jonsson, J. Ponten, and J. Thorell, *Diabetologia* **2**, 157 (1966).
35. H. Goldman and E. Colle, *Science* **192**, 1014 (1976).
36. A. Agren, A. Andersson, C. Bjorken, C. G. Groth, R. Gunnarsson, C. Hellerstrom, G. Lindmark, G. Lundqvist, B. Petersson, and I. Swenne, *Diabetes* **29** (suppl. 1) 64 (1980).
37. M. Kostianovsky, P. E. Lacy, M. H. Greider, and M. F. Still, *Lab. Invest.* **27**, 53 (1972).
38. A. Andersson and C. Hellerstrom, *Diabetes* (suppl. 2) **21**, 546 (1972).
39. C. Hellerstrom, N. J. Lewis, H. Borg, R. Johnson, and N. Freinkel, *Diabetes* **28**, 769 (1979).
40. J. Ono, R. Takaki, H. Okano, and M. Fukuma, *In Vitro* **95**, 95 (1979).
41. H. Ohgawara, R. Carroll, C. Hofmann, C. Takahashi, M. Kikuchi, A. Labrecque, Y.

Hirata, and D. Steiner, *Proc. Natl. Acad. Sci. USA* **75**, 1897 (1978).

42. T. E. Mandel, L. Hoffman, S. Collier, W. M. Carter, and M. Koulmanda, *Diabetes* (suppl. 4) **31**, 39 (1982).

43. A. Anderson, H. Borg, C. Gustav-Groth, R. Gunnarsson, C. Hellerstrom, G. Lundgren, T. Westman, and J. Ostman, *J. Clin. Invest* **57**, 1295 (1976).

44. J. H. Nielsen, J. Brunstedt, A. Andersson, and C. Frimodt-Moller, *Diabetologia* **16**, 97 (1979).

45. W. L. Chick, A. A. Like, and V. Lauris, *Science* **187**, 847 (1975).

46. A. Rabinovitch, B. Blondel, T. Murray, and D. H. Mintz, *J. Clin. Invest.* **66**, 1065 (1980).

47. A. Rabinovitch, C. Quigley, T. Russell, Y. Patel, and D. H. Mintz, *Diabetes* **31**, 160 (1982).

48. A. Rabinovitch, C. Quigley, and M. M. Rechler, *Diabetes* **32**, 307 (1983).

49. J. Punter, F. Wengenmayer, K. Engelbart, and H. Rolly, *In Vitro* **18**, 291 (1982).

50. J. T. Braaten, M. J. Lee, A. Schenk, and D. H. Mintz, *Biochem. Biophys. Res. Commun.* **61**, 476 (1974).

51. W. L. Chick, A. A. Like, and V. Lauris, *Endocrinology* **96**, 637 (1975).

52. S. F. Gilbert and B. R. Migeon, *Cell* **5**, 11 (1975).

53. B. Blondel and C. B. Wollheim, *Experientia* **30**, 700 (1974).

54. P. Meda, E. Kohen, C. Kohen, A. Rabinovitch, and L. Orci, *J. Cell Biol.* **92**, 221 (1982).

55. G. E. Paget, *Stain Technology* **34**, 223 (1959).

56. L. G. Caro, R. P. van Tubergen, and J. A. Kolb, *J. Cell Biol.* **15**, 173 (1962).

57. R. G. Worton and C. Duff, *Methods Enzymol.* **58**, 322 (1979).

58. D. L. King, K. C. Kitchen, and W. L. Chick, *Endocrinology*, **103**, 1321 (1978).

J

CRYOPRESERVATION OF THE FETAL PANCREAS
Rat, Pig, Human

JOSIAH BROWN

Department of Medicine, University of California, Los Angeles, California

WILLIAM R. CLARK AND JOHN A. DANILOVS

Department of Biology (Immunology) and the Molecular Biology Institute, University of California, Los Angeles, California

YOKO S. MULLEN

Dental Research Institute, University of California, Los Angeles, California

317

1. INTRODUCTION

In 1974 our laboratories published the first report showing that the fetal pancreas could be used as a donor organ to reverse diabetes in an adult animal treated with streptozotocin (1). It quickly became apparent to us that the advantages of the fetal pancreas in organ transplantation could best be exploited if a means of long-term preservation of donor tissue could be established. We thus worked with Peter Mazur of the Oak Ridge Laboratories to extend his technology for cryopreservation of mouse blastomeric embryos (2) to more complex tissue structures. In a series of papers published beginning in 1976, we reported the first successful cryopreservation of a histologically complex organ—the fetal rat pancreas (3–6).

The advantages of cryopreservation of fetal pancreas tissue for transplantation are obvious: increased availability of donor tissues; prospective HLA matching of donor and recipient; ease of transportation of donor tissues to distant transplant centers; and the ability to cryopreserve in parallel other donor tissues, such as liver cells, for use in possible tolerance-inducing regimens. The problems have proved to be remarkably few. The principal objective is to remove heat in a controlled fashion from islet structures scattered throughout the pancreas without causing osmotic or ice crystal damage to individual islet cells. These types of damage are minimized by the use of an appropriate cryopreservative agent such as dimethyl sulfoxide (DMSO) and slow cooling rates. DMSO is quite toxic to tissues and must be used with great care. Manipulation of these two variables (cooling rate and controlled delivery of the cryoprotective agent) is the major technical problem to be dealt with. These variables, which differ for the various fetal pancreata we have cryopreserved to date (rat, pig, and human), are discussed in the following sections.

This work was supported by NIH grants AM-17980 and 20827, the Kroc Foundation and the N.E. Treadwell Foundation. Special thanks are appropriate to Morton W. Barke, M.D., Chief of Staff, to the Staff of the Inglewood Hospital, and to Anne Sheng, who provided skilled technical assistance.

2. PREPARATION OF TISSUES

Fetal pancreata are dissected away from surrounding gut tissues and transferred to sterile tissue culture dishes containing balanced salt solution, where they are further cleaned of adherent connective tissue and membranes. Fetal rat pancreata of 17 days gestation or earlier are used intact; all other pancreata are dissected into $1-2$-mm^3 fragments. In the case of human fetal pancreata we have had good results cryopreserving strips of tissue $1-2$ mm in diameter and up to $7-8$ mm long (ref. 7). Apparently, penetration of DMSO, is sufficient to give good cryoprotection.

We are able to expose fetal rat pancreas tissue to DMSO directly after dissection and to freeze it immediately thereafter. When we attempted this with human fetal pancreas, we were unable to recover viable tissue after thawing. We found, quite by accident, that if human fetal pancreas tissues are first cultured overnight ($12-16$ hr), they can then be cryopreserved using a protocol similar to that for rat. The reason for this is unclear. It may be related to the fact that the human tissues are processed $1-3$ hr after removal from the mother, whereas the rat pancreata are processed immediately. The human tissues may be somewhat traumatized and need a period of recovery before being able to withstand the additional trauma of freezing. With pig fetal pancreas we also routinely culture tissues overnight before exposure to DMSO and freezing. Both human and pig pancreas fragments are incubated overnight in RPMI containing HEPES buffer and 10 percent fetal calf serum (FCS) at 37°C in 5 percent CO_2/95 percent air. The tissue is placed in the bottom of a 35-mm plastic culture dish, to which is added 0.75 mL medium, just sufficient to coat the fragments by surface tension. They are thus effectively cultured at an air–liquid interface.

3. EXPOSURE TO DMSO

Exposure of tissues to be frozen to DMSO is one of the most critical steps in the freezing procedure. Both the concentration of DMSO used and the length of time the tissues are exposed are critical.

Our initial studies with rat fetal pancreas utilized a rather complex protocol for exposure to DMSO. The intact pancreata or fragments were exposed first to 0.2 mL of 1.0 M DMSO in saline at room temperature for 60 min. An equal volume of 3.0 M DMSO was added to bring the samples to 2.0 M, and the tubes were incubated in an ice bath for an additional 15 min. The tissues are always left in the final cryopreservative solution for the remainder of the freezing protocol.

The protocol for exposure of human fetal pancreas to DMSO was patterned largely on the rat procedure, except that, as noted above, the tissues were cultured overnight prior to exposure to DMSO. Best results were obtained with a single 60-min room temperature exposure to 1.5 M DMSO in saline.

We experienced more difficulty with the pig fetal pancreas, which in our hands appears to be more sensitive to DMSO than pancreata from the other two species. The optimal treatment for this tissue is a single 5–8-min exposure to 2.1 M DMSO in saline at room temperature. We have not tried this procedure (shorter exposure to a higher DMSO concentration) with human fetal pancreas.

4.   FREEZING PROCEDURE

We have from the beginning found that a simple freezing apparatus of our own construction, patterned after that used by Peter Mazur, is superior to most commercially available programmable freezers. It consists of a 2-L, double-walled, evacuated glass Dewar flask immersed in a larger Dewar flask containing liquid nitrogen. The inner dewar flask contains absolute ethanol, although any of a variety of other solvents (acetone, for example) may be used as well. Simply by varying the ratio of the volumes of the two liquids that are in contact with each other (across the double walls of the inner dewar flask), it is possible to control in a very precise fashion the flow of heat out of the ethanol bath. Rates of flow less than 1°C/min are easily attained and can be controlled to within 0.1°C.

Sample tubes (either glass or plastic, 10 mm in diameter), containing two to three tissue samples in 0.2 mL of the final DMSO solution, are placed in a constant temperature ethanol bath at −8°C to −10°C and allowed to equilibrate for 3 min. A small ice crystal is introduced into the super-cooled solution, usually on the tip of a Pasteur pipette, to initiate rapid and homogeneous crystallization of extracellular liquid. After a further 5 min samples are transferred to the inner dewar flask of the freezing apparatus, the initial temperature of which is also −8°C to −10°C.

The temperature within the ethanol bath is monitored by a copper-constantin thermocouple bound to one of the sample tubes and read on a calibrated recorder chart. The rate of heat removal in our system is reasonably constant across the range −8°C to −50°C, but decreases dramatically between −50°C and the end of the run (usually −75°C). The optimal freezing rate for rat fetal pancreas between −8°C and −50°C was found to be 0.30°C/min. The best freezing rate across this same range for pig fetal pancreas is 0.24°C/min, and for human fetal pancreas, 0.22°C/min.

In keeping with the findings of others with simpler cell aggregates, we find that the thawing rate of cryopreserved fetal pancreas is considerably less crucial than the freezing rate. In fact, our routine thawing procedure consists of nothing more than removal of samples from liquid nitrogen storage and exposure to room temperature air until the freezing buffer is partially liquid. The samples are then transferred to room temperature balanced salt solutions containing serum or other suitable additives. In our initial work with fetal rat pancreas we used a complex series of washings with sucrose buffer (6). More recent experience, particularly with fetal pig pancreas, suggests this may not be necessary. Simply incubating the thawed tissue in medium or salt solution containing 10 percent serum seems to work very well. After about 15 min the solution is removed from the tissue and replaced with fresh. Fifteen minutes later the tissues are washed once and are ready for transplantation or for long-term tissue culture.

5. TESTS FOR VIABILITY OF CRYOPRESERVED PANCREATA

Cryopreserved animal tissues have the advantage of being transplantable in order to assess functional viability. In our experience, cryopreserved fetal rat pancreas stored for periods of up to at least 8 months (the longest we have attempted) is as efficacious as freshly dissected tissue in reversing diabetes in adult rats. On the other hand, transplantation into a diabetic recipient and long-term observation of the results is a rather tedious and time-consuming procedure for use as a routine viability assay. We have therefore developed several alternative assay methods, which we now describe.

5.1. Incorporation of Radioactive Amino Acids into TCA-Precipitable Protein

In the first method freeze-recovered and fresh control pancreata are incubated for 4 hr at 37°C in medium plus 10 percent fetal calf serum, 10 percent Trasylol (a protease inhibitor), and 5 μCi/mL [^{14}C]-labeled amino acids. Control tissues are treated with DMSO exactly as the cryopreserved samples, reduced in temperature to -8°C to -10°C (but not seeded), and then immediately put through the standard thawing regimen. Labeled pancreatic rudiments are washed three times and disrupted by freeze-thawing and sonication. Three 0.2-mL aliquots from the sonicate of each pancreas are transferred to strips of No. 17 Whatman filter paper. A fourth 0.2-mL aliquot is saved for measurement of total protein. The paper strips are placed successively in 10 percent (w/v) trichloroacetic acid (TCA) for 30 min at 4–6°C, 5 percent TCA for 15 min at 80°C, and 5 percent TCA for 15 min at room temperature and then are given two 15-min washes in 95 percent ethanol at room temperature. The strips are then dried and radioactivity measured in a liquid scintillation system. The protein is measured in the fourth aliquot by the Lowry assay. Survival values of cryopreserved fetal pancreases are expressed as cpm/per microgram of protein and typically range from 80 to 100 percent of control values obtained using fresh (unfrozen) fetal pancreata. In the rat, viability as judged by this means is a good indicator of functional integrity upon transplantation into diabetic recipients. In the human, survival by this method correlated well with function of the tissue in organ culture (see below).

5.2. Gross Histological Observation in Organ Culture

Until we appreciated the greater sensitivity of pig fetal pancreas to DMSO, we had considerable difficulty obtaining a reliable correlation between amino acid incorporation and survival in culture. We thus developed a method of close monitoring of the gross histological appearance of cryopreserved tissues in organ culture after thawing. Pancreatic fragments are cultured in RPMI medium containing 10 percent fetal calf serum at 37°C in a 5 percent CO_2/95 percent air atmosphere and observed daily for 2–3 days or more. Successfully freeze-recovered tissues show clearly defined limiting edges with a well-organized structure visible via transmitted light. Such structure is lacking or deteriorates rapidly in nonviable tissues. Viability as judged by these criteria appears, from preliminary experiments, to be a good predictor of survival upon transplantation. We have not yet reestablished the amino acid incorporation assay in the pig, although we expect to do so shortly.

5.3. Secretion of Immuno-Reactive Insulin *in Vitro*

We have assessed the functional integrity of freeze-recovered human fetal pancreas by the ability to secrete insulin in response to an appropriate stimulus *in vitro*. Two to three nonfrozen positive controls, freeze-recovered samples, or freeze-killed negative controls (three cycles of rapid freeze-thawing in liquid nitrogen) are incubated at the air–medium interface on a stainless steel wire mesh screen covered with Millipore ultrathin filter (THWP 102FO) in a multiwell tissue culture plate. Each well contains approximately 1 mL of Dulbecco's Modified Eagle's medium (DMEM), an antibiotic/antimycotic solution, 10 percent FCS, and 5 percent Kallikrein inactivator (20,000 U/mL). Glucose is present at 1000 mg/L (5.6 mM). This is referred to as maintenance medium. Culture conditions are 37°C, humidified incubator with 7 percent Co_2 and 93 percent air.

Every 24 hr the maintenance medium is removed from each group and replaced with stimulation medium, which is maintenance medium supplemented with 25 mM glucose or 25 mM glucose plus 10 mM theophylline. Serum is omitted during stimulation. After 4 hr medium is removed from each well and stored for assay. All rudiments are returned to culture in maintenance medium for 24 hr, after which time the maintenance medium is again removed and replaced with the stimulation medium. These culturing and stimulation cycles are repeated three to four times. The collected test media are assayed for insulin using the double antibody radioimmunoassay. As we have reported previously (8), cryopreserved human fetal pancreata survive well in organ culture and respond to high glucose plus theophylline by secreting immunoreactive insulin.

5.4. Transplantation into Nude Rats

The functional viability of cryopreserved fetal rat pancreas can be assessed conveniently by direct transplantation into a diabetic recipient (4). This procedure is something less than convenient for pig fetal pancreas and impossible for the human. We have therefore examined functional survival in the latter two cases by transplanting freeze-recovered tissues into nude rats (rnu). Fragments of appropriate sizes are implanted under the kidney capsule because this site is easily accessible throughout the experiment and provides immediate and rich vascularization for transplanted tissues.

We have noted in the course of these studies that there may be an upper age limit on fetuses from which pancreas can be safely transplanted. Because the recipients are immuno-incompetent, failure to survive and function cannot be attribute to immunological transplant rejection. We find that pancreata from pig fetuses over 9 weeks of age do not survive well (as judged by gross and microscopic histological appearance) after transplantation into nude rats. Based on our experience with transplantation of fetal rat pancreata into adult syngeneic recipients, we would guess that this failure to survive may be related to an advanced state of differentiation of the exocrine pancreas, although we have no clear evidence that this is so. Although one cannot extrapolate results in nude rats to the situation that may obtain in clinical transplantation of fetal human pancreata, our results nonetheless indicate a careful evaluation of fetal donor age and transplant survival when clinical trials begin in the near future.

6. DISCUSSION

Our experience with cryopreservation of fetal pancreata is still evolving. Each species has presented its own unique challenges, causing us to constantly refine our techniques. Our most recent efforts have focused on cryopreserving the fetal pig pancreas. We find in this case that better survival is achieved when tissues are exposed to higher concentrations of DMSO for shorter periods of time. We will apply this method to the human fetal pancreas in the near future and compare it with the method described in the previous section. The rather complicated sucrose washes applied to thawed rat and human fetal pancreas was suggested by Peter Mazur's previous experience with mouse blastomeric embryos. We found this method not to be necessary with pig fetal pancreas and will soon test the pig method with human fetal pancreas. Also, our recent experience with testing the secretory response of freeze-recovered fetal pig pancreas to theophylline suggests that the procedure described for the human can be simplified. We culture several fragments of pig pancreas in "maintenance" or "stimulation" medium in 35-mm culture dishes with 0.75 mL of medium, rather than on the more cumbersome stainless steel screen–Millipore filter apparatus.

Cryopreservation of complex (albeit very small) biological structures, lacking a precise theoretical basis, is thus a highly empirical technological exercise. We do not yet know, for example, what the upper size limit is on fragments that can be successfully cryopreserved. As with other empirical approaches, there is a tendency to stick to what works. But beyond any doubt, fetal pancreata (and perhaps other diffuse fetal structures) can be cryopreserved virtually indefinitely and function fully upon transplantation.

REFERENCES

1. J. Brown, I. G. Molnar, W. Clark, and Y. Mullen, *Science* **184**, 1377–1379 (1974).

2. D. G. Whittingham, S. Seibo, and P. Mazur, *Science* **178**, 411 (1972).

3. P. Mazur, J. Kemp, and R. Miller, *Proc. Natl. Acad. Sci. U.S.A.* **73**, 4105 (1976).

4. J. A. Kemp, P. Mazur, Y. Mullen, R. H. Miller, W. Clark, and J. Brown, *Transplantation Proceedings* **9**, 325–328 (1977).

5. J. Brown, W. Clark, I. G. Molnar, J. Kemp, P. Mazur, and Y. S. Mullen, "Functional Capacity and Cryopreservation of Fetal Rat Pancreas in Streptozotocin-Diabetes," in *Proceedings of the 9th Congress of International Diabetes*, FEBS, J. S. Bajaj (ed.), Excerpta Medica, Amsterdam, 1977, pp. 167–175.

6. J. A. Kemp, Y. Mullen, H. Weisman, D. Heininger, J. Brown, and W. R. Clark, *Transplantation* **26**, 260–264 (1978).

7. J. Brown, J. A. Kemp, S. Hurt, and W. R. Clark, *Diabetes* **29**, (suppl. 1), 70–73 (1980).

8. J. A. Kemp, S. N. Hurt, J. Brown, and W. R. Clark, *Transplantation* **32**, 10–15, (1981).

K

MORPHOLOGY OF ISLET BLOOD SUPPLY

TSUNEO FUJITA

Department of Anatomy, Niigata University, School of Medicine, Niigata, Japan

The pattern of the blood supply to the pancreatic islet is studied by two varieties of the vascular injection method. One is the dye injection technique for light microscopy and the other is the resin cast preparation for scanning electron microscopy.

1.   DYE INJECTION TECHNIQUES

1.1.   India Ink Injection

India ink is a most suitable material for demonstration under the light microscope of the pancreatic microcirculation, including the finest capillaries (1; page 472 in ref. 2). One does not need to exercise care with the temperature of the injection material; the colloid particles of India ink will not easily diffuse into the tissue parenchyme; they are topographically fixed in blood vessels when gelatin contained in the ink is chemically fixed by formaldehyde.

The best way to prepare the ink is to gently rub down the India ink stick into physiological saline or Ringer's solution. More simply, one may dilute commercial thickened ink with 3–4 volumes of saline. Pelikan's "Tusche" can be used. Although gelatin is inherent in every India ink preparation, one may add a certain amount of gelatin liquified by warming. It is recommended that the injected material be filtered so that the coarse particles will be eliminated (2).

The India ink thus prepared is injected with a syringe and cannula system into the arteries supplying the pancreas or into the aorta in smaller animals. In the pancreas or a portion removed surgically, the severed ends of the arteries must be sought for injection. Venous injection (from the portal vein) is also worth investigating; the result may supplement that obtained by arterial injection (3).

The injection is performed gently but quite forcefully. Measurement of the injection pressure is usually useless because the pressure at the injection site does not always reflect the pressure at the peripheral vascular bed. It is, on the other hand, very important to control the injection pressure by carefully observing the grade of blackening and swelling of the tissue by perfusion. The caval vein or right auricle is cut to let out the blood and perfusate, and the pancreas is thoroughly perfused (Fig. 1).

Next the main veins emerging from the pancreas and associated viscera as well as the artery used for injection are ligated in order to prevent leakage of the ink. The pancreas, with associated viscera, is now excised and dipped in greater than 10 volumes of 10 percent formalin. After two or three days one may cut out pieces of the organ to be examined.

According to the classic method, the tissue pieces are embedded in paraffin or celloidin to be cut into considerably thick (20–40 μm), preferably serial, sections (3–5). One can obtain beautiful preparations with this method, especially when the sections are stained by hematoxylin or carmine, but it is difficult to visualize the three-dimensional extensions and connections of fine vessels even if one overcomes the tedious work of reconstructing a montage of the images in serial sections.

In order to avoid this difficulty, a much simpler method is recommended (6):

1. The India ink is injected and the tissue fixed in formalin, as explained above.
2. The pancreas is cut into blocks.

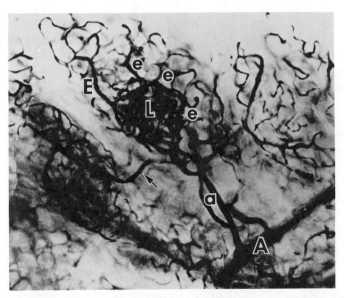

FIGURE 1. Microcirculation in the rat pancreas as demonstrated by the India ink injection method. An intralobular artery (A) gives two vasa afferentia (a) to the islet (L), which issues larger (E) and smaller (e) vasa efferentia to the vascular bed of the exocrine tissue. An arteriole directly supplying the exocrine tissue is seen (arrow).

3. The tissue blocks are dehydrated in a series of ascending concentrations of ethanol and xylene and then cleared in methyl salicylate. Usually 12 hr are necessary for the tissue blocks to become transparent and appropriately hard. One may keep them in methyl salicylate for months to years.

4. The blocks are sliced with a razor blade. It is recommended that one carefully observe the courses of the main blood vessels under the dissecting microscope to decide the direction and thickness of the slicing.

5. The slice, immersed in several drops of methyl salicylate, is observed under a light microscope. For lower magnification, the specimen is covered by a coverslip, but for higher magnification it is observed without a coverslip, the objective lens being directly dipped in the methyl salicylate immersing the specimen.

1.2. Other Injection Methods

India ink can be replaced by other chemical dyes such as Berlin blue, trypan blue, and lithium carmine (3). Latex is also suitable for injection. In this case the specimen is better observed under the incident light, after being made transparent.

Microradiography of the pancreas after arterial injection of contrast media can be used to study the microcirculation of the organ (7).

2. RESIN CASTING FOR SCANNING ELECTRON MICROSCOPY

Vascular casts of resin have long been used for light microscopic observation, but the results obtained by this method are limited because of the small depth of focus and low resolution. Since the advent of the scanning electron microscope, attempts have been made to apply it to the more precise and convincing demonstration of vascular casts.

Among the methods thus introduced, the cast preparation technique of Murakami (8–11) described below is most highly recommended and, in fact, most used worldwide.

Methyl methacrylate monomer (100 mL) is added to 1–1.5 mL 2,4-dichlorobenzoyl peroxide (catalyst) and warmed to 60–65°C. As polymerization occurs, the temperature will spontaneously reach 85–90°C in a few minutes. This half-polymerized resin is quickly cooled to a temperature lower than 30°C, and then 1.5–2 g benzoyl peroxide is added with gentle stirring. In 5–10 min the resin becomes adequately viscous (slightly less viscous than glycerin). At this time 1.5 mL dimethyl aniline (accelerator) is added. The resin is now ready to be used.

Recently a partially polymerized methacrylate medium suited for vascular casting has become commercially available (Mercox; Japan Vilene Chemical and Hospital, Tokyo).

In the animal or the organ the pancreas is arterially perfused with Ringer's solution with gradually increasing temperatures (37–50°C) and then the injection-ready resin is introduced into the perfused organ with an adequate pressure, also under visual control. The animal or the excised pancreas is then immersed in a warm water bath (60–70°C) and placed in an oven at the same temperature for 24 hr, so that the resin in the organ can become polymerized. The pancreas is then macerated with 20 percent NaOH and the resin cast is washed.

The resin cast is usually divided into smaller pieces with forceps, a razor blade, or small scissors. This should be done carefully under a dissecting microscope. Islets, for example, can be recognized in this preparation. Sometimes it is helpful to correctly trim the cast by shaving with a blade for embedding in ice.

The resin casts are sputter coated with metals for observation under the scanning electron microscope. The metal coating should be made carefully and sufficiently as the casts of fine and dense arborizations of blood vessels easily cause charging in the electron microscope. A good method to avoid the charging is to place the casts in osmium gas for several hours. Casts obtain excellent electric conductivity and give beautiful images in the electron microscope even without metal coating (12).

Microdissection of the casts in or out of the scanning electron microscope can be performed in order to expose or isolate a specific part of the cast (Figs. 2 and 3).

3. RESULTS

The following observations on the microcirculation of the pancreas may be expected from the India ink-injected pancreas or from the resin casts (3–6, 10, 13).

1. The arteries run interlobularly and intralobularly. The veins take their course mainly interlobularly.

2. The intralobular arteries give one, or sometimes two, of their branches (arterioles) to each islet. This *vas afferens* breaks up to form the capillary network of the islet and, in turn, issues numerous capillaries which radiate to connect with the capillary bed of the exocrine pancreas. These radiating vessels are called insuloacinar portal vessels and are regarded as the routes conveying the hormones and transmitters released from the endocrine cells and nerves in the islet to their vicinal target, the exocrine pancreas (6, 10, 14–17).

3. Parallel to the above-described blood route via the insuloacinar portal system, a few branches of the intralobular arteries are found directly bound to the exocrine pancreas. The blood flow through this route seems to exceed that through the insuloacinar portal system in some animals like the rat and rabbit (13, 18, 19), whereas in other animals, including the horse (5, 6), circulation via the portal vessels predominates.

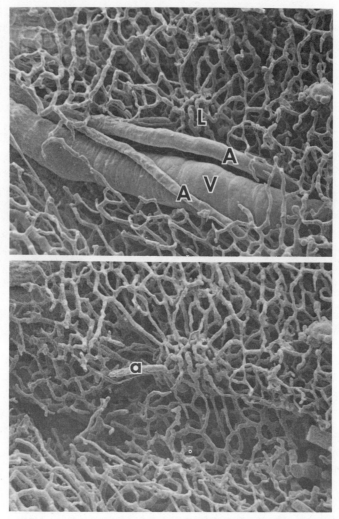

FIGURE 2.   Methacrylate cast of rhesus monkey pancreas. Figure 2-1(A) is a scanning electron micrograph with the capillary glomus of an islet (L) in the center. Interlobular arteries (A) and vein (V) hinder the view of the islet, and were removed by microdissection. Figure 2-2B shows the view of the same site after microdissection. An arteriole, vas afferens (a) entering the islet and many vasa efferentia radiating from it are demonstrated. Figure 2-3C is a closer view of the cast of islet vessels. Figure 2-1A and 2-2B × 200; Fig. 2-3C: × 400. [Reproduced from T. Fujita and T. Murakami, *Arch. Histol. Japon.* **35**, 255–263 (1973).]

    4.   Large islets in the rat (19) and guinea pig, some snake species, and birds may have *vasa efferentia* which are partially drained directly by veins which do not pass through the capillary network of the exocrine pancreas.

    5.   Islets of the rat located interlobularly often give their *vasa efferentia* to the capillary network surrounding the interlobular ductules. These connections have been designated as insuloductular portal vessels (13).

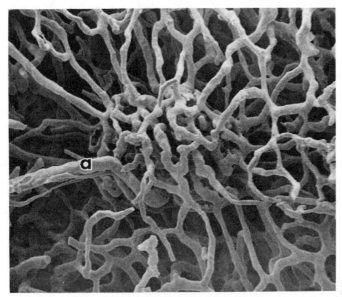

FIGURE 3

6. The *vas afferens* arborizes in the periphery of the islet in those animals in which the α and δ cells are located at the periphery of the islet (rat, mouse, and rabbit), whereas it enters into the center of the islet before branching in those animals in which α and δ cells are located in the islet center (horse and monkey). The *vas afferens* breaks up at more random sites in animals in which α, β, and δ cells are mingled irregularly (man and dog). This relationship seems to be accounted for by the fact that glucagon released from the α cells stimulates insulin secretion from the β cells, whereas somatostatin from the δ cells inhibits the release of insulin (6, 10, 13, 15).

4.   *IN SITU* OBSERVATION OF THE PANCREAS

It seems worthwhile to add here that the microcirculation of the pancreas can and should also be investigated by microscopic observation of the vasculature in the organ of living animals. Rats, mice, and young rabbits are suited for these studies since their pancreata are relatively confined. Practice is needed in order to position the animal on the stage of the microscope, which is equipped with fiberoptic light sources and saline immersion objective lenses. The blood stream in the pancreas, exposed and transilluminated, may be observed visually and also can be recorded in motion pictures or videotape. Actual blood flow through the insuloacinar portal vessels has been demonstrated in the pancreas *in situ* in mice (20), rabbits (21), and rats (19).

Ohtani (19) recommends injection of fluorescent tracer (brilliant sulfoflavin or fluorescein isothiocyanate) through the tail vein in the rat and observation of the pancreatic blood stream under incident ultraviolet illumination. Ohtani (19) recently studied the same pancreatic islets, both with light fluorescent microscopy while the animals (rats) were alive and also with scanning electron micrographs of resin casts of the vascular bed.

The microcirculation of the pancreas is a highly important field of study, and recent physiological studies have indicated the significance of the endocrine–exocrine axis in this organ. It is hoped that investigations in this field will be advanced by the application of the methods introduced in this article.

REFERENCES

1. K. Taguchi, *Arch. Mikrosk. Anat.* **31**, 565 (1938).

2. B. Romeis, *Mikroskopische Technik* R. Oldenbourg, München, 1948.

3. G. Wharton, *Anat. Rec.* **53**, 55 (1932).

4. M. Tohyama, *Japan J. Med. Sci. Anat.* **5**, 61 (1935).

5. A. Thiel, *Z. Zellforsch* **39**, 339 (1954).

6. T. Fujita, *Arch. Histol. Japon.* **35**, 161 (1973).

7. N. Hayasaka and N. Sasano, *Tohoku J. Exp. Med.* **100**, 327 (1970).

8. T. Murakami, *Arch. Histol. Japon.* **32**, 445 (1971).

9. T. Murakami, M. Miyoshi, and T. Fujita, *Arch. Histol. Japon.* **33**, 179 (1971).

10. T. Fujita and T. Murakami, *Arch. Histol. Japon.* **35**, 255 (1973).

11. T. Murakami, *Arch. Histol. Japon.* **35**, 323 (1973).

12. T. Murakami, M. Unehira, K. Kawakami, and A. Kubotsu, *Arch. Histol. Japon.* **36**, 119 (1973).

13. O. Ohtani and T. Fujita, *Biomed. Res.* **1**, 130 (1980).

14. J. R. Henderson, *Lancet*, 7618 (1969).

15. T. Fujita and Y. Watanabe, "The Effects of Islet Hormones upon the Exocrine Pancreas," in *Gastro-entero-pancreatic Endocrine System—A Cell-Biological Approach*, T. Fujita (ed.), Igaku shoin Ltd., Tokyo, 1973, pp. 164–173.

16. T. Fujita and S. Kobayashi, *Arch. Histol. Japon.* **42**, 277 (1979).

17. T. Fujita, S. Kobayashi, S. Fujii, T. Iwanaga, and Y. Serizawa, "Langerhans Islets as the Neuro-paraneuronal Control Center of the Endocrine Pancreas," in *Cellular Basis of Chemical Messengers in the Digestive System*, M. I. Grossman, M. A. Brazier, and J. Lechago (eds.), Academic Press, New York, 1981, pp. 231–242.

18. N. Lifson, K. G. Kramlinger, R. R. Mayrand, and E. J. Lender, *Gastroenterology* **79**, 466 (1980).

19. O. Ohtani, *Arch. Histol. Japon.* **46**, 315 (1983).

20. R. S. McCuskey and T. M. Henderson, *Am. J. Anat.* **126**, 395 (1969).

21. P. A. Fraser and J. R. Henderson, *Quart. J. Exp. Physiol.* **65**, 151 (1980).

L

A SIMPLE TECHNIQUE FOR VISUALIZATION OF THE PANCREATIC ISLETS AND ITS APPLICATION TO MEASUREMENTS OF ISLET BLOOD FLOW WITH THE MICROSPHERE METHOD

LEIF JANSSON AND CLAES HELLERSTRÖM
Department of Medical Cell Biology, University of Uppsala, Uppsala, Sweden

1. INTRODUCTION

The hormone release from the islets of Langerhans may be regulated not only by nutrients, nervous signals, or biologically active factors in the immediate vicinity of islet cells, but also by changes in the rate of islet blood flow. Studies of the blood flow to the islets and its regulation are, however, hampered by the small total volume of the islet organ and its distribution within the pancreas as a large number of minute cell aggregates. Intravital microscopy has been attempted for such studies, but the information obtained is difficult to quantify and the risk of artifactually changing the blood flow by the methodological manipulations is considerable. The introduction of the microsphere technique (1) for studies of both whole organ blood flow and intraorgan distribution of flow, however, offers a possibility of measuring islet blood flow separately from that of the acinar part of the pancreas. A prerequisite for this approach is a method for detecting and counting microspheres in the islets as distinct from those in the surrounding exocrine parenchyma. In the following section we will describe a relatively simple method for separate measurements of islet and acinar blood flow using nonradioactive microspheres after visualization of islets by freezing and thawing of the pancreas.

2. PRINCIPLES OF THE MICROSPHERE METHOD AND CALCULATIONS OF THE BLOOD FLOW

The method for measurement of organ blood flow with the aid of microspheres is based on the observation that spherical plastic particles of suitable size and density, which are injected intra-arterially, will mix uniformly with the blood and distribute throughout the arterial system in proportion to the blood flow. Due to their size and rigidity, the particles become entrapped in arterioles and capillaries during their first passage through these vessels where they can be enumerated either by direct visual inspection or, if they are labeled with a radioactive γ-isotope, by their radioactivity. A quantitative measure of the blood flow through the organ is obtained by the use of the so-called reference sample method in which an artificial external organ is created by the attachment of a syringe to a catheter placed in the abdominal aorta. When the microspheres are injected into the arterial circulation, a simultaneous blood sample is drawn with the syringe at a known and constant flow rate. The number of microspheres in the reference sample is thus representative of the flow to the syringe, and

The technical assistance of Mrs. Elisabet Wennberg and Mrs. Astrid Nordin is gratefully appreciated. Financial support was obtained from the Swedish Diabetes Association, The Clas Groschinsky Foundation, the Medical Faculty of Uppsala University, and the Swedish Medical Research Council (Grant 12X-109). We thank Mrs. Agneta Snellman for valuable help in typing the manuscript.

if the total number of microspheres in the organ is known, the blood flow to that organ can be calculated according to the formula

$$Q_{org} = \frac{N_{org} \times Q_{ref}}{N_{ref}}$$

where Q_{org} is the organ blood flow (mL/min); Q_{ref} is the flow of reference sample (mL/min); N_{org} is the number of microspheres present in organ; and N_{ref} is the number of microspheres present in reference sample.

If the number of injected microspheres is known, the cardiac output can also be calculated according to the formula

$$CO = \frac{Q_{ref} \times N_{inj}}{N_{ref}}$$

where CO is the cardiac output (mL/min); Q_{ref} is the flow of the reference sample (mL/min); N_{inj} is the number of microspheres injected; and N_{ref} is the number of microspheres in the reference sample (for review see 2).

Studies of the blood flow to the islets of Langerhans involve the measurements of blood flow both to a whole organ and within an organ. This necessitates a method of either determining the exact position of each microsphere within the organ or separating the compartments of the organ (i.e., islets and acini) followed by counting of the microspheres in each compartment. The latter alternative is unrealistic since even the most careful isolation of islets will yield only a fraction of the total number of islets. The identification of the location of each microsphere in the pancreas is, therefore, the method of choice. Although this could be achieved with routine histological sectioning of the pancreas, this would be very tedious and time consuming and in addition would introduce the risk of displacement of the microsphere due to the preparation of the specimens, for example by the action of the microtome knife. It would be preferable to identify the islets and localize the microspheres in relation to these structures within the intact pancreas. Such identifications have been achieved by the use of two techniques, one in which the pancreas is perfused with a dye to stain the islets followed by clearing in methyl salicylate (3) or glycerol (4) and another in which the islets are identified by freezing and thawing the pancreas (5). The latter method will be described in detail below.

3. SURGICAL PROCEDURE

The following description refers to experiments performed in the rat. Anesthesia is induced with thiobutabarbital sodium (Inactin, Byk Gulden, Konstanz, FRG;

125 mg/kg body weight i.p.) about 10 min before surgery. This drug appears to have particularly small effects on the circulation in the rat and allows extensive surgery to be carried out over several hours. The animal is placed on its back, a thermistor temperature probe (YSI 402 Yellow Springs Instrument Co., Yellow Springs, OH) is inserted into the rectum and the body temperature recorded throughout the experiments. The left femoral vein and artery are freed from the surrounding tissue by blunt dissection and 200 IU heparin (Heparin 5000 IU/mL, Lövens Läkemedel, Malmö, Sweden) are injected intravenously with a 1-mL syringe. A polyethylene catheter with an inner diameter of 0.58 mm (heated and drawn to a diameter of about 0.35 mm) is inserted into the artery and advanced approximately 1 cm. The catheter in the left femoral artery is connected to a pressure transducer (PDCR 75/1, Druck Ltd., Groby, Leicestershire, UK) and the blood pressure registered on a pressure arterial module (SEM-422-01, SE-Labs Ltd., Feltham, Middlesex, UK). Another arterial catheter is inserted in the right femoral artery and advanced into the lower part of the abdominal aorta (i.e., approximately 3 cm). This catheter is connected to a programmable syringe (Microlab M Dispenser, Hamilton Bonaduz AG, Bonaduz, Switzerland). The tube connecting the dispenser and the artery is previously weighed to the nearest milligram. An incision is made on the right side of the neck and about 2 cm of the right carotid artery is carefully freed from its surrounding tissue. Special care is taken to avoid injury to the vagus nerve and the sympathetic trunk. Another catheter is inserted into the right carotid artery and is advanced to the heart (about 4 cm). As the catheter is advanced, a slight resistance is felt when the catheter tip reaches the aortic root just prior to entering into the left ventricle. Care must be taken at this point to avoid perforating the aortic wall. When the tip of the catheter is successfully located in the left ventricle, the entire catheter exhibits rhythmic movements corresponding to the beating of the heart. If the placement of the catheter in the heart remains unsuccessful, the catheter tip may be left at the aortic root. We have been unable to detect any differences in flow values between the two catheter positions.

When the above procedures have been completed, usually within 15 min, the animals are allowed to equilibrate, under a lamp to keep them warm, for 20 min, or until the blood pressure becomes stabilized. Since the risk of respiratory acidosis increases with time under anesthesia it is preferable to minimize the time necessary for the surgical procedures prior to the injection of the microspheres. Prolonged experiments require tracheal intubation or assisted ventilation.

In preparation for the microsphere injection, nonradioactive microspheres with a diameter of approximately 10 μm (New England Nuclear Boston, MA) are suspended in saline (0.9 percent NaCl w/v) containing 0.002 percent of Tween 80. The microspheres are uniformly suspended by vigorous shaking for 10 min with the aid of a whirl mixer and 0.3 mL of the suspension (containing between 1.2 and 1.5 × 10^5 microspheres as determined by counting in a hemocytometer) is injected via the carotid catheter during a 20–25-sec period.

Immediately after the injection the catheter is flushed with 0.2 mL of physiological saline. For a total of 90 sec, beginning 5 sec before the injection of
microspheres, the reference sample is withdrawn, from the catheter in the
right femoral artery at a constant rate of 0.60 mL/min with the aid of the
programmable dispenser. When the reference sample has been collected, blood
samples for the determination of serum glucose and serum hormone concentrations are obtained from the arterial catheter. About 3 min after the injection
of the microspheres the animal is killed by cervical dislocation. The pancreas,
the adrenals, and the lower lobe of the left lung are quickly removed through
a midline incision and placed in Hanks' balanced salt solution until further
processing (see below). The polyethylene tube containing the reference sample
is weighed to ascertain the exact volume of the sample which must be known
to calculate the blood flow. To prevent clotting, 200 IU of heparin is added
to the blood which is stored at 4°C until counting of its microsphere content
(see below). After removal of the organs the positions of the arterial catheters
are verified by dissection.

4. METHODS FOR VISUALIZATION OF THE ISLETS AND COUNTING OF THE MICROSPHERES

Immediately after removal the pancreas is dissected free of fat and connective
tissue, blotted, and weighed. The gland is cut into pieces, each weighing 10–
20 mg (about 5 mm in diameter), which are placed on microscope slides with
about five pieces on each slide. A small piece of adhesive tape (thickness
approximately 50 μm) is applied to each end of the slide and the preparation
is covered with another slide. The slides are pressed firmly together and held
by further strips of tape at both ends, resulting in a flattening of the pancreatic
pieces in the space between the slides. The slides, usually 15 per animal, are
frozen and stored at $-20°C$. Storage for more than 4 days, however leads to
some drying of the tissue, which may hamper the identification of the islets.
Counting of microspheres is performed immediately after the preparations
have thawed and reached room temperature. For this purpose the pancreas is
viewed in a Wild M3 stereo microscope (Wild Heerbrug Ltd., Heerbrug,
Switzerland) equipped with both bright-field and dark-field illumination. When
the frozen/thawed pancreas is viewed under dark field, each islet stands out
as a distinct white spot against the translucent acinar part of the gland (5; see
also Figs. 1 and 2). Since the microspheres can be seen more distinctly under
bright-field illumination, it is of importance that the microscope is equipped
with both these types of condensers. In counting the microspheres they are
first localized under bright field (40 × magnification) and the microscope condenser is then switched to the dark-field position to determine whether the
sphere is located in an islet or in the exocrine parenchyma. The resolution and
focal depth of the microscope usually permits a precise localization of a microsphere within or outside an islet. In the few instances when it is doubtful

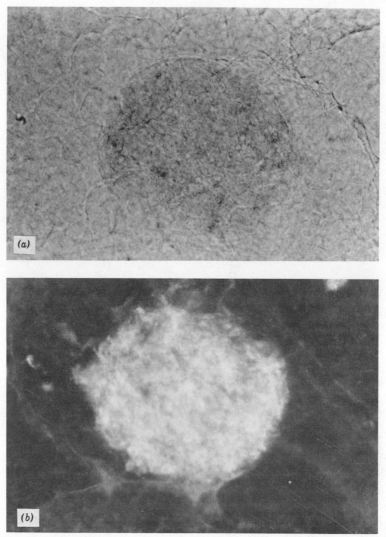

FIGURE 1.   An islet as it appears in bright-field (*a*) and dark-field (*b*) illumination (magnification 160×).

whether a sphere is located in the acinar part above or below an islet, the preparation is inverted and the spheres localized and counted again. The mean value of the two counts is then used in the calculation of the blood flow.

The number of microspheres present in the reference sample is determined by distributing 40–50 μL portions of the sample on glass microfiber filters (GF/A 2.5 cm, Whatman Ltd., London, UK) with a pore size less than 10 μm. Thus, 20–25 filters are needed for a reference sample of 0.90 mL. Each

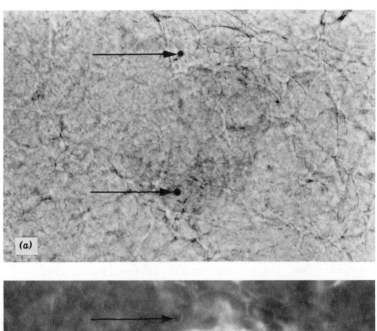

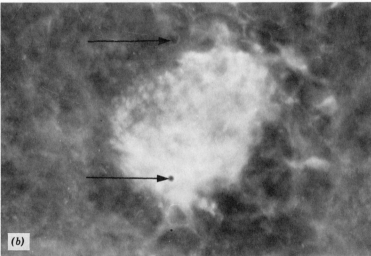

FIGURE 2.   Two microspheres (arrows), one in an islet and the other in the exocrine parenchyma, visualized with bright-field (*a*) and dark-field illumination (*b*). Note that the microspheres are more easily identified under bright field (magnification 160 ×).

filter is placed on a glass microscope slide and counted under bright-field illumination in the stereo microscope (magnification 40 ×). Shunting of spheres is checked by counting the number of microspheres in preweighed portions of the lung and the homogeneous distribution in the blood by counting the spheres in paired organs like the adrenals (see below). Identification of spheres can be made directly when pieces of these organs are compressed between glass microscope slides as described above, but for convenience each preparation is treated identically to the pancreas, that is, frozen and thawed prior to counting the microspheres.

5. SOURCES OF ERROR

The microsphere technique depends on the validity of several assumptions regarding the behavior of the microspheres in the circulation: (ii) The spheres are completely mixed with the blood at the arrival to the target organ. (ii) They show the same flow properties in the circulation as an erythrocyte. (iii) They are completely trapped in the target organ without any recirculation. (iv) They do not disturb the blood flow to or within the organ. (For review see ref. 2.) A rapid and complete mixing of the spheres with the blood is facilitated by adding a detergent like Tween 80 to the vehicle in which the spheres are suspended. Ideally, the injection of the spheres should take place in the left atrium of the heart (6), but this is difficult to achieve in the rat without extensive equipment. The experience the authors (7) and others (8–10), however, suggests that reliable results are obtained when injections are performed in the left ventricle or at the aortic root. A measure of the uniformity of mixing of microspheres in blood may be obtained by counting the number of spheres in paired organs, for example the adrenals. Similar numbers of spheres in the two organs indicate even mixing, at least at the origin of the arteries supplying the organs with blood.

The flow properties of the microspheres appear to be a function of their size. Studies *in vivo* (11) and *in vitro* (12) have demonstrated a size-dependent skimming of spheres, suggesting that the larger ones tend to travel more centrally in the blood stream giving rise to a nonhomogenous distribution. In studies of pancreatic and islet blood flow $10\mu m$ appear to be an optimal size (7, 13, 14). Bypass (A–V shunting) and recirculation of spheres will take place unless they are totally trapped at the first passage through the microcirculation bed. To determine the degree of shunting (i.e., nonentrapped spheres), the number of microspheres present in the lungs may be used as a control. In doing so the accumulation of spheres due to the normal bronchial circulation (2–3 percent of the cardiac output) must be taken into account. It should be noted, moreover, that evaluation of microsphere shunting through the splanchnic area, including the pancreas, poses particular problems since spheres passing through that area may be trapped in the liver (14). Of further importance is the possibility of displacement of spheres when the tonus in the vascular wall decreases after the death of the animal. This has been observed in the intestine, where microspheres may move from the submucosal area to the mucosal (15, 16). However, this source of error appears to be of significance mainly when vesseis are connected in series. This may thus be of little relevance to the islets of Langerhans as it has been suggested that these receive blood from afferent arterioles connected in parallel to those supplying the acinar part, at least in the rat (17). Administration of microspheres should result in as little perturbations of blood flow as possible. For this purpose the total number of microspheres injected should be kept below an upper limit of 200,000 in the rat. Thus, we have regularly observed marked decreases in blood pressure when this number have been exceeded and we usually inject not more than 150,000 spheres per animal. It is, on the other hand, important to maintain the injected spheres at a number sufficient enough to retrieve a significant number in the reference sample and in the organs. The statistical background of the methods has been treated by several authors who agree that a certain minimal number of spheres is required to attain an acceptable accuracy. This number is usually given as about 400 (18, 19), but in the rat 200 has been found to be enough (8, 20). With the method described the number of microspheres in the reference sample and the whole gland is well above 400 while that in the islets is usually 150–170. In our experience, however, quite reproducible results are observed even with the latter number of spheres as evidenced by the low standard errors of the means recorded in our measurements (7). Not mentioned above but of importance is also the correct position of the tip of the catheter used to provide the reference sample from the abdominal aorta (21) and the withdrawal rate which should not be too low (22).

REFERENCES

1. A. M. Rudolph and M. A. Heymann, *Circulat. Res.* **21**, 163 (1967).
2. M. A. Heymann, B. D. Payne, J. I. E. Hoffman, and A. M. Rudolph, *Progr. Cardiovasc. Dis.* **20**, 55 (1977).
3. K. G. Kramlinger, R. R. Mayrand, and N. Lifson, *Stain Technol.* **54**, 159 (1979).
4. H. H. Meyer, F. Vetterlein, G. Schmidt, and A. Hasselblatt, *Am. J. Physiol.* **242**, E298 (1982).
5. L. Jansson and C. Hellerström, *Acta Physiol. Scand.* **113**, 371 (1981).
6. S. Kaihara, P. D. van Heerden, T. Migita, and H. N. Wagner, Jr., *J. Appl. Physiol.* **25**, 696 (1968).
7. L. Jansson and C. Hellerström, *Diabetologia* **25**, 45 (1983).
8. S. Ishise, B. L. Pegram, J. Yamamoto, Y. Kitamura, and E. D. Frohlich, *Am. J. Physiol.* **239**, H443 (1980).
9. D. G. McDewitt and A. S. Nies, *Cardiovasc. Res.* **10**, 494 (1976).
10. P. Wicker and R. C. Tarazi, *Cardiovasc. Res.* **16**, 580 (1982).
11. R. H. Phibbs and L. Dong, *Can. J. Physiol. Pharmacol.* **48**, 415, (1970).
12. E. S. Øfjord, G. Clausen, and K. Aukland, *Am. J. Physiol.* **241**, H342 (1981).
13. N. Lifson, K. G. Kramlinger, R. R. Mayrand, and J. E. Lender, *Gastroenterology* **79**, 466 (1980).
14. N. Lifson, "Use of Microspheres to Measure Intraorgan Distribution of Blood Flow in the Splanchnic Circulation," in *Measurement of Blood Flow. Applications to the Splanchnic Circulation*, D. N. Granger and G. B. Bulkey (eds.), Williams & Wilkins, Baltimore/London, 1981, p. 177.
15. C. A. Greenway and V. S. Murthy, *Br. J. Pharmac.* **46**, 177 (1972).

16. L. C. Maxwell, A. P. Sheperd, and G. L. Riedel, *Am. J. Physiol.* **243**, H123 (1982).

17. S. Bonner-Weir and L. Orci, *Diabetes* **31**, 883 (1982).

18. G. D. Buckberg, J. C. Luck, D. B. Payne, J. I. E. Hoffman, J. P. Archie, and D. E. Fixler, *J. Appl. Physiol.* **31**, 598 (1971).

19. W. P. Dole, D. L. Jackson, J. I. Rosenblatt, and W. L. Thompson, *Am. J. Physiol.* **243**, H371 (1982).

20. M. Tsuchiya. R. A. Ferrone, G. M. Walsh, and E. D. Frohlich, *Am. J. Physiol.* **235**, H357 (1978).

21. J. Idvall, K. F. Aronsen, L. Nilsson, and B. Nosslin, *Eur. Surg. Res.* **11**, 423 (1979).

22. C. D. Moore, B. L. Gewertz, H. T. Wheeler, and W. J. Fry, *Microvasc. Res.* **21**, 377 (1981).

M

MORPHOLOGY
AND BLOOD FLOW
OF THE ISLET ORGAN

NATHAN LIFSON AND CHRISTINE V. LASSA
*Department of Physiology, University of Minnesota Medical School,
Minneapolis, Minnesota*

1. INTRODUCTION

The methods to be described deal with aspects of the morphology and blood flow of the islet organ (ensemble of the islets of Langerhans in a pancreas) in which the islet is taken as a unit. Intraislet morphology or intraislet distribution of blood flow will not be considered. The method employed here for quantitative morphology of the islet organ of rabbits and rats is one in which measurements are made on unsectioned tissue and thus do not require stereological formulas, because the pancreata of these animals are thin. The pancreas is stained postmortem by intra-arterial perfusion of hematoxylin (1). Pieces of pancreatic tissue are then cleared in methyl salicylate for microscopic examination. The procedure preferentially stains islets, making it possible to count the islets and to determine the frequency distribution of their diameters and other derived morphometric values.

Measurement of the perfusion of the islet organ presents difficulties due to its disseminated nature and the microscopic or semimicroscopic size of most of its units. Only recently has this difficulty been surmounted at least in principle by administration of microspheres followed by a method by which spheres in islets and nonislet tissue can be distinguished (2–4). These measurements provide estimates of the percentage distribution of the pancreatic blood flow to the exocrine and endocrine portions of the gland. If the tissues have been stained as described above, it also becomes possible to obtain estimates of the relationship between islet size and islet blood flow. The methods as most recently carried out on rabbits and rats will be described.

2. METHODS

2.1. Experiments on Rabbits

Unfasted New Zealand white rabbits weighing about 2 kg were used. They were anesthetized by intravenous injection of a combination of 30 mg/kg of

sodium pentobarbital (Nembutal) and 5 mg of diazepam (Valium). Body tem-
controlled by a rectal thermister probe. "Carbonized" nonradioactive polystyrene microspheres 10 μm in diameter (Nuclear Products Division, 3M
Company, St. Paul, MN) were suspended in 0.9 percent NaCl containing
0.0075 percent Tween 80 [polyoxyethylene (20) sorbitan monooleate]. The
suspension was held in an ultrasonic sonicator for 3 min and gently mixed
before injection into the left ventricle of the heart through a catheter (PE 90)
inserted via the left common carotid artery. The blood pressure in the catheter
was monitored by a pressure transducer and recorder to ascertain ventricular
positioning of the catheter. Duration of the injection was about 10 sec, and
the volume injected was 1 mL/kg. The sphere injectate was followed by a
flush of 2–3 mL of heparinized saline. The injectate contained 10 mg of spheres
(1.5×10^7) per mL. Blood pressure was recorded except during the injections.

A value for the rate of blood flow per sphere was obtained by the reference
organ method. A blood sample was withdrawn into a syringe (containing 0.5
mL of heparin, 1000 USP units/mL) by pump from the lower abdominal aorta
at a constant rate of 5 mL/min via a cannula (PE 60) inserted into the femoral
artery. The blood sample was transferred to a tube containing 0.5 mL of
heparin and immediately examined under the microscope for clumping of
spheres, and with a few exceptions essentially none was seen. (If the microspheres in a suspension made up in the manner described were not satisfactorily
dispersed as single spheres, the batch was returned to the supplier.) The experiments with clumped spheres were disregarded. The total number of spheres
in the blood sample was obtained by counting the number of spheres in aliquots
of a well-mixed sample placed on a slide and covered with a glass coverslip.
The syringe is in effect an organ of known flow which completely traps the
spheres and which is assumed to receive blood identical with respect to bead
content to the blood received by the region under investigation. Then the rate
of blood flow per sphere becomes the rate of withdrawal divided by the number
of spheres in the total withdrawn blood sample. After the microsphere injection
and femoral arterial blood collection, the rabbits were sacrificed by injection
of a saturated KCl solution into the carotid cannula.

The abdomen was opened by a midline incision. Both ends of the loop of
small intestine whose mesentery contained the pancreas were ligated, as were
the renal pedicles and the abdominal aorta above the origin of the celiac artery.
A polyethylene cannula (PE 160) was inserted into the aorta below the kidney
and tied in place. After a large hemostat had been clamped across most of the
intestinal mass not involved with the pancreas, the tissues were perfused by
syringe via the catheter in the aorta in the following sequence:

1. Isotonic (0.9 percent) NaCl containing 10 units of heparin per mL
   (about 30–50 mL);
2. 25 percent formalin (4 parts of formaldehyde solution N.F. 37 percent,
   1 part ethanol, 1 part H_2O) (30 mL);

   3. Fresh Harris' hematoxylin (4–5 mL) filtered through a Millipore filter
   (Type RA, 1.2 μm) (this filtering was found to be very important); and

   4. Distilled water (60 mL). All perfusion solutions were at room temperature
   (24–26°C).

The rates of injection were on the order of 0.5 mL/sec. About halfway through
the formalin injection, the portal vein or liver was cut to allow continued free
drainage from the perfused regions. The hematoxylin was injected only until
the pancreas was seen to stain a moderately dark orchid color. Following the
final perfusion step, the pancreas was removed with its surrounding intestine,
placed in 75 percent ethanol for about 1 hr, and then in 100 percent ethanol.
One or more pieces of pancreatic tissue, typically about 2 cm² in area, were
cut out from selected sites. The tissue was teased under a dissecting microscope
to remove most gross fat and mesentery. The specimen was flattened and gently
stretched so that there were practically no overlapping lobules. It was then
cleared in methyl salicylate. Because the rabbit pancreas is so thin, clearing
usually requires less than 15 min. The pieces, still in methyl salicylate, were
placed on a microscope slide and covered with a glass coverslip for measurement
by use of a standard compound microscope with an eyepiece graticule. Values
were determined for the number of islets, the diameter of each islet, the number
of spheres in each islet, and the total number of spheres and their distribution
between islets and nonislet tissue. Spheres were assigned to islets by careful
focusing. Those judged to be in islets or touching the islet perimeter (a small
minority) were taken as islet spheres. The magnification was customarily 200 × ,
but it was increased as necessary to facilitate identification of such spheres.
If an islet was seen as essentially circular in area, its volume was calculated
as a sphere. If the islet area was not circular, its volume was calculated as
that of an ellipse rotated about its long axis (prolate spheroid) and assigned
the diameter that a sphere of equal volume would have. The appearance of the
pancreas is illustrated in Kramlinger, Mayrand, and Lifson (1).

   The wet weight of the tissue examined was not measured directly when it
was removed from the animal. The reason for this was that the tissue had been
subjected to the intra-arterial perfusion fluids and was subsequently teased as
described above. Instead, the tissue actually viewed was dried to constant
weight at 100–110°C, and the desired fresh wet weight was calculated by
multiplying the dry weight by 5.92. This factor had been established by suitable
control determinations on rabbit pancreata similarly treated. Where the dry
weight was less than 5 mg, the value was determined on a Cahn electrobalance.
To obtain the total weight of the pancreatic tissue, the remainder of the pancreas
was treated like the above pieces and dried to constant weight. No distinction
was made between weight and volume; that is, the density of tissue was taken
as 1 g/mL.

   The morphological values provided by the above measurements included
the parameters and shape of the frequency distributions of islet diameter and

volume, volume of the islet organ as a percentage of the pancreatic volume, and total volume of the islet organ.

Blood flow determinations were made on a given piece of a pancreas as follows:

1.   The total blood flow to the area was calculated from the product of the number of spheres in it and the reference blood value for flow per sphere.

2.   Values for the intensity of perfusion of pancreatic organ tissue ($mL \cdot min^{-1}$ per g or mL of pancreas; units, min^{-1}) were calculated from the blood flow to the area divided by its volume.

3.   The percentages of the flow to islets and acini were calculated from the percentages of the spheres in the two locations.

4.   Mean single islet flow in an area was calculated by multiplying the mean number of spheres per islet by the reference organ value of flow per sphere.

5.   Mean intensity of perfusion of the islet organ (units, min^{-1}) was calculated by dividing the value of mean single islet flow by the mean single islet volume of the area. (This is the same as total islet blood flow divided by total islet volume.)

To obtain values for the relationship between single islet volume and single islet blood flow or islet intensity of perfusion, it was necessary to combine results from several animals and to normalize the values to adjust for animal-to-animal variability. For this purpose, the intensity of perfusion of the islets of a given class interval of single islet volume in each pancreas was expressed as a percentage of the mean intensity of perfusion of the islet organ of that pancreas.

2.2.   Experiments on Rats

The procedures carried out on rats were similar to those on rabbits, modified chiefly for the smaller size of the rats. Holtzman rats weighing some 500–600 g were used. They were anesthetized by an intraperitoneal injection of sodium pentobarbital (Nembutal), 50 mg/kg of body weight. The femoral arterial cannula was PE 10, but we have most recently changed to 28-gauge lightweight spaghetti teflon tubing (outside diameter, 0.015 in.; inside diameter, 0.027 in.); the carotid cannula was PE 50, inserted via the right common carotid artery into the left ventricle or in some cases to a point just above the aortic valve. The trachea was cannulated to avoid respiratory distress. The volume of injectate was 0.5 mL/kg. The rate of withdrawal of the reference organ blood sample was 340 μL/min.

3. DISCUSSION

3.1. Staining Procedure

When tissue was stored in formalin, the staining remained essentially unchanged for several months. When stored in methyl salicylate, islet staining becomes more diffuse in a matter of days. As in the rabbit, the staining of the pancreas in the rat made it possible to count and measure the diameters of the islets and to locate spheres in them as well as in the nonislet tissues ("acini"). The rat pancreas is thicker and required more thorough teasing to prepare it for quantitative microscopy. When viewed, there were differences between the results of the staining procedure in the rabbit and rat pancreata:

1. Obviously fewer islets per unit area were seen in the rat.
2. In the rat pancreata the afferent vessel of the islet was less frequently seen, the internal structure of the islet vasculature was less clear, and the boundaries of the islets were less certain.
3. Not uncommonly conglomerations of islet tissue were seen.

These presented the problem of deciding whether they were a single large islet or whether they consisted of 3–15 islets of ordinary size. Four of these problem conglomerates of islet tissue were removed, sectioned, and stained with hematoxylin and eosin. Without exception, acinar tissue was seen to separate the candidate islets. For this reason, these conglomerates were taken to be made up of individual islets, rather than a single large islet. This issue requires further work.

The intensity of staining of islet and acinar capillaries increased when the volume of stain injected in step 3 (Section 2.1) was 40 mL instead of 4–5 mL, and diffuse staining of the acinar tissue occurred especially near the islets. Intense staining of the islets makes seeing the spheres in them more difficult; it might be advantageous for other purposes. The islet dimensions as measured are subject to possible systematic error due to shrinking or swelling during the staining and clearing procedures. These effects have not as yet been evaluated, but they should be similar to those produced by conventional histological processing except for the embedding and slicing steps. Relative values among tissues treated similarly should of course be more reliable than absolute ones.

Such a wide range of values has been reported for even simple aspects of the morphology of the islet organ and a comparison with accepted values is not possible. For example, the islet organ in rats about 300 g in weight has been found to be some 0.16 percent of the pancreas (5–7) or 1.4 percent (8); and the number of islets per gram, some 1700 versus 12,000–20,000 in the two series.

The most comprehensive measurements available for any species are those of Tejning, Hellman, Hellerstrom, and colleagues on the islet organ of Wistar rats [reviewed by Hellerstrom (9)]. These were made on tissue slices with the application of stereological formulas. When the results of the intra-arterial hematoxylin staining method were compared with those of Hellman (5–7) for adult rats (480 days old; average weight, 403 g), statistically significant differences were found for number of islets per gram and mean single islet volume (Table 1); but these differences do not seem large compared to the range reported in the literature. The finding that about 50 percent more islets per gram were measured by the intra-arterial hematoxylin method suggests that this procedure is not underestimating the islet number by failure of staining. The diameter-by-diameter percentage frequency distributions of islet size were similar, with one exception: Instead of an approximately lognormal shape found by the present method for both rats and rabbits, these investigators found the mode to be at the class interval with the smallest diameter and the frequencies to decrease exponentially with increasing islet diameter. Part (but not all) of this difference is due to the exclusion of islets less than 47 μm in diameter by these investigators. With the intra-arterial stain, all islets identifiable as such were recorded, the smallest of which was 22 μm in diameter. The frequency distributions of islet volumes in the dog, monkey, and human suggest lognormality (10). However, the distributions documenting this observation were obtained from only 100 islets in a single pancreas of each species. Figure 1 compares the percentage volume distribution of islet tissue as a function of islet diameter as obtained by Hellman and the present method. (The units on the abscissa are the single islet diameter class intervals of Hellman (5), slightly modified as specified in the figure legend.) The general similarity of the findings by the two methods is evident.

3.2. Blood Flow Procedure

A general account of the measurement of blood flow by the use of microspheres will be found in Heyman et al. (11). The validity of the technique for measuring

TABLE 1. Comparison Between Some Mean ($\pm$ SE) Morphological Values for Rat Pancreas as Found by Intra-arterial Staining with Hematoxylin and by Hellman (5–7) by Measurements on Tissue Sections

	Intra-arterial Values ($N = 8$)	Hellman Values ($N = 15$)
Body weight, (g)	554 ± 16	403
Pancreas weight (g/100 g of body weight)	0.33 ± 0.02	0.34
Number of islets/g of pancreas	3750 ± 600	2437 ± 135^a ($p < 0.03$)
Mean SIV (nL)	0.79 ± 0.09	1.03 ± 0.05^a ($p < 0.03$)
Islet volume as % of pancreas	0.30 ± 0.06	0.25

^{a} Islets less than 47 μm in diameter not included.

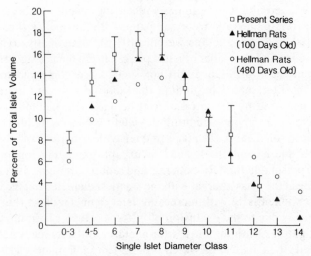

FIGURE 1. Volume distribution of islet tissue as a function of islet diameter. Comparison between values from intra-arterial staining with hematoxylin of rat pancreata and values of Hellman (5–7). Interval for single islet diameter classes 0 to 3 is 0–78.1 μm; for classes 4 to 5, 78.1–109.4 μm; for each of the following classes, the class interval is 31.25 μm wide; class interval is 359.4–390.6 μm.

blood flow to the pancreas and its intraorgan distribution by the present method with nonradioactive spheres has been discussed elsewhere (2, 12, 13). The basic assumptions are that the spheres are delivered to and are trapped in the part under investigation in proportion to the blood flow to the part. Spheres 10 μm in diameter are recommended here on the basis of the results in the rabbit with a range of sphere sizes; and Jansson and Hellerstrom (4) have concluded that spheres of this size were suitable for the rat pancreas.

Measurements of regional intraorgan blood flow by the microsphere technique are more subject to error than measurements of total organ blood flow. Even if the sphere localization and counting procedures were perfect, the intrapancreatic distribution of spheres as calculated may not represent the distribution of pancreatic blood flow at the time of injection of the spheres due to (i) invalidity of the assumptions underlying the microsphere method, (ii) perturbing effects of the injectate, and (iii) inherent statistical effects. In addition, the experimentally measured flows, even if accurate, may be different from the preexperimental flows we wished to measure due to the procedures involved in preparation for the injection, particularly anesthesia and surgery. Inherent statistical variability does not introduce systematic error; the other three items could do so. For the described procedures the injectate and inherent statistical effects require special consideration.

Given that all assumptions of the microsphere approach are valid and that spheres are accurately counted in a group of islets, the percentage coefficient of variation (CV) of repeated determinations of the number of microspheres

N in identical experiments would be the Poisson distribution value of $1/\sqrt{N}$. Hence, for $N = 25$, 100, and 400, respectively, the CV is 20, 10, and 5 percent respectively. Similar considerations apply to each individual value involved in a calculation. For example, to the value of mean single islet blood flow, inherent statistical variability is contributed by the values of the number of islets counted, the number of islet spheres counted, and of the number of reference blood spheres that were counted to obtain the value for flow per sphere—all counts being perfect.

The inherent statistical variability in counting the spheres in the pieces of pancreas can be reduced by increasing the dose of spheres and/or increasing the size of the sample (tissue or bloood) being counted. However, with increasing dose, the injected spheres can perturb the circulation by acting as emboli. They can also produce artifactual dissociation of microsphere and blood flow by interacting with one another. As the tissue sample becomes progressively larger, the number of islets to be measured becomes very great and increasingly time consuming to count. In the way the single islet flow and especially the relationship between single islet flow and single islet volume were actually measured, a compromise was made from the standpoint of these considerations. The dose of spheres and the sample sizes were such that the inherent statistical variability, even though large by usual standards, was small relative to the animal-to-animal variability. Nevertheless, the dose was large enough to noticeably affect the blood pressure in some animals, as implied by statements in the literature for spheres in the range from 9 to 11 μm in diameter injected into rabbits or rats (3, 4, 14, 15). However, the extent to which the blood pressure changes (or other concomitant circulatory alterations) affect pancreatic perfusion measurements is not known. The large animal-to-animal variability typically encountered for both morphology and perfusion makes it difficult to establish statistically significant differences in group comparisons unless they are gross or the number of animals is impractically great for most purposes.

An additional source of error of the microsphere method in these particular experiments which is not present in the usual microsphere measurements of blood flow is the staining procedure. One cannot be sure that the postmortem flows of perfusion fluids in the procedure have not moved microspheres. One reason for believing that such an effect has not been large is that the postmortem perfusion of the intestinal wall with silicone latex did not cause detectable differences in the distribution of microspheres in the intestinal tissue layers (12). Another reason is that when the fluid draining from the portal vein during the staining procedure was collected and examined for its content of microspheres, it was found that the total of these spheres were a minor percentage of those remaining in the tissues (2).

Meyer et al. (3) and Jansson and Hellerstrom (4) have recently reported measurements of pancreatic blood flow and its percentage distributions to the exocrine and endocrine pancreas of anesthetized rats by the microsphere procedure. Meyer et al. stained the islets *in vivo* with diphenylthiocarbazone (dithizone) and cleared them in glycerol for postmortem microscopic examination. Jansson and Hellerstrom cleared the pancreas by freeze-thawing, after which the islets and spheres could be indentified by dark-field microscopy. Islet numbers or dimensions were not reported in either of these investigations. In the studies thus far carried out, importantly different values for percentage of pancreatic flow received by the islets have been obtained by the three

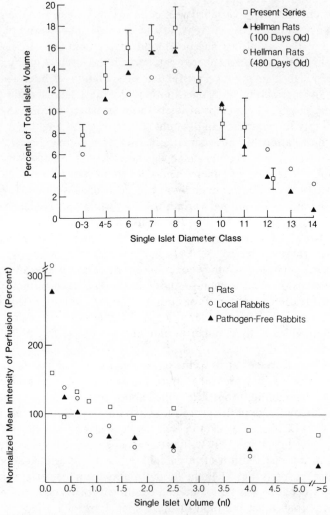

FIGURE 2. Relationship between normalized intensity of perfusion and single islet volume for two series of rabbits and a series of rats. For each pancreas the mean intensity of perfusion (nL·min^{-1}/nL of islet volume) of islets of a class interval of volume was normalized by expressing it as a percentage of the intensity of perfusion of the islet tissue of the pancreas. The plotted points are the mean values for the animals of the series (9 local rabbits; 18 pathogen-free rabbits; 8 normal rats).

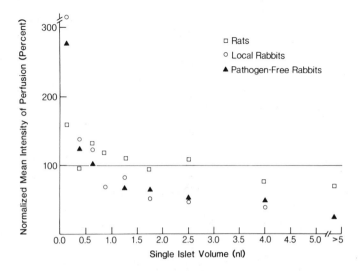

FIGURE 2. (*Continued*)

procedures used: intra-arterial hematoxylin, dithizone, freeze-thawing. It remains to be determined whether these discrepancies are due to the use of animals of different size and strain, to procedural aspects other than the methods of identifying spheres in islet tissue, or to these methods proper. This issue is discussed by Jansson and Hellerstrom (4).

So far as we are aware, the data obtained by the procedures described here are the first relating single islet blood flow and intensity of perfusion to single islet size and number (13, 16; others, in preparation). The reservations indicated with respect to their validity are stronger for absolute values than for relative ones, which reduce the animal-to-animal variability and the effects of systematic errors. The reliability of the findings for normalized single islet perfusion as a function of single islet volume is supported by the similarity of the results for local rabbits, pathogen-free rabbits, and normal rats (Figure 2).

REFERENCES

1. K. G. Kramlinger, R. R. Mayrand, and N. Lifson, *Stain Technol.* **54**, 159–162 (1979).

2. N. Lifson, K. G. Kramlinger, R. R. Mayrand, and E. J. Lender, *Gastroenterology* **79**, 466–473 (1980).

3. H. H. Meyer, F. Vetterlein, G. Schmidt, and A. Hasselblatt, *Am. J. Physiol.* **242** (Endocrinol. Metab. 5), E298–E304 (1982).

4. L. Jansson and C. Hellerstrom, *Diabetologia* **25**, 45 (1983).

5. B. Hellman, *Acta Endocrinol.* **31**, 91–106 (1959).

6. B. Hellman, *Acta Endocrinol.* **32**, 63–77 (1959).

7. B. Hellman, *Acta Endocrinol.* **32**, 78–91 (1959).

8. R. E. Haist, and E. J. Pugh, *Am. J. Physiol.* **152**, 36–41 (1948).

9. C. Hellerstrom, "Growth Pattern of Pancreatic Islets in Animals," in *The Diabetic Pancreas*, B. W. Volk and K. F. Wellman (eds.), Plenum Press, New York, 1977, pp. 61–97.

10. W. R. Thompson, R. Tennant, and R. Hussey, *Science* **78**, 270 (1933).

11. M. A. Heyman, B. D. Payne, J. I. E. Hoffma , and A. M. Rudolph, *Progr. Cardiovasc. Dis.* **20**, 55–79 (1977–78).

12. N. Lifson, B. Sircar, D. G. Levitt, and E. J. Lender, *Microvasc. Res.* **17**, 158–180 (1979).

13. N. Lifson, "Use of Microspheres to Measure Intraorgan Distribution of Blood Flow in the Splanchnic Circulation," in *Measurement of Blood Flow: Applications to the Splanchnic Circulation*, D. N. Granger and G. B. Buckley (eds.), Williams and Wilkens, Baltimore, 1981, pp 179–194.

14. L. Bankir, N. Farman, J.-P. Grunfeld, E. Huet de la Tour, and J.-L. Funk-Bretano, *Pflugers Arch.* **42**, 111–123 (1973).

15. J. Sabto, L. Bankir, and J.-P. Grunfeld, *Clinical Exptl. Pharmacol. Physiol.* **5**, 559–565 (1978).

16. N. Lifson, C. V. Lassa, and P. K. Dixit, *Fed. Proc.* **42**, 505 (1983).

V

ETIOLOGY, COMPLICATIONS, AND ANIMAL MODELS

A

PREPARATION AND ANALYSIS OF GLOMERULAR BASEMENT MEMBRANE

MARGO P. COHEN

The University of Medicine and Dentistry of New Jersey, Department of Medicine, Division of Endocrinology and Metabolism, Newark, New Jersey

EDWARD C. CARLSON

The University of North Dakota, Department of Anatomy, School of Medicine, Grand Forks, North Dakota, and California Primate Research Center, University of California, Davis, California

1. INTRODUCTION

Basement membranes (BMs) are specialized connective tissue matrices that lie outside the plasma membrane and characteristically separate parenchymal cells from the adjacent connective tissue space. On electron microscopy (Fig. 1), they appear as amorphous material with a central region of marked electron density (lamina densa) that is bordered by less electron-dense material (laminae rarae). The latter is closely approximated to the cell surface, and there are interactions between, and possible sharing of, certain cell surface and BM components such as proteoglycans and attachment proteins. Thus, the precise localization of where one ends and the other begins may not be as straightforward as previously thought, and may require redefinition. BMs provide scaffolding, support, and orientation for tissues and serve as barriers between cells of different tissues. Although considered inert until recently, it is now clear that they have important filtration, adhesion, and attachment functions and help maintain the integrity of tissue boundaries.

BMs are relatively insoluble, rich in carbohydrate, and contain unique collagenous and noncollagenous proteins. The carbohydrate moieties predominantly consist of glucosyl-galactose disaccharide units linked to hydroxylysine residues of collagen components; smaller amounts of other sugars such as mannose and hexosamine are present as heteropolysaccharide units linked to asparaginyl residues in noncollagenous domains or comprise the carbohydrate portion of unique noncollagenous glycoproteins. Additionally, BMs contain glycosaminoglycans, of which heparan sulfate is the principal species, as polysaccharides linked to the peptide core of proteoglycans. The collagenous components resemble procollagen in several respects including size, the presence of sulfhydryl linkages, the presence of α-chainlike segments associated with noncollagenous regions, and a partial susceptibility to proteases. BM procollagens are either not converted to collagen chains or are incompletely cleaved and are incorporated as such into the extracellular matrix, and their susceptibility to limited pepsin digestion derives from interruptions in the triple helix of the collagen portion as well as retention of noncollagen extension sequences or domains of procollagen. Unique noncollagenous components of BMs include the glycoproteins laminin and entactin, and one or more proteoglycans. These components have been isolated from aberrant cell lines (EHS sarcoma, embryonal endodermal carcinoma) that produce BM-like matrices, and their identification in glomerular BMs has been largely by immunofluorescent techniques. While the information obtained from studies with these and other tumors and cell

The authors wish to express gratitude to Mr. Walter J. Berger III and Ms. Janice Audette for expert technical assistance and to Ms. Lisa Eiteljorge, who typed the manuscript. This work was supported in part by a grant from the American Diabetes Association, North Dakota Affiliate, Inc.

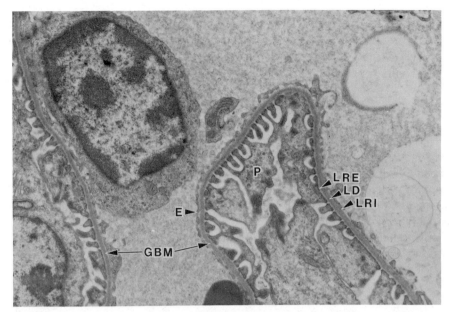

FIGURE 1. Transmission electron micrograph of blood–urine barrier in rat renal glomerulus. The glomerular BM (GBM) intervenes between fenestrated endothelium (E) and visceral epithelial cells or podocytes (P). The GBM is comprised of a lamina rara interna (LRI), lamina densa (LD), and lamina rara externa (LRE). ×4600.

lines that elaborate BM components has greatly advanced understanding of BM biochemistry, synthesis, and organization, it is not clear to what extent this information is directly applicable to the renal glomerular and other natural BMs which have been difficult to study in view of their insolubility, susceptibility to proteolysis, and, in many instances, inaccessibility. Many excellent publications providing in-depth discussion of the biochemistry, immunology, function, and intermolecular organization of BMs have appeared in recent years (1–5).

The renal glomerular BM has been one of the most intensively studied natural BMs. In part this derives from its unique anatomic relationship wherein it intervenes between two cell layers from which it can be dissociated with relative ease, as well as the abundant availability of renal cortex from many animals. It is also of special interest because of its important functional role as the only continuous structure between circulatory and excretory systems, and its ability to provide a size- and charge-selective filtration barrier. Furthermore, the glomerular BM is a structure in which complications of diabetes mellitus characteristically occur and is associated with pathologic and functional changes in diabetes that can lead ultimately to renal failure. This chapter surveys methods for preparation and analysis of glomerular BM that are useful for morphologic, biochemical, and comparative studies of normal and diabetic samples. For this purpose the definition of glomerular BM that we employ is utilitarian and simply refers to that material prepared according to the described techniques that has the morphologic and copositional features associated with BM.

2. DISSOCIATION OF GLOMERULI FROM RENAL TISSUES

The method used for isolation of glomeruli is a modification of the sieving technique of Krakower and Greenspon (6). The renal capsule is first removed from freshly isolated kidneys, which are then cut into thin slices. Fine scissors are used to separate the lighter-colored cortex from the darker medulla. Alternatively, curved forceps may be employed to "pinch" the softer cortex from the underlying tougher "core" of medulla. The cortex is then minced with razor blades or scissors into pieces <1 mm^3.

Pieces of this cortical mince are further reduced in size on a large-diameter mesh stainless steel screen (250–350 μm; W. S. Tyler Inc., Mentor, OH) supported on the rim of a 500-mL glass beaker. A spoon-blade spatula or the bottom of a small beaker or Erlenmayer flask is used to force approximately 1-gm portions of mince through the sieve. The preparation is then gently washed through the screen with a stream of cold, neutral-buffered saline (20–50 mL/portion), and the material remaining on the sieve is discarded. The filtrate is centrifuged at low speed (350g) for 5 min in a clinical centrifuge; this is repeated twice to eliminate cellular debris.

Glomeruli are separated from other cortical tissues by resuspending the pellets in saline, followed by pouring and washing the suspension through a series of graded nylon or stainless steel sieves (6–8). The nylon screening (Tetco, Elmsford, NY) can be supported in embroidery hoops. Pore sizes vary for different species. For human and adult rat tissue, sequential screens of 150, 230, and 63 μm are employed. The first two sieves, which can be placed in tandem, retain vascular elements, tubules, and connective tissue fragments. The filtrate is collected, repelleted as above if necessary, and then passed through the final sieve, which retains glomeruli >63 μm but <149 μm in diameter. Using a Pasteur pipette and small amounts of buffered saline, glomeruli are collected from this sieve by repeated rinsing and aspiration, followed by brief centrifugation. The preparations are usually 90–95 percent pure (Fig. 2), and retain metabolic activity when samples are processed rapidly and in the cold. Purity of the glomerular preparation can be further improved through low-speed differential centrifugation. Since glomeruli contain red blood cells and are denser than most noncellular debris or tubules, pellets obtained after centrifugation of the material collected from the final sieve appear stratified, with the lower, reddish layer composed mostly of glomeruli. The overlying whitish layer is mostly debris and can be carefully pipetted off.

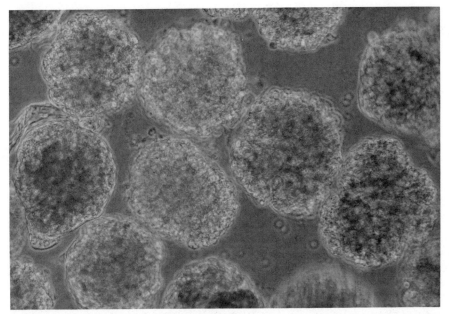

FIGURE 2. Phase-contrast photomicrograph of rat renal glomeruli dissociated from cortical tissues by differential sieving on nylon screens. ×240.

A modification of this procedure involves the separation of iron-containing glomeruli from renal tubules by bar magnets (9). This technique results in a purified preparation of glomeruli which is 99 percent free of tubular contamination. The descending aorta of anesthetized rats is ligated above and below the renal arteries prior to cannulation of the aorta just above the inferior ligation site. The vena cava is then severed and the kidneys perfused with 20 mL of Earle's balanced salt solution (EBSS; 116 mM NaCl, 16 mM KCl, 1 mM NaH$_2$PO$_4$·H$_2$O, 0.8 mM MgSO$_4$·7H$_2$O, 5.6 mM glucose, 1.8 mM CaCl$_2$) buffered with HEPES, (pH 7.4) fortified with 0.01 percent bovine serum albumin, followed by 10 mL of iron oxide (0.072 percent) in the same buffer with 4 percent polyvinylpyrolidone. The kidneys are removed and the cortex is dissected, minced, and homogenized with five up-and-down strokes in a hand-held tissue grinder (Arthur H. Thomas) with a Teflon pestle specially machined to a teardrop shape (9). The homogenate is passed through a 210-μm mesh nylon sieve with a buffer spray. This is followed by sequential sieving through 153-, 110-, and 64-μm mesh screens. The residue on the final sieve contains iron-containing glomeruli and tubular fragments. This is suspended in buffer and placed on a permanent bar magnet. The iron oxide particles within glomerular vascular channels cause them to aggregate while nonmagnetic material is decanted off with several buffer washings.

Another method for isolation of renal glomeruli entails the use of a Ficoll gradient for their separation from vascular and tubular elements during centrifugation. This procedure, detailed in ref. 10, is reported to yield glomeruli of purity comparable to that obtained with the foregoing methods. It offers the advantage of not excluding glomeruli on the basis of size, such as may occur with the differential sieving technique.

3.   ISOLATION OF THE GLOMERULAR BASEMENT MEMBRANE

Most investigators have employed sonic disruption (7, 11) or sequential detergent treatment (9, 12) to remove cellular elements from isolated glomeruli with the aim of preparing pure samples of glomerular BM.

If the purified glomerular BM is to be used for chemical analysis only, isolation by sonication is a useful technique that provides adequate yields and excellent purity. There is some concern, however, that integral components are partially lost or destroyed due to the harshness of the sonication treatment. Certainly there is fragmentation and loss of spatial arrangement of the BMs purified by ultrasonic disruption. With this method, the isolated glomeruli are suspended in ice-cold saline buffered with 25 mM Tris to pH 7.2, adjusted to 1 M sodium chloride, and containing protease inhibitors (25 mM EDTA, 1 mM benzamidine hydrochloride, 1 mM phenylmethylsulfonylfluoride, and 10 mM N-ethylmaleamide). They are disrupted in 10 to 20 mL aliquots in a small beaker immersed in a bucket of ice. The sonicating probe should provide about 300 W of energy delivered in 1-min bursts. Care should be taken that the material being vibrated is not overheated. Usually a total of 6–10 min of sonic vibration with a cooling time of one minute between each burst is adequate to disrupt the cells. Preparations are monitored with light or phase-contrast microscopy to ensure optimum glomerular disruption. Optimally, glomerular BM should appear as refractile loops or plates with few or no cells attached. The sonicated material is briefly centrifuged at about 800g to sediment the BMs. These are carefully washed with 1 M NaCl that contains protease inhibitors, followed by several washes with distilled water. Alternatively, the sonicated material can be passed over a 250-μm mesh nylon sieve to remove undisrupted glomeruli, tubules, or vascular fragments before collection of the filtrate by centrifugation and washing.

When investigations of isolated glomerular BM include observations of the preparation by light or electron microscopy, or in studies where a combination of chemical and morphological analyses are planned, excellent results are achieved by passing the dissociated glomeruli through a series of detergents and treating with endonuclease to solubilize cellular components while leaving the BMs intact (9, 12). With this method the inevitable fragmentation produced by high-frequency vibration can be avoided and BMs of individual glomeruli maintain their convoluted spheroidal shapes (Fig. 3).

This procedure is begun by stirring or shaking gently the dissociated glomeruli in a large volume (50:1) of distilled water containing the above protease inhibitors for 2–4 hr to osmotically shock the cells. Alternatively, 1–5 mM EDTA may be added to bind calcium, which is required for maintenance of intercellular junctions. Either suspension should contain 0.05 percent sodium azide. The partially disrupted glomeruli are pelleted, resuspended, and stirred in a solution of 3 percent Triton X-100 with 0.05 percent sodium azide for 2–4 hr. The pellet obtained following centrifugation is extensively washed (three to five times) in distilled water prior to resuspension and incubated for 1–2 hr in 40 mL of 1 M NaCl containing 0.05 percent deoxyribonuclease (Sigma, type I). The suspension is again centrifuged and resuspended in 4 percent sodium deoxycholate (DEOC) containing 0.05 percent sodium azide and stirred for 2–4 hr. The DEOC treatment should be carried out at room temperature (viscosity increases with decreasing temperature) and preferably in a polypropylene container to prevent the BMs from adhering to its surface. The BMs derived from this procedure are collected by centrifugation and washed three times to remove adhering DEOC. When relatively small numbers of glomeruli (<1 × 10^6) are used as starting material, the DNase treatment can be omitted (13). With larger amounts of tissue, this step assures preparations devoid of nuclear materials.

As mentioned above, a major advantage of the detergent extraction procedure is the preservation of morphologic integrity and *in vivo* histoarchitecture. This

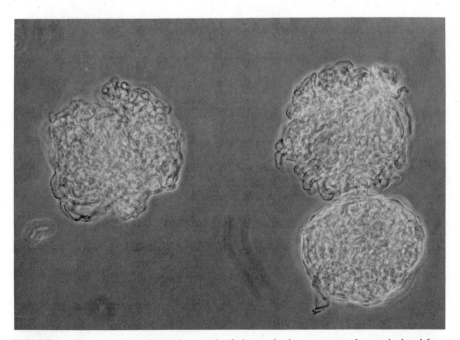

FIGURE 3. Phase-contrast photomicrograph of glomerular basement membranes isolated from dissociated glomeruli (see Fig. 2) by detergent washings as described in the text. × 290.

is particularly true of glomerular BMs which possess striking intrinsic structural rigidity (14). Although their orderly lobulated structure is easily demonstrable when isolated glomeruli are used as starting material, it is occasionally advantageous to observe them by either light or transmission electron microscopy *in situ*. This is accomplished by treating samples of minced renal cortex with detergents (14) or by rendering the entire kidney acellular by vascular perfusion with the same reagents (15).

To prepare acellular renal cortex, freshly isolated kidneys are placed in cold (4°C) Earle's balanced salt solution buffered with 50 m*M* Tris at pH 7.4 (Fig. 4). Renal capsules are incised and dissected free along with associated perirenal fat and connective tissue. The renal sinus is cleared of its vascular and ureteric structures. Transverse slices (<2 mm thick) are made from each kidney using a single-edge razor blade or scalpel. The cortex (outer 2 mm for rats) is removed from each slice and the medullary portion discarded. The cortical slices are further minced to form tissue blocks <1 mm^3. If it is important to study the microvascular architecture of the renal cortex, several thin (<1

PREPARATION OF ACELLULAR RENAL CORTEX

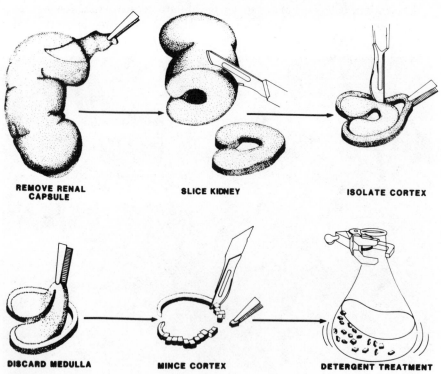

REMOVE RENAL   SLICE KIDNEY   ISOLATE CORTEX
CAPSULE

DISCARD MEDULLA   MINCE CORTEX   DETERGENT TREATMENT

FIGURE 4. Technique for preparation of acellular renal cortex from freshly isolated kidney (see text for details).

mm) slices of unminced cortex should be retained for stereo dissection microscopy following detergent extraction.

Cortical sections or minced blocks are transferred to a large volume (100:1) of 1–5 mM EDTA containing 0.1 percent sodium azide and gently stirred or shaken for 48 hr in the cold. Several changes of solution should be made during this initial period of osmotic shock. The tissues are then passed over a 210-μm mesh nylon sieve and extensively rinsed with distilled water. The residue is carefully collected with a spoon-shaped spatula and suspended in 3 percent Triton X-100 with 0.1 percent sodium azide and stirred or shaken for 8–12 hr at room temperature. Tissues are again rinsed extensively (sieve method) with distilled water until no soapy froth is evident, and then resuspended in 0.025 percent DNase in 1 M NaCl for 2–4 hr with stirring or shaking at room temperature. Tissues are again collected on a 210-μm nylon sieve and resuspended in 4 percent DEOC with 0.1 percent sodium azide. This treatment is carried out for 8–12 hr at room temperature. DEOC is removed by final washes with large volumes of distilled water. Acellular tissue blocks derived from this procedure are stored at 4°C in 0.25 mM Tris-buffered saline (pH 7.2) with protease inhibitors. If morphological integrity is important, the samples should not be frozen.

In circumstances where it is advantageous to determine the precise location from which an acellular tissue block is derived, vascular perfusion of kidneys with detergents can be carried out to prepare intact acellular kidneys prior to dissection. The procedure was originally described by Brendel and co-workers (16) and was designed for permeability studies of glomerular BMs with electron-dense tracers. More recently we described a similar procedure (15) using a specially modified disposable renal perfusion cassette (Waters Instruments Co.). The following method was designed to be used with rabbit kidneys, which are a convenient size for excellent perfusion results. We have, however, utilized the same procedure for rat, cat, guinea pig, dog, rhesus monkey, and human, altering the times and volumes of solutions in proportion to the relative wet weights of their respective renal tissues.

Rabbits are injected initially with 1 percent procaine hydrochloride (1.0 mL), 50 mg/mL sodium pentobarbital (2.0 mL), 0.2 mg/mL isoproterenol (0.5 mL), 5 mg/mL isoxsuprine (0.5 mL) and 1 mL heparin via the marginal ear vein. Approximately 10–15 min later a lethal dose (~ 3 mL sodium pentobarbital, 50 mg/mL) is given. The abdominal cavity is incised and the left renal vein is ligated adjacent to the inferior vena cava. A saline-filled polyethylene canula (1.22 mm outside diameter) is inserted into the left renal artery and doubly ligated with braided silk. The ureter, renal vein, and artery (proximal to the cannulation point) are severed and the cannula is attached to a 40-mL syringe containing 47.5 mL 0.9 percent saline, 0.5 mL 1 percent procaine hydrochloride, 0.5 mL isoxsuprine (5 mg/mL), and 1 mL heparin. This solution is advanced through the renal vascular tree.

The kidney and cannula are transferred to the perfusion apparatus, which is equipped with a three-way valve to permit voiding the perfusate or conducting it to a prepump reservoir for recirculation. The apparatus is driven by a Harvard peristaltic pump, which has been primed and cleared of all bubbles.

The pump is activated and the cannula connected to the apparatus while the initial fluid is circulating. The flow rate and pressure are adjusted to approximately 5 mL/min and 90/80 mm Hg, respectively. The schedule of solution changes is as follows:

1. Nonrecirculatory (NR): 4 L 0.9 percent saline with 4 mM EDTA.
2. NR: 2 L distilled water.
3. NR: 4 L 0.5 percent Triton X-100.
4. NR: 4 L, 0.5 percent Triton X-100, 5 mM CaCl$_2$, 5 mM MgSO$_4$.
5. Recirculatory (R): 300 mL, 3 percent Triton X-100, 5 mM CaCl$_2$, 5 mM MgSO$_4$ (4 hr).
6. R: 300 mL, 3 percent Triton X-100, 1 M NaCl, 5 mM MgSO$_4$ (16 hr minimum).
7. NR: distilled water until no bubbles appear.
8. R: 500 mL, 0.025 percent deoxyribonuclease, pH 5, in sodium acetate buffer (4 hr).
9. NR: 1 L, distilled water.
10. R: 600 mL, 4 percent DEOC, (300 mL for 5 hr, change to fresh solution and run additional 5 hr).
11. NR: distilled water, minimum 12–16 hr.

The above times and volumes apply to two rabbit kidneys perfused simultaneously. All perfusions are carried out at room temperature. This technique yields a completely acellular kidney, which can be dissected before or after fixation for microscopy.

4. MORPHOLOGICAL ANALYSIS OF ISOLATED GLOMERULAR BM OR ACELLULAR RENAL TISSUE BLOCKS

The development of the detergent method for BM isolation has provided an impetus for morphological investigation of these sheets of extracellular matrix. This is particularly true of glomerular BMs where microscopic observation of materials prepared by ultrasound previously provided only incomplete information on the starting material used in compositional analyses.

To prepare isolated glomerular BM for light and transmission electron microscopic studies, a small aliquot of the material is pelleted in a 1.5-mL microfuge tube and the suspension medium (usually 0.25 mM Tris-buffered saline with protease inhibitors) is carefully withdrawn with a Pasteur pipette.

The glomerular BMs are gently resuspended in Karnovsky's (17) paraform-aldehyde-glutaraldehyde fixative buffered at pH 7.4 with 0.2 M sodium caco-dylate/HCl. Fixation lasts 1 hr and is followed by postfixation in 1 percent buffered OsO_4. In our hands electron density of the acellular glomerular BMs is increased when 0.2 M s-collidine/HCl is employed as the buffer for the osmium. Contrast is further enhanced when postfixed samples are rinsed in 0.2 M sodium cacodylate/HCl buffer, treated for 1 hr in tannic acid (1 percent in 0.1 M sodium cacodylate/HCl buffer), rinsed again in buffer and stained 90 min *en bloc* in 0.5 percent aqueous uranyl acetate (18). Isolated glomerular BMs are briefly pelleted and resuspended at each solution change. They are dehydrated in a graded series of ethanols and propylene oxide and embedded in a mixture of Araldite and Epon (18). Curing is ordinarily carried out in two stages: 24 hr at 37°C and an additional 48 hr at 60°C.

When acellular tissue blocks (prepared either by immersion or vascular perfusion) are used as starting material for morphological investigations, they are carried through the same series of reagents as described above for isolated glomerular BMs. Since the blocks tend to be somewhat larger, however, ($\sim$2 mm^3), they sediment fairly quickly in the microfuge tubes, and most solutions can be changed without prior centrifugation.

For light microscopy 1-μm thick sections of glomerular BM pellets or blocks of acellular renal cortex are cut using glass or diamond knives. These are mounted on glass slides and stained with toluidine blue (1 percent in 1 percent sodium borate). Light microscopic observation shows that isolated glomerular BMs are remarkably resilient and remain faithful to their *in vivo* shapes (Fig. 5). Likewise, the acellular renal cortex maintains its histoarchitecture and all major renal BM types are recognizable within a single section (Fig. 6).

For transmission electron microscopy, thin sections are cut and mounted on naked 200- or 300-mesh copper grids and stained with lead citrate (18). These are observed at original magnifications of approximately 2000–50,000 diameters at an accelerating voltage of 60–80 kV (Fig. 7).

One of the attractive features of morphologically intact isolated glomerular BMs is that they are easily subjected to experimental manipulation prior to preparation for microscopy. Treatment of isolated glomerular BMs with pro-teolytic enzymes (19), denaturing agents (20), cytochemical "stains" (21), and immunochemical markers followed by transmission electron microscopic studies offer exciting possibilities for demonstrating glomerular BM hetero-geneity in normal, pathological, experimental, and developmental conditions.

Recently, techniques have been developed for dissection and preparation of glomerular BMs for scanning electron microscopy. Isolated glomerular BMs are allowed to sediment (usually overnight) in a small plastic beaker provided with a strip of double-sided cellophane tape extending from the rim down across the bottom and back up to the opposite rim. The BMs attached to the tape are fixed and postfixed as described above and may be air dried from acetone or critical-point dried in a conventional critical point drier (e.g.,

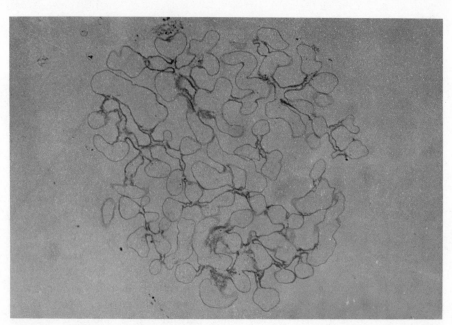

FIGURE 5. Photomicrograph of toluidine blue-stained section of isolated glomerular basement membrane similar to those shown in Figure 3. Lobulated peripheral basement membrane radiates from clearly identifiable mesangial regions. × 950.

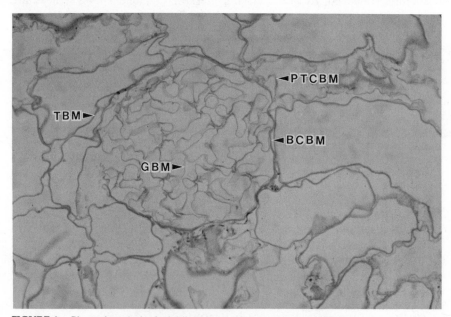

FIGURE 6. Photomicrograph of toluidine blue-stained section of rat acellular renal cortex prepared by the method illustrated in Figure 4. By this technique all major renal basement membranes can be identified in the same section. GBM, glomerular basement membrane; TBM, tubular basement membrane; BCBM, Bowman's capsule basement membrane; PTCBM, peritubular capillary basement membrane. × 880.

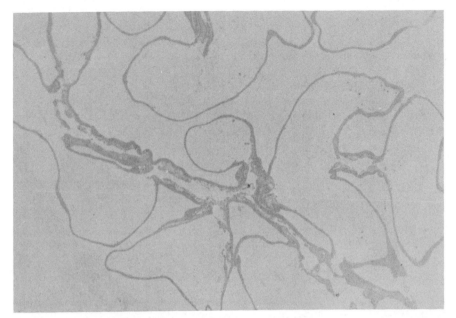

FIGURE 7. Transmission electron micrograph of isolated glomerular basement membrane similar to that shown in Figure 5. Despite the absence of cells, the basement membrane retains its *in vivo* histoarchitecture. ×4300.

Tousimis Sam-Dri). Alternatively, fixed isolated glomerular BMs can be placed in fine 63-μm nylon mesh bags or containers constructed of lens paper. These are placed in a plastic embedding (Beem) capsule with a perforated cover and carried through the critical point drying procedure. The dried samples are mounted on aluminum specimen stubs and coated with a thin layer of gold in a sputter coater.

It has been our experience that glomerular BMs located at the surface of acellular renal tissue blocks often show optimal preservation and are easiest to observe by scanning electron microscopy (15). Tissue blocks may be rendered acellular either by immersion or vascular perfusion. The entire block is fixed, dehydrated, and critical-point dried prior to coating with gold for observation (Fig. 8).

If it is advantageous to obtain SEM images of the inner surfaces of isolated glomerular BMs, cryofracturing is the method of choice (15). It is best to use somewhat larger (~3 mm³) acellular renal cortical blocks for this procedure. These are fixed and postfixed and dehydrated to absolute ethanol as described above. The samples are then transferred to freon 22 and cooled to liquid nitrogen temperature. This is followed by plunging the blocks to be fractured directly into liquid nitrogen where they are cleaved with a cold single-edged razor blade while they are still submerged. The samples are then returned to

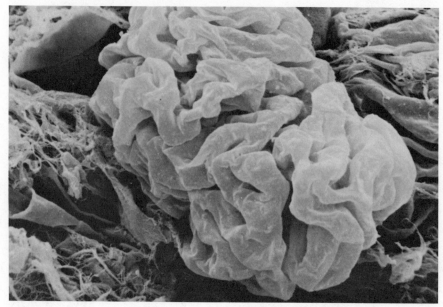

FIGURE 8. Scanning electron micrograph of rat renal glomerular basement membrane on the surface of an acellular cortical tissue block. Peripheral lobes of basement membranes maintain their *in vivo* conformations and the overall spheroidal shape of the glomerulus is retained. × 2200.

absolute ethanol. The critical-point drying procedure is carried out as described above. Individual fractured blocks are mounted on aluminum specimen stubs under a stereo dissection microscope (fracture surface up) and coated with gold. SEM observation of fractured surfaces frequently shows opposing surfaces of glomerular BMs as well as mesangial matrix material (Fig. 9).

5. BIOCHEMICAL ANALYSIS

Purification and analysis of individual components of glomerular BM has been extremely difficult because of the complex, multicomponent, highly cross-linked, insoluble nature of this extracellular matrix. Limited pepsin digestion has been widely employed to liberate collagen from isolated glomerular BM or from kidney cortex (22, 23). This technique rests on its ability to degrade cross-linked regions of native collagen molecules and presumes resistance of the collagen triple helix, as occurs in interstitial collagens, to this procedure. The triplet sequence Gly-X-Y, which confers pepsin resistance, is interrupted in BM collagens, however, and there are deletions of single glycine residues as well as interruptions by stretches of nonhelical sequences (24, 25). Thus, although collagen chains of good purity can be obtained from pepsin digests, they represent fragments of authentic components, and yields of intact native moieties are low.

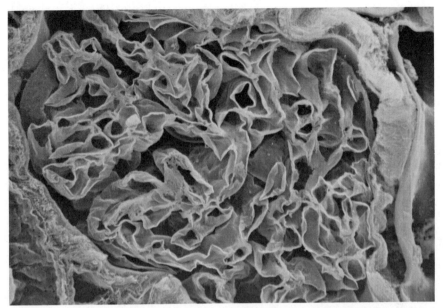

FIGURE 9. Scanning electron micrograph of cryofractured glomerular basement membrane. By this technique internal and external surfaces of peripheral glomerular basement membrane can be observed and compared. The mesangial matrix appears as a system of fenestrated plates and branching trabecula. × 1800.

Limited pepsin digestion is conducted at 4°C in 0.5 M acetic acid for 16–24 hr with an enzyme-to-tissue ratio of about 1:10 and continuous stirring. The digest is centrifuged at 18,000g for 1 hr, and the collagen in the extract can be purified by sequential selective salt precipitation, followed by separation and characterization of the collagen chains with ion exchange and molecular sieve chromatography. These procedures are described in detail in Volume 82 of *Methods in Enzymology* (26).

Another technique traditionally employed for solubilization of BM components entails reduction and denaturation in sodium dodecyl sulfate (SDS). Since this method avoids pepsin digestion, better preservation of high molecular weight collagen moieties would be expected. This can be accomplished when the glomerular BMs are prepared rapidly and in the cold, but is not the universal experience. Lyophilized glomerular BM is reduced and denatured by heating at 100°C for 2 min in 2 mL of 1 percent (wt/vol) SDS and 5 percent (v/v) β-mercaptoethanol in 0.1 M sodium phosphate buffer, pH 7.4. Samples are then incubated for 2 hr at 37°C and dialyzed at room temperature against two changes of 500 mL of 0.1 percent SDS in 0.1 M sodium phosphate buffer. Unsolubilized material is removed by centrifugation at 3000g for 10 min. Further analysis of the solubilized material can be accomplished following gel filtration, ion exchange chromatography, and SDS-polyacrylamide gel electrophoresis.

Modifications of this procedure allow differential solubilization of noncollagen and collagen components. Initial extraction of purified glomerular BM with 8 M urea solubilizes material that is devoid of hydroxyproline and hydroxylysine (27) and contains a high molecular weight species associated with glycosaminoglycan that represents heparan sulfate-containing proteoglycan. Extraction with 4 M guanidine-HCl also solubilizes proteoglycan that may represent two protein cores, one associated with heparan sulfate and the other with chondroitin sulfate (28). Urea extraction is conducted for 6–18 hr at 4°C in 0.05 M Tris, pH 8.6, containing 8 M urea and protease inhibitors in the concentrations given earlier. Guanidine extraction is conducted at 4°C for 24 hr with 4 M guanidine-HCl containing 0.01 M sodium EDTA, 0.01 M sodium acetate, pH 5.8, 0.1 M 6-aminohexanoic acid, 0.005 M benzamidine-HCl, and 0.001 M phenylmethylsulfonylfluoride. With both methods unextracted residue is pelleted by centrifugation. About 35 percent of the mixture of noncollagen and collagen components remaining after urea extraction can be solubilized by reduction and alkylation. This is performed under a nitrogen atmosphere at room temperature for 4–6 hr after suspending the sample in the solution used for urea extraction containing 0.05 M dithiothreitol. The pH of the solution is then adjusted to 8.0 with sodium hydroxide, and iodoacetic acid added to a final concentration of 0.11 M. Alkylation is performed in the dark for 40 min at room temperature and terminated by the addition of excess β-mercaptoethanol. Components solubilized by reduction and alkylation are separated from the insoluble material by centrifugation. About 60 percent of the latter, which contains high molecular weight aggregates and BM procollagen, can be solubilized with 1 percent SDS (29). Further analysis of the material solubilized by these procedures is accomplished by traditional techniques including gel filtration, SDS-polyacrylamide gel electrophoresis, affinity chromatography, and immunoassay, all of which are described in detail in recently published procedural manuals (4, 30).

Two additional areas of glomerular BM biochemistry deserve comment since they have generated special interest in recent years in view of a possible role in the pathogenesis of diabetic nephropathy. These are the glycosaminoglycans, which constitute anionic sites and are believed to contribute to the charge- and size-selective nature of the glomerular filtration barrier, and the nonenzymatic glycosylation of free amino groups at the N-terminus or ϵ-amino groups of lysine and hydroxylysine residues of proteins.

For isolation of glycosaminoglycans, samples are digested with 0.5 percent papain for 24 hr at 60°C in 0.1 M acetate buffer, pH 5.5, containing 5 mM EDTA and cysteine (31, 32). For more extensive digestion half the amount of papain can again be added and the incubation continued for another 24 hr. The digest is made 1 percent in cetylpyridinium chloride (CPC), and the resulting precipitate dissolved in 2 M NaCl and reprecipitated with two volumes of absolute ethanol. This precipitate is dissolved in 0.05 M Tris containing calcium, made 0.5 percent in pronase, and incubated at 37°C for 24 hr. Residual protein and nucleic acid substances are removed by precipitation after making the suspension 10 percent in trichloroacetic acid (TCA). The supernatant is extracted twice with two volumes of ether to remove TCA, and the glycosaminoglycans in the aqueous solution are precipitated with 1 percent CPC and washed with absolute ethanol. Identification of the glycosaminoglycans can be accomplished with cellulose acetate electrophoresis coupled with response to enzymatic digestion. Samples (1–10 μg) are spotted on cellulose acetate strips and electrophoresced in 0.1 M calcium acetate buffer, pH 4.0 (32). The strips are stained with alcian blue in 50 mM sodium acetate buffer, pH 5.8, containing 50 mM MgCl$_2$ and destained in 50 mM acetate, 50 mM MgCl$_2$ (33). Alternatively, strips can be stained with 0.5 percent alcian blue in 0.3 percent acetic acid and destained with 0.3 percent acetic acid. Known standards are run simultaneously. Identity can be corroborated by susceptibility to enzymatic digestion and/or nitrous acid oxidation, performed on duplicate aliquots prior to application to cellulose acetate strips. Specificity of digestion or oxidation is documented by subjecting glycosaminoglycans standards to the same procedure with appropriate controls in buffer alone. Chondroitinase ABC digestion (5 U/mL) is conducted in 0.1 M Tris, pH 8.0 (34); hyaluronidase digestion (3 mg/mL) is conducted in acetate or phosphate buffer, pH 5.4 (35). For nitrous acid oxidation (for heparan sulfate), samples are incubated at room temperature with a solution prepared by mixing equal volumes of 5 percent sodium nitrite and concentrated acetic acid (36).

Nonenzymatic glycosylation of proteins in purified glomerular BM can be determined by measuring the amount of chromogen produced by the reaction of 5-hydroxymethylfurfural (HMF) with thiobarbituric acid (TBA). This method detects carbohydrate bound by ketoamine linkage to proteins and depends on the generation of HMF from the carbohydrate moieties upon heating under acid conditions (37). Pure 5-hydroxymethylfurfuraldehyde is used as standard. BM samples, homogenized in 1.0 mL of Tris-buffered saline or solubilized in 0.1 N NaOH with heat, are hydrolyzed with 1.0 mL of 1.0 M oxalic acid for 5 hr at 100°C (38). After precipitation by addition of 1.0 mL of 40 percent trichloroacetic acid, 1.5 mL of the clear supernatant is reacted with 0.5 mL of 0.05 M TBA for 30 min at 40°C and the absorbance measured at 443 nm.

Affinity chromatography on a column of phenylboronate resin will separate glycosylated from nonglycosylated residues and is particularly useful when sample size is too limited for accurate measurement by the TBA colorimetric procedure (sensitive to 1–2 nmol HMF). Acid-hydrolyzed samples are applied to a 0.8 × 10-cm column of m-amino-phenylboronic acid linked to agarose or immobilized on Bio-Gel P-6 equilibrated with 50 mM HEPES buffer, pH 8.5, containing 10 mM MgCl$_2$. This resin selectively retains glycosylated amino acids and peptides (39–41). After washing with the alkaline HEPES buffer to remove nonglycosylated residues, the glycosylated products are eluted with 0.1 M acetic acid. Effluent is monitored for ninhydrin positivity and, when radiolabeled by reduction with tritiated sodium borohydride, for radioactivity in a liquid scintillation counter. Using an aliquot of the initial hydrolyzed sample for direct amino acid analysis, and a ninhydrin standard curve with lysine and/or hydroxylysine, μmol equivalents of glycosylated amino acid per residue of lysine or hydroxylysine can be calculated. Subsequent application of the phenylboronate-absorbed material to the amino acid analyzer identifies the actual amount and kind of glycosylated amino acid, using tritiated glycosylated amino acids as standards. The latter are prepared by incubating the respective amino acid with excess glucose concentration and reducing with sodium borohydride (42, 43). Either the amino acid or the sugar may be radiolabeled. The α-amino groups of lysine and hydroxylysine should be protected when preparing ε-amino-glycosylated standards of these amino acids (44). Excess borohydride and unreacted sugar are removed with Dowex 50 Wx8, from which products are eluted with $0.5\ N$ NH$_4$OH (43, 45). The glycosylated products are further freed of contaiminating free sugar and nonglycosylated amino acid reactant by passage through a column of Bio-Gel P-2 and application to a phenylboronate affinity resin column (41, 43).

REFERENCES

1. P. Bornstein and H. Sage, *Ann. Rev. Biochem.* **49**, 957 (1980).
2. N. A. Kefalides and C. C. Clark, *Int. Rev. Cytol.* **61**, 164 (1979).
3. E. D. Hay (ed.), *Cell Biology of Extracellular Matrix*, Plenum Press, New York, 1981.
4. H. Furthmayr (ed.), *Immunochemistry of the Extracellular Matrix*, CRC, Boca Raton, Florida, 1982.
5. K. M. Yamada, *Ann. Rev. Biochem.* **52**, 761 (1983).
6. C. A. Krakower and S. A. Greenspon, *Arch. Pathol.* **51**, 629 (1951).
7. R. G. Spiro, *J. Biol Chem.* **242**, 1915 (1967).
8. M. P. Cohen and C. V. Klein, *J. Exp. Med.* **149**, 623 (1979).
9. E. C. Carlson, K. Brendel, J. T. Hjelle, and E. Meezan, *J. Ultrastruct. Res.* **62**, 26 (1978).
10. M. E. Grant, R. Harwood, and I. F. Williams, *Eur. J. Biochem.* **54**, 531 (1975).
11. N. G. Westberg and A. F. Michael, *Biochemistry* **19**, 3837 (1970).
12. E. Meezan, J. T. Hjelle, K. Brendel, and E. C. Carlson, *Life Sciences* **17**, 1721 (1975).
13. M. P. Cohen, A. Dasmahapatra, and V. Y. Wu, *Nephron* **27**, 146 (1981).
14. E. C. Carlson and M. C. Kenney, *Renal Physiol.* **3**, 280 (1980).
15. E. C. Carlson and D. Hinds, *J. Ultrastruct. Res.* **82**, 96 (1983).
16. K. Brendel, E. Meezan, and R. Nagle in *Biology and Chemistry of Basement Membranes*. N. A. Kefalides (ed.), Academic Press, New York, 1978, pp. 177–193.
17. M. J. Karnovsky, *J. Cell Biol.* **27**, 137a (1965).
18. E. C. Carlson and D. Hinds, *J. Ultrastruct. Res.* **77**, 241 (1981).
19. E. C. Carlson, E. Meezan, K. Brendel, and M. C. Kenney, *Anat. Rec.* **200**, 421 (1981).
20. E. C. Carlson, K. Brendel, and E. Meezan, in *Biology and Chemistry of Basement Membranes*, N. A. Kefalides (ed.), Academic Press, New York, 1978, pp. 33–41.
21. Y. S. Kanwar and M. G. Farquhar, *Proc. Natl. Acad. Sci. USA* **76**, 4493 (1979).
22. K. Tryggvason and K. I. Kivirikko, *Nephron* **21**, 230 (1978).
23. S. N. Dixit, *FEBS Lett.* **106**, 379 (1979).
24. D. Schuppan, R. Timple, and R. W. Glanville, *FEBS Lett.* **115**, 297 (1980).

25. R. W. Glanville and A. Rauter, *Physiol. Chem.* **362**, 943 (1981).

26. E. J. Miller and R. K. Rhodes, in *Methods in Enzymology*, Vol. 82, L. W. Cunningham and D. W. Frederiksen (eds.), Academic Press, New York, 1982, pp. 33–64.

27. M. P. Cohen, V. Y. Wu, and M. L. Surma, *Biochim. Biophys. Acta* **678**, 322 (1981).

28. Y. S. Kanwar, V. A. Hascall, and M. G. Farquhar, *J. Cell Biol.* **90**, 527 (1981).

29. M. P. Cohen and V. Y. Wu, *Renal Physiol.* **4**, 112 (1981).

30. L. W. Cunningham and D. W. Frederiksen (eds.), *Methods in Enzymology*, Vol. 82, Academic Press, New York, 1982.

31. A. Linker and P. Hovingh, *Carbohyd. Res.* **29**, 41 (1973).

32. A. Linker and P. Hovingh, in *Methods in Enzymology*, Vol. 28, Victor Ginsburg (ed.), Academic Press, New York, 1972, pp. 902–911.

33. P. Whiteman, *Biochem. J.* **131**, 351 (1973).

34. H. Saito, T. Yamagata, and S. Suzuki, *J. Biol. Chem.* **243**, 1536 (1968).

35. T. W. Wight and R. Ross, *J. Cell Biol.* **67**, 660 (1975).

36. J. A. Cifonelli, *Carbohydr. Res.* **8**, 233 (1968).

37. R. Fluckiger and K. H. Winterhalter, *FEBS Lett.* **71**, 356 (1976).

38. R. E. Pecoraro, R. J. Graf, J. B. Halter, H. Beiter, and D. Porte, *Diabetes* **28**, 1120 (1979).

39. M. Brownlee, H. Vlassara, and A. Cerami, *Diabetes* **29**, 1044 (1980).

40. H. Vlassara, M. Brownlee, and A. Cerami, *Proc. Natl. Acad. Sci. USA* **78**, 5190 (1981).

41. M. P. Cohen and V. Y. Wu, *Exp. Gerontol.*, in press (1983).

42. A. J. Bailey, S. P. Robins, and M. J. A. Tanner, *Biochim. Biophys. Acta* **434**, 51 (1976).

43. M. Brownlee and A. Cerami, *Diabetes* **32**, 499 (1982).

44. B. Trueb, G. J. Hughes, and K. H. Winterhalter, *Analyt. Biochem.* **119**, 330 (1981).

45. B. A. Schwartz and G. R. Gray, *Arch. Biochem. Biophys.* **181**, 542 (1977).

B

MICROANALYTICAL CHARACTERIZATION OF COLLAGENS DERIVED FROM PURIFIED MICROVESSEL BASEMENT MEMBRANE

EDWARD C. CARLSON AND JOHN C. SWINSCOE

The University of North Dakota, Department of Anatomy, School of Medicine, Grand Forks, North Dakota and California Primate Research Center, University of California, Davis, California

1.   INTRODUCTION

Microvascular basement membrane (BM) thickening is widely accepted as the morphological hallmark of diabetic microangiopathy (1). This condition has been observed in human diabetics in the renal glomerulus (2) and the capillaries of the retina (3), central nervous system (4), skin (5), heart (6), and skeletal muscle (7). Although microvessel BM thickening is neither constant nor specific for diabetes, it is undoubtedly most common and most exaggerated in this state. The causes, specific compositional alterations, and significance of diabetic BM disease, however, are not clear.

   Since a significant proportion of BM protein is collagenous (8), recent advances in the preparation and characterization of distinct collagen types (9) have contributed substantially to the understanding of microvessel BM composition. Much of the new information has been derived from highly vascular organs such as placenta where it is assumed that the majority of BM collagen extracts are derived from large and small blood vessels (10). Biochemical analysis of BMs from tissue-specific microvessels, however, are few. This is due largely to the difficulty of obtaining sufficient quantities of purified capillary BMs to utilize as starting material. The purpose of this chapter is to describe several methods for isolation of homogeneous samples of microvessels, purification of their BMs, and microanalytical characterization of their BM collagenous peptides.

2.   ISOLATION OF MICROVESSSELS

Since the purpose of the current report is to describe some methods by which tissue-specific BMs may be analyzed for their collagenous peptides, micro-

The authors gratefully acknowledge the technical assistance of Janice Audette and Kristene Surerus in this project. Thanks are also extended to Lisa Eiteljorge for typing the manuscript. The work was supported in part by a grant from the American Diabetes Association North Dakota Affiliate, Inc. and NIH Grant EY05106-01.

vascular beds which may be purified rapidly and efficiently and which are subject to diabetic BM thickening should be considered excellent candidates for starting material. These criteria are perhaps best met by vessels isolated from the retina or of the cortical gray matter of the brain. Isolation procedures for purified preparations of both vessels types have been developed (11, 12) and thickening of their BMs in the diabetic state, at least in humans, is well documented (3, 4). Accordingly, the following discussion will present details of the procedures generally applicable to isolation of these vessel types, the purification of their respective BMs, and characterization of their BM collagenous components.

2.1. Preparation of Purified Retinal Vessels

Retinal vessels from laboratory animals and humans can be prepared by the methods originally described by Meezan and co-workers (11) for bovine retinas. Indeed we have found the bovine model to be excellent because the eyes are readily obtainable, relatively inexpensive, and large enough to offer ease of retinal vessel isolation. Moreover, sufficient quantities of tissue can be prepared from about five pairs of eyes for several collagen assays, including SDS-polyacrylamide gel electrophoresis and [^{125}I] two-dimensional mapping. The methods described below, therefore, relate to bovine eyes obtained from a local slaughterhouse and are essentially those previously described (13). By appropriate downsizing of materials and equipment, we have employed similar methods for isolating retinal vessels from humans, rhesus monkeys, kittens, and rats.

Since BMs are proteinaceous and are therefore subject to endogenous protease digestion, eyes to be used as a source for these structures should be enucleated as soon as possible following slaughter. They are transported on ice to the laboratory and the isolation procedure is immediately begun. Bovine eyes are conveniently held firmly with gloved hands in a 100 mm glass Petri dish containing a small amount of $0.15\ M$ NaCl (all solutions are made up in 0.05 percent sodium azide unless otherwise indicated) to keep the external surface moist. A small (~ 1.0 cm) slit is made in the wall of the globe at about the equator. The opening is then carried around the periphery of the eye with a sharp-nosed scissor, bisecting the globe. The anterior half is discarded and the vitreous gently rolled from the posterior shell with gloved fingers.

The neuroretina is easily separated from the retinal pigmented epithelial layer by directing a fine stream of $0.15\ M$ NaCl at its cut edge. It is then freed from its attachment at the optic papilla with fine-pointed scissors and collected in chilled saline.

For optimum dissociation of retinal vessels, approximately 12 bovine retinas are pooled, transferred to a tissue grinding vessel (Thomas, type B) and disrupted with 20 up-and-down strokes of a specially machined teardrop-shaped (small end directed upward) Teflon pestle with serrated tip (14). The homogenate is poured over a 210 μm mesh nylon screen (Tetko, Inc., Elmsford, NY) held taut by 6 in. concentric plastic embroidery hoops and placed directly on the rim of a 2 L Nalgene plastic beaker. The screen must be wetted with saline prior to use to prevent tissues from tightly adhering to the nylon.

The larger retinal vessels (arterioles and venules) remain on the 210 μm mesh screen following extensive rinsing with 0.15 M NaCl ($\sim$ 250 mL). A stream of saline is directed from a plastic squirt bottle at first at the periphery of the screen. The screen is slowly rotated while the residue is washed toward the center of the screen where it tends to blanche (as red blood cells and neural elements are rinsed away) and form an aggregate. The vessels are harvested with an angled flat spatula.

As described by Meezan and co-workers (11), an extremely pure homogeneous population of retinal capillaries can be prepared from the filtrate of the 210 μm mesh sieve by passing it over an 88 μm sieve (Tetko, Inc.), rinsing (250–500 mL saline) as described above and harvesting the residue. Purity is confirmed by phase-contrast microscopy (Fig. 1).

2.2.   Preparation of Purified Brain Microvessels

A major breakthrough in the isolation of intact, metabolically active brain microvessels was achieved by Brendel and co-workers (12) using techniques similar to those described for retinal vessels. By this method cerebral microvessels can be prepared selectively for *in vitro* studies (15) or for isolation of their associated BMs (13).

Whole brains are removed from the cranial vault and the cerebellum, brain stem, and olfactory bulbs are severed to facilitate the stripping away of pia and arachnoid membranes and the associated extracerebral vasculature.

Pieces of gray matter pinched with forceps from the cerebral cortex are homogenized with a Teflon tissue homogenizer similar to that described above for isolation of retinal microvessels. Cortical tissues are placed in the grinding vessel with a small volume of 0.15 M NaCl and ground to liquidity (5–10 up-and-down strokes). The homogenate is poured over previously wetted nylon sieves of descending mesh size with careful washing of the residue at each step with 0.15 M NaCl. The mesh size of the initial screen varies with the animal species. As examples, for bovine brain, 153 μm mesh is optimal for the initial sieving (12) while 86 μm is most appropriate for rats, rabbits, or guinea pigs (14). It is often advantageous to subject isolated vessel elements to a second homogenization prior to further sieving on smaller (or identical) mesh size screens. Usually an 86 μm mesh size is sufficiently discriminating to retain capillary size vessels. Careful washing of this final residue with monitoring by phase-contrast microscopy results in homogeneous preparations of brain microvessels.

3.   ISOLATION OF MICROVESSEL BASEMENT MEMBRANE

In early chemical and fine structural studies of isolated BM, ultrasonic vibration was adopted as a nearly universal procedure for disrupting the cells and loosening

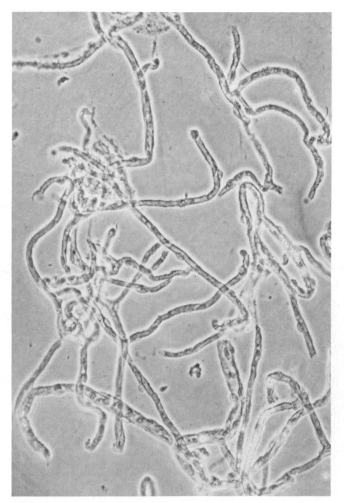

FIGURE 1. Phase-contrast photomicrograph of dissociated bovine retinal microvessels prepared by differential sieving. × 290.

them from their associated extracellular matrices (16). This technique has the advantage of being a nonchemical method which relies solely on physical forces to remove cellular materials from the BM. However, ultrasonic fragmentation is nonselective and BMs as well as cellular components are physically disrupted by the procedure. Therefore, although BMs have been defined historically by morphological criteria, these could not be applied to most BMs prepared by ultrasound. Such problems are minimized when single sheets of BM (e.g., posterior lens capsule, Descemet's membrane) are the choice for study. On the contrary complex BMs which exhibit several extracellular matrix components (e.g., renal glomerular BM, retinal vessel BM) are difficult to interpret morphologically following the ultrasonic method of BM isolation.

Many of the technical difficulties described above can be obviated by applying sequential detergent extraction to preparations of isolated microvessels (13). The technique is similar to that described for isolated glomeruli (see Vol. IC, VA) and involves osmotic lysis of microvessel cells followed by detergent solubilization of lipoprotein membranes and DNA disruption with endonoclease.

Isolated microvessels are first stirred (shaken) gently in a large volume (100:1) of distilled water (with 0.05 percent sodium azide) for several hours at 4°C. In some cases EDTA (1–5 mM) is added to the solution to facilitate breakdown of calcium-requiring intercellular junctions. The samples are then centrifuged (10,000 rpm, 10 min), the supernatant discarded, and the pellet suspended in a solution of 1–3 percent Triton X-100 (with 0.05 percent sodium azide) and stirred gently for 2–4 hr at room temperature. The preparations are recentrifuged and washed several times to remove completely the Triton X-100 prior to incubation of the pellet (1–2 hr at room temperature) in 1 M NaCl containing 0.025 percent deoxyribonuclease (type I, Sigma). If the Triton X-100 is not completely removed from the samples, the DNase is inactive and undigested DNA will cause clumping of the sample in final extraction step. The volume of DNase solution does not seem critical, but we routinely use approximately 40 mL for the microvessels derived from 50 bovine retinas. The vessel preparations are again centrifuged to a firm pellet followed by resuspension in 4 percent sodium deoxycholate (with 0.05 percent sodium azide) for 2–4 hr with stirring. The deoxycholate extraction should be carried out at room temperature because the viscosity of the solution rapidly increases as the temperature is reduced. The suspension is pelleted and washed extensively with distilled water prior to further analysis.

The final pellet derived from the detergent extraction technique consists principally of microvessel BM which, at the level of transmission (Fig. 2) or scanning electron microscopy (Fig. 3) is free of plasmalemmae and other cellular contaminants. Therefore this isolation procedure is the method of choice when morphologically intact BMs are necessary or desirable.

The foregoing extraction technique can be applied with equal efficacy to vessels dissociated from brain or retina (13). However, because the intact retina can be physically separated with ease from the internal surface of the posterior ocular hemisphere, retinal BM can be prepared from whole retinas without first isolating the vessels (17). The major disadvantages to this procedure are that BMs associated with vessels (or a particular diameter vessel, e.g., capillaries) cannot be prepared selectively, and preparations may be contaminated with small amounts of non-BM extracellular components such as fibrillar collagen and/or elastin. Nevertheless, except for the internal limiting membrane (which is a BM at the interface between the anterior surface of the retina and the vitreous), all retinal BMs are associated with its microvasculature. Accordingly, chemical studies of whole-retina BM have been taken as representative of retinal vessesl BM (17).

To solubilize the cellular constituents of the intact retina, the retina is removed as described above and immersed in 5 mM EDTA and 0.05 percent

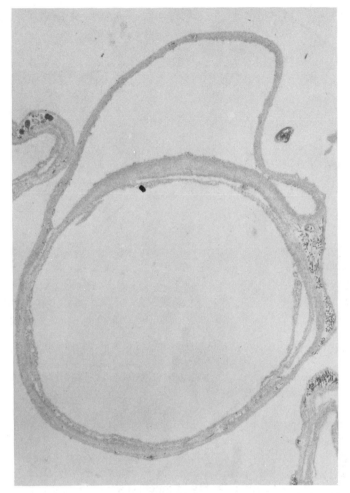

FIGURE 2. Transmission electron micrograph of basement membrane isolated by detergent washings from retinal vessels similar to those shown in Figure 1. × 10,300.

sodium azide in distilled water (50 mL centrifuge tube) and gently shaken 2– 4 hr at 4°C. Centrifugation between extraction steps is optional but not recommended if detailed morphological studies of the retinal vasculature is to be performed. The liquid is carefully removed with a drawn Pasteur pipette. Following osmotic shock the retina is treated sequentially with the same reagents and times as described above for isolated microvessels. Shaking or rotation of the samples reduces treatment times. This procedure results in a network of arborizing acellular retinal vessel BMs (Fig. 4), which at the level of transmission electron microscopy are identical to those isolated from previously dissociated vessels (see Fig. 2).

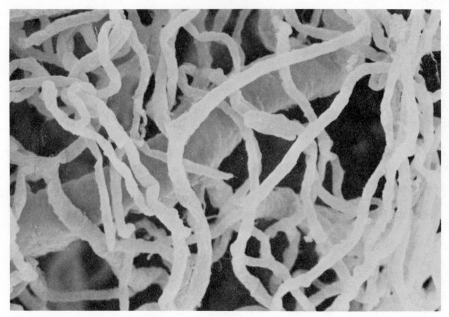

FIGURE 3.   Scanning electron micrograph of isolated bovine retinal microvessel basement membrane. ×630.

4.   BIOCHEMICAL ANALYSIS OF MICROVESSEL BASEMENT MEMBRANE COLLAGENS

The major components of vertebrate BMs are collagenous and noncollagenous glycoproteins (8, 18). The ultrastructural lamina densa (Fig. 2) comprises an organized network of collagen molecules identified as type IV collagen, represented by at least two distinct chains, $\alpha1(IV)$ and $\alpha2(IV)$. Heparan sulfate proteoglycan, laminin, and possibly fibronectin are the major noncollagenous components of the lamina rara. The biochemical procedures we describe utilize either pepsin digestion or strong denaturing agents to solubilize the BM, producing collagenous (pepsin-resistant) peptides, or a mixture of procollagen molecules and noncollagenous glycoproteins respectively. Characterization by the several microanalytical techniques will apply to all protein components of microvessel BM regardless of their origin but will be specifically addressed to the collagen peptides.

4.1.   Isolation of Basement Membrane Collagenous Peptides

A general procedure is to use the enzyme pepsin at a concentration of 0.5–1.0 mg/mL in 0.5 M acetic acid (HAc) with a digestion period of not less than 12 hr at 4°C (19, 20). Routinely we digest microvessel BM with 0.5 mg/mL of pepsin in 0.5 M HAc for 24 hr at 4°C followed by a second similar digestion

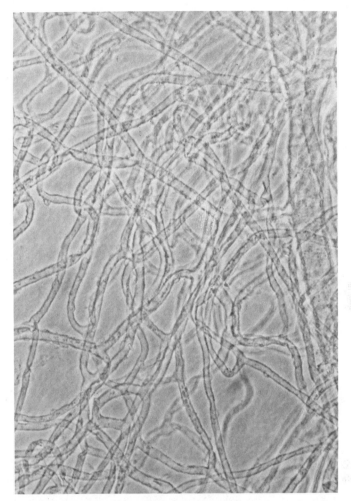

FIGURE 4. Phase-contrast photomicrograph of bovine retinal microvascular basement membranes in detergent-treated whole intact retina. Basement membranes appear as network of arborizing translucent tubes.

for a further 24 hr. It is important to stir the digestion mixture throughout the incubation. An insoluble residue remains and is pelleted by centrifugation at 10,000g for 30 min. Much of the residue can be solubilized by boiling in Laemmli (21) sample buffer (see Table 1) and should be retained for the eventual purification of the proteins retained in this fraction by preparative acylamide gel electrophoresis. The supernatants from both pepsin digests are pooled and may be treated in one of two ways: (i) immediately lyophilize and store at −20°C to await characterization and (ii) neutralize with 5 N NaOH using phenol red as indicator and dialyze into 1 M NaCl, 50 mM Tris, pH 7.2, at 4°C. Protein is then precipitated by the slow addition of solid NaCl to 4 M

TABLE 1. SDS-PAGE Reagents[a]

A. Running (separation gel)

Gel	15 percent	7.5 percent	10 percent	12.5 percent	15 percent
Bis-acrylamide (30:0.8)	5.0 mL	7.5 mL	10.0 mL	12.5 mL	15.0 mL
1.5 M Tris, pH 8.8	7.5	7.5	7.5	7.5	7.5
10 percent SDS[b]	0.3	0.3	0.3	0.3	0.3
TEMED[a]	0.01	0.01	0.01	0.01	0.01
10 percent Ammonium persulfate	0.30	0.30	0.30	0.30	0.15
Water	17.0	14.5	12.0	9.5	7.0

B. Stacking (upper) gel

Gel	5 percent
Bis-acrylamide (30:0.8)	2.5 mL
0.5 M Tris, pH 6.8	3.8
10 percent SDS[b]	0.15
TEMED[c]	0.005

C. Sample Buffer

0.5 M Tris, pH 6.8	10.0 mL
10 percent SDS[b]	20.0
Glycerol	5.0
0.1 percent Bromophenol blue	1.0

10 percent Ammonium persulfate	0.30
Water	8.80

D. Electrophoresis (running) Buffer

1.5 M Tris, pH 8.8	64.0 mL
Glycine	47.6 g
10 percent SDS[b]	40.0 mL
Water	To 4 L

E. Staining Solution

Stock Soln. A	Stock Soln. B
60 percent Methanol	25 percent 2-propanol
10 percent Acetic acid	10 percent Acetic acid
	65 percent Water

0.04 percent Coomassie-blue
30 percent Water
Mix 25 mL solution A with 225 mL Solution B

F. Destaining Solution

10 percent Methanol
7 percent Acetic acid
83 percent Water

G. Bis-acrylamide

30 percent Acrylamide
0.8 percent Bis[d]
10 percent Glycerol
60 percent Water

[a] After ref. 21.
[b] Sodium dodecyl sulfate.
[c] N,N,N¹,N¹,-tetramethylenediamine.
[d] N,N-Methylene-bis-acrylamide.

and the solution left standing at 4°C overnight. The precipitate is collected by centrifugation, dissolved in 0.5 M HAc, and protein reprecipitated by adding solid NaCl to 1.5 M at 4°C, and left standing at 4°C overnight. The precipitate is again collected by centrifugation, resuspended in cold 0.5 M HAc and dialyzed extensively against 0.5 M HAc at 4°C. The dialyzate is then lyophilized and stored at −20°C. This second precipitation results in a slightly purer preparation of total collagenous peptides.

4.2.   Isolation of Basement Membrane Procollagen

Other isolation procedures have recently been devised in order to study newly synthesized collagen (pre-collagen) mRNA transcripts. Certain BM sources such as fetal membranes (22) and EHS sarcoma (a mouse tumor) (23) do not require vigorous treatment for collagen extraction. This is not so, however, for the more highly organized BM structures such as glomerular BM and microvessel BM. One such nonproteolytic method for glomerular BM disruption has been devised by Hudson and co-workers (24). The BM is isolated in the presence of protease inhibitors (25). Purified BM is resuspended in 8 M urea (0.5 g/mL), 0.01 M Tris-HCl, pH 8.5, and incubated for 6 hr at 37°C with stirring. The insoluble material is collected by centrifugation at 10,000g for 15 min, resuspended in 8 M urea, and the process repeated. A third urea extraction is similarly performed. All steps are carried out in the presence of protease inhibitors PMSF (phenylmethylsulfonylfluoride), NEM (N-ethyl-maleimide), and EDTA (ethylenediaminetetraacetic acid), all at 10 mM. The precipitate which remains consists mainly of highly cross-linked procollagen and can be solubilized by reduction and alkylation of disulfide bonds in denaturing agents: 8 M urea, 0.3 M Tris, pH 8.5, under nitrogen with 1 percent β-mercaptoethanol for 12 hr at 37°C. The free sulfhydryl groups are alkylated with a threefold excess of iodoacetamide for 2 hr at room temperature. The resultant procollagen molecules may then be analyzed by SDS-PAGE.

4.3.   Chemical Characterization of Microvessel BM Collagens

There are two major factors which complicate the biochemical identification of collagen proteins purified from isolated microvessel BM. First, available quantities of pure protein are usually limited to only a few hundred micrograms. Second, type IV collagen (the only apparent collagen of this BM) is uncharacteristically susceptible to further cleavage by pepsin, generating a number of peptides with apparent molecular weights ranging from 140,000 to 25,000 daltons. This heterogeneity has made chain identification difficult and also reduces the absolute amounts of each available collagen peptide. While several of the currently available chemical techniques for collagen characterization apply to microvessel BM collagen identification, others, such as column chromatography (sieve and ion exchange) and salt fractionation do not. Some of the existing methodology has been refined over the last several years with a concomitant increase in sensitivity, while a few new techniques have been introduced. In the following sections we will describe several methodologies which apply to the identification of microvessel BM collagen.

4.3.1. SDS-POLYACRYLAMIDE GEL ELECTROPHORESIS (SDS-PAGE)

This procedure is considered an analytical tool and has been the basis of collagen identification for many years. We use the method also as a preparative tool. A presumptive identification of collagen types can be made based on the banding pattern of extractable proteins in SDS gels (reduced and unreduced). While a Tris-borate gel system may suffice (26) and is simple to use, we prefer the Laemmli (21) gel system (Table 1) since it gives better resolution especially between proteins with apparent molecular weights of 100,000 and 25,000 daltons. The running gel is a 7.5 percent acrylamide solution (acrylamide to bis-acrylamide ratio, 30:0.8) in a Tris buffer, pH 8.6. The upper sample gel is a 5 percent acrylamide solution in 0.5 M Tris buffer, pH 6.8. Although this system can be applied to disc (tube) gels, we prefer to use slab gels of size 18 × 14 cm with a 10-well Teflon comb. The Teflon thickness is 1.5 mm. The lower gel is poured to a height of 8 cm, overlaid carefully with water, and allowed to polymerize (approximately 5 min). The overlying liquid is removed, the upper gel solution poured on top, and the appropriate comb inserted to a depth of 2 cm leaving approximately 1.5 cm of upper gel. The upper gel is allowed to polymerize. Protein samples are usually prepared from lyophilized protein by the addition of 50–150 μL of sample buffer (see Table 1) with or without added β-mercaptoethanol. Alternatively, sample buffer may be added to protein in acetic acid (1:1, vl/vl). The sample is then denatured by placing in a boiling water bath for 5 min and cooled. With the gel clamped to the electrophoresis chamber the sample is applied to a well through the running buffer by means of a micropipette and the gel is run at 90 V until the sample has stacked on top of the running gel (about 1 hr). The voltage is then increased to 150 V (constant voltage) until the tracking dye reaches the bottom (about 2.5 hr). The gel is removed, placed in stain (0.04 percent Coomassie blue in 6 percent methanol, 10 percent HAc, and 25 percent 2-propanol for several hours and destained in 10 percent methanol–7 percent HAc.

4.3.2. PREPARATIVE SDS-PAGE

This same system is employed as a preparative gel to purify somewhat larger quantities (several 100 μg) of protein. In this instance no comb is used and the sample to be run is laid across the entire upper gel. Protein bands may be identified and removed from the gel either by lightly staining the entire gel in Coomassie blue stain for 15 min followed by destaining for 15 min or by similarly staining three narrow zig-zag strips removed from the gel and reinserting them into their original positions in order to locate and remove the protein in the unstained portion of the gel (27). The gel that is removed is cut into small pieces, packed into a small glass column (we use a shortened 5-mL pipette plugged with glass wool), and electroeluted into a dialysis bag tied to the pipette. The regular slab gel electrophoresis apparatus is used with a filter paper wick running into the top of the pipette column. Laemmli running buffer is used throughout, and the dialysis bag rests in the lower reservoir buffer. The column is held in position by high-vacuum grease. It is necessary to purge the column of large air bubbles. The protein is electroeluted at 350 V for 3–4 hr after which the sample is removed and dialyzed against an appropriate buffer (we uses 0.02 percent SDS) and lyophylized.

4.3.3. COLLAGENASE DIGESTION

Since all collagenous peptides are susceptible to degradation by bacterial collagenase, this enzyme is used to distinguish between collagen and noncollagen proteins. The enzyme requires Ca^{2++} for activation. Noncollagen proteins are not sensitive to highly purified bacterial collagenase (Sigma, type VII, or Advanced Biofactures, Lynbrook, NY). Generally, collagen protein (20–40 μg) is dissolved in a collagenase buffer consisting of 0.2 M HEPES buffer, pH 7.4, with added $CaCl_2$ (10 mM) and NEM (10 mM). Purified bacterial collagenase dissolved in 10 mM Tris, pH 7.4, containing 15 mM $CaCl_2$ is added to the mixture with an enzyme-to-substrate ratio of 1:1. Digestion is carried out at 37°C for 1 hr, after which the sample is heated to 60°C for 2 min and lyophilized. The produces are analyzed by SDS-PAGE.

Alternatively, BM proteins may be identified as largely collagenous in nature by measurement of their hydroxyproline content. Ordinarily a colorimetric method is performed on total hydrolysates (28).

Having established which BM-derived proteins are collagenous, a more precise assignment of the individually purified protein to both its collagen type and chain is required. A number of methods are available for such studies which *in total* require less than 500 μg of pure starting material. Cyanogen bromide cleavage and amino acid composition each utilize between 100–150 μg of sample per analysis. *Staphylococcus aureus* V8 protease digestion and mast cell protease digestion each utilize approximately 40 μg of sample. Two-dimensional [125I]peptide mapping and one-dimensional [125I]CNBr mapping utilize from 1 to 10 μg of sample. We have estimated that retinal microvessel BM from approximately 500 bovine eyes provides sufficient purified protein for one of each of the above mentioned determinations, although obviously the radioactive procedures will allow for several analyses.

4.3.4. CYANOGEN BROMIDE CLEAVAGE

As a routine procedure we reduce each collagen sample prior to chemical cleavage in order to convert methionine sulfoxide residues to methionine. This is accomplished by dialysis in 0.2 M NH_4HCO_3 containing 0.15 M β-mercaptoethanol, at 40°C for 24 hr (29). This is followed by lyophilization. The residue is redissolved in 1 mL of distilled water and again lyophilized. One milliliter of 70 percent formic acid saturated with nitrogen is then added followed by solid CNBr (equivalent to a 10:1 excess, w/w), and each tube is gassed with a steady stream of nitrogen for 3 min, closed with a tight fitting cap, and sealed with parafilm. Incubation proceeds at 30°C for 4 hr. The reaction is stopped by the addition 10 volumes of distilled water, the sample shell-frozen and lyophilized overnight. The small residue which remains is carefully dissolved in Laemmli sample buffer, boiled for 3 min and electrophoresced using a Laemmli 7.5–15 percent discontinuous gel (Table 1). Voltage is maintained at 100 V for 12 hr after which time the gel is removed and CNBr peptides visualized with Coomassie blue stain. This technique creates unique peptide banding patterns for the various collagen types and their individual chains (Fig. 5).

4.3.5. STAPHYLOCOCCAL V8 PROTEASE DIGESTION

Heat-denatured collagen samples (60 μg) dissolved in 0.05 M Tris, pH 6.8, are subjected to limited proteolysis by incubation with V8 protease (Miles Laboratories) at an enzyme-to-substrate ratio of 1:20 for 30 min at 37°C. The reaction is stopped by the addition of SDS to 0.1 percent. After lyophilization

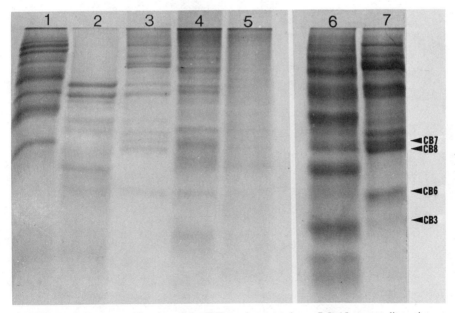

FIGURE 5. Collagen peptides cleaved by CNBr and separated on a 7.5–15 percent discontinuous SDS-polyacrylamide gel. Lane 1: bovine vitreus Type II; lane 2: bovine Descemet's membrane collagen; lane 3: bovine cornea type I; lane 4: human placenta type V; lane 5: human placenta type IV; lane 6: bovine skin type III, lane 7: bovine skin type I. The cyanogen bromide peptides indicated by arrows represent the (α_1) chain of type I.

the dried samples are redissolved in Laemmli sample buffer (Table 1) with added β-mercaptoethanol, heated (100°C, 1 min), and applied to a SDS-PAGE slab gel (7.5–15 percent discontinous gel) (Fig. 6). Electrophoresis is performed for 1 hr at 90 V (stacking) followed by 4 hr at 150 V (constant voltage).

4.3.6.   MAST CELL PROTEASE DIGESTION

This enzyme is not available commercially and is usually prepared from rat skeletal muscle (30). The lyophilized sample (25–40 μg) is digested with mast cell protease by adding the enzyme in a buffer consisting of 0.15 M NaCl, 50 mM Tris, pH 7.5 (1 mg/mL), at an enzyme-to-substrate ratio of

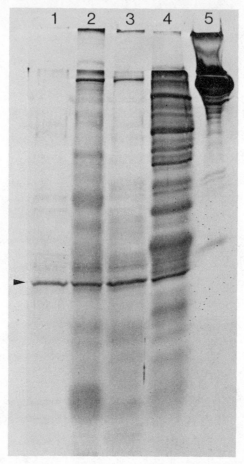

FIGURE 6.   Staphylococcal V8 protease digests of collagens. Peptides were separated on a 7.5–15 percent discontinuous SDS-polyacrylamide gel. Lane 1: bovine Descemet's membrane collagen; lane 2: bovine skin type III; type III: lane 3: bovine vitreus type II; lane 4: bovine skin type I; lane 5: undigested bovine skin type I. Arrow marks the position of the V8 enzyme.

1:100 (w/w). The reaction proceeds at 37°C for 5–60 min (or 22°C for 48 hr) and is terminated by cooling to 0°C followed by the addition of an equal volume of Laemmli sample buffer (Table 1) and 50 mM dithiothreitol. The cleavage products are then analyzed by SDS-PAGE on a 10 percent slab gel (31, 32).

4.3.7. TWO-DIMENSIONAL [^{125}I]PEPTIDE MAPPING

Radioiodination of proteins followed by a two-dimensional separation technique is not a new procedure. A methodology was devised by Elder and co-workers (33) using the chloramine-T iodination system with Na[^{125}I] which efficiently iodinated protein in gels. This technique has been used successfully to distinguish between peptides, in particular *in vitro* protein translation products. Subsequently, it has undergone various refinements in a number of laboratories. One such modification is that of Sage and co-workers (34) to study collagen polymorphism. Their method uses a relatively mild protein esterification step with the Bolton–Hunter [^{125}I] p-hydroxyphenylpropionic acid, N-hydroxysuccinimide ester reagent (New England Nuclear or Amersham) and can be used to label proteins in gels (dry or wet) or in solution. The technique is relatively simple, sensitive, and appears to be consistent, but the reagent is somewhat expensive. We have taken the same general principle to devise another modification which is rapid, sensitive, consistent, and relatively inexpensive.

Sage-Pritzl–Bornstein (34) Method. The Bolton–Hunter reagent is supplied in vials of 0.25-mCi aliquots dissolved in benzene. One vial is used per reaction. The benzene is removed by evaporation under nitrogen in a fume hood and the vial placed on ice. The collagen sample (1–10 µg), previously dialyzed into 0.1 M calcium acetate, pH 8.5 (adjusted with 0.2 M sodium borate, pH 9.0) at 4°C is injected into the vial. The reaction is allowed to proceed on ice for 2 hr with constant shaking. Glycine (0.1 mL, 0.2 M) in 0.1 M calcium acetate buffer, pH 8.5, is then added and the mixture shaken on ice for a further 30 min. The solution is then removed and dialyzed against 0.05 percent HAc at 4°C and lyophilized. The [^{125}I]collagen is then dissolved in Laemmli sample buffer (Table 1) with added β-mercaptoethanol and electrophoresed on a 5–7.5 percent discontinuous Laemmli gel. Proteins are stained with Coomassie blue stain and the bands of interest are cut from the gel. The stain can be removed by the method of Elder and co-workers (33) which involves washing with 2 mL of 25 percent isopropanol four times followed by 2 mL aliquots of 10 percent methanol three times, with vigorous shaking. We have shown, however, that the stain does not interfere with subsequent analyses (unpublished data). The gels are then lyophilized and stored at −20°C prior to enzyme digestion. Alternatively, unlabeled protein can be cut from gels and the gel slices iodinated as described above. The radioiodinated slices are then incubated with 20 µg of proteinase K (Fungal protease XI, Sigma) in

0.05 M NH$_4$HCO$_3$, pH 8.0, for 20 hr at 37°C in siliconized glass tubes. After digestion the sample is lyophilized and stored at −20°C.

Two-dimensional peptide mapping is performed on 10 × 10-cm cellulose-coated plastic plates without fluorescent indicator (EM Biochemical, Brinkman, NY, or American Scientific Products). The first dimension is electrophoresis in acetic acid–formic acid–water (15:5:80) as described by Elder and co-workers (33). The lyophilized sample is dissolved in 10 μL of running buffer, centrifuged briefly and counted. Approximately 1 × 10^5 cpm are spotted in a lower corner of the plate and bromophenol blue dye is spotted on an upper corner. A suitable electrophoresis chamber (Desaga-Brinkman or Gelman) is used to support the plate horizontally and the sample is electrophoresed at 400 V for approximately 60 min at room temperature. The plate is then removed, dried at room temperature, and run in a second dimension in an appropriate chromatography chamber equilibrated with n-butanol–pyridine–acetic acid–water (32.5:25:5:20) containing 7 percent 2,5-diphenyloxazole (w/v) (33). Chromatography is finished when the solvent front has migrated 8 cm. The plate is removed, dried at room temperature, and exposed to Kodak XAR-5 X-ray film with Dupont Chronex Lighting plus intensifying screens at −70°C (35) for 4–24 hr. This technique has been used in support of collagen identification by the other more conventional methods.

Swinscoe–Carlson Method. We have utilized a recent iodination procedure (36) which uses Na [^{125}I] and iodogen (1,3,4,6-tetrachloro-3, 6-diphenylglycoluril) (Pierce Chemical Co.) as catalyst. We have found this to be a very suitable mild iodination reaction and efficient (1 × 10^5 cpm/μg protein). Iodination is performed on collagen peptides either lyophilized out of HAc or electroeluted from acrylamide gels with or without Coomassie blue stain. The electroeluted samples are dialyzed against 0.02 percent SDS, lyophilized, and stored at −20°C before iodination. Collagen peptide (1–10 μg) is dissolved in 0.5 mL iodination buffer (60 mM triethanolamine–1 percent SDS, pH 8.0) and heated to 60°C for 5 min. The sample is then placed on ice. Potassium iodide (10 μL, 5 mM) containing 40 μCi ^{125}I is added to the sample, which is then transferred to another test tube (soda lime) coated with iodogen (36). The reaction is allowed to proceed on ice for 15 min with an occasional gentle rotation of the tube. The sample is then transferred to a microfuge tube containing 50 μL of a 3.0 M solution of potassium acetate, vortexed, and left on ice for 30 min. The SDS–protein precipitate is pelleted by a 2-min centrifugation and the supernatant, containing over 90 percent of unreacted ^{125}I, is discarded as radioactive waste. The pellet is resuspended in 1 mL of 0.05 percent HAc, placed in a dialysis bag, and dialyzed against 0.05 percent HAc for 24 hr (two 5-L changes) at 4°C. The iodinated sample is then lyophilized and ready for protease digestion. Reaction conditions described in the "Sage-Pritzl-Bornstein Method" (see above) are used to digest the sample, which is first divided into halves; one-half is treated with proteinase K (20 μg), the other with trypsin (20 μg) (Sigma type III). After incubation the lyophilized samples are stored at −20°C for mapping.

It is not always possible to control the amount of salt and SDS carried through to the final lyophilized sample. If this quantity is considerable, it will result in streaking of the ^{125}I spots during electrophoresis. To overcome this inconsistency we routinely presoak each map (with spotted sample) in a solvent mixture of *n*-butanol ethanol-H_2O (56:36:8) for 30 min. This procedure eliminates the streaking of spots without changing the pattern. Each map is then processed as described above and developed with Kodak XAR-5 X-ray film.

By these procedures we are able to generate collagen peptide maps specific for two separate enzyme digests. It should be mentioned that the proteinase K maps produced by our technique (Fig. 7) are not identical to those of the previous protocol (34) because the former method radioiodinates modified amino groups while the latter appears to incorporate ^{125}I into tyrosine, histidine,

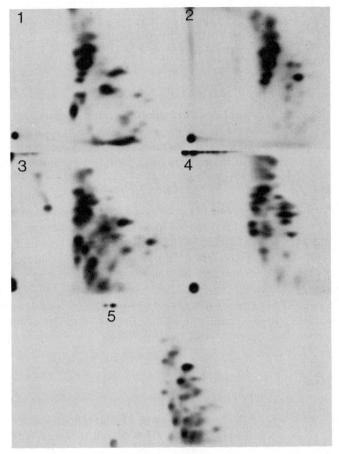

FIGURE 7. Two-dimensional [^{125}I]peptide maps generated from collagens using proteinase K. Electrophoresis is from left to right; chromatography is from bottom to top of each map. (1) Rat tail tendon type I; (2) bovine vitreus type II; (3) human placenta type III; (4) human placenta type IV; (5) human placenta type V.

methionine residues in particular, and other as yet unidentified residues with less efficiency.

4.3.8. ONE-DIMENSIONAL MAPPING OF IODINATED CYANOGEN BROMIDE PEPTIDE FRAGMENTS [^{125}I]PROTEINS

Aliquots of protein (10 μg), which have been iodinated in the manner described above, are desulfoximated and cleaved with CNBr (29). The cyanogen bromide fragments are separated on a 7.5–15 percent discontinuous Laemmli gel. The gel is then blotted onto a nitrocellulose filter. We use a Bio-Rad electroblotting apparatus in which peptides are transferred to nitrocellulose quantitatively by applying a constant current of 180 mA for 6 hr. However, in order to reduce the background level of ^{125}I, the gel is first blotted for 1 hr, after which the filter is removed (and discarded) and a fresh prewetted filter is placed against the gel and the blotting allowed to proceed for 6 hr. The buffer used in this procedure consists of 57.6 g glycine, 12.1 g Tris, in 4 L of 10 percent methanol. The dried nitrocellulose filter is developed against Kodak XAR-5 X-ray film plus intensifying screen for 2–3 days.

4.3.9. AMINO ACID COMPOSITION

Microvessel BM collagens are purified from Laemmli preparative gels using the electroelution techniques described previously. We consider it important to acid-wash all glassware and to charcoal the gel reagents and filter them before use. Gloves are also worn during the entire procedure. The sample is dialyzed first against 0.02 percent SDS, then against distilled water, and placed into a Pyrex glass hydrolysis tube and lyophilized. Constant boiling (0.5 mL 6 N) HCl is added and the tube sealed *in vacuo*. Hydrolysis is performed at 110°C for 20 hr and the HCl is removed in a vacuum dessicator with acid trap. Several drops of double-distilled water are added and the sample dried *in vacuo*. This process is repeated until all traces of acid are removed. The final dried hydrolysate is then analyzed on an appropriate amino acid analyzer. We use a Durrum D-500 autoanalyzer utilizing a single-column procedure. Pierce (Pierce Chemical Co.) chemical buffers give excellent peak resolution and low background. Hydroxyproline and aspartic acid residues coelute but can be resolved on a short column using a second Pierce buffer system (37).

REFERENCES

1. J. R. Williamson and C. Kilo, *Diabetes* **25** (suppl. 2), 925 (1976).
2. R. Osterby, H. J. G. Gundersen, A. Horlyck, J. P. Kroustrup, G. Nyberg, and G. Westberg, *Diabetes* **32**, 79 (1983).
3. N. Ashton, *Brit. J. Opthal.* **58**, 344 (1974).
4. P. C. Johnson, K. Brendel, and E. Meezan, *Arch. Pathol. Lab. Med.* **106**, 214 (1982).

5. B. B. Banson and P. E. Lacy, *Am. J. Pathol.* **45**, 41 (1964).

6. M. D. Silver, V. F. Huckell, and M. Larber, *Pathology* **9**, 213 (1977).

7. J. R. Williamson and C. Kilo, *Diabetes* **32**, 96 (1983).

8. N. A. Kefalides, R. Alper, and C. C. Clark, *Int. Rev. Cytol.* **61**, 167 (1979).

9. P. Bornstein and H. Sage, *Ann. Rev. Biochem.* **39**, 957 (1980).

10. R. Rhodes and E. Miller, *Biochemistry* **17**, 3442 (1978).

11. E. Meezan, K. Brendel, and E. Carlson, *Nature* **25**, 65 (1974).

12. K. Brendel, E. Meezan, and E. Carlson, *Science* **185**, 953 (1974).

13. E. C. Carlson, K. Brendel, J. T. Hjelle, and E. Meezan, *J. Ultrastruct. Res.* **62**, 26 (1978).

14. R. J. Head, J. T. Hjelle, B. Jarrott, B. Berkowitz, G. Cardinale, and S. Spector, *Blood Vessels* **17**, 173 (1980).

15. T. Hjelle, J. Baird-Lambert, G. Cardinale, S. Spector, and S. Udenfriend, *Proc. Natl. Acad. Sci. USA* **75**, 4544 (1978).

16. R. G. Spiro, *J. Biol. Chem.* **242**, 1915 (1967).

17. R. C. Duhamel, E. Meezan, and K. Brendel, *Exp. Eye Res.* **36**, 257 (1983).

18. M. E. Grant, J. G. Heathcote, and R. W. Orkin, *Bioscience Reports* **1**, 819 (1981).

19. N. A. Kefalides, *Biochem. Biophys. Res. Commun.* **45**, 226 (1971).

20. T. F. Kresina and E. J. Miller, *Biochemistry* **18**, 3089 (1979).

21. U. K. Laemmli, *Nature (London)* **227**, 680 (1970).

22. K. Tryggvason, P. G. Robey, and G. R. Martin, *Biochemistry* **19**, 1284 (1980).

23. R. Timpl, G. R. Martin, P. Bruckner, G. Wick, and H. Wiedemann, *Eur. J. Biochem.* **84**, 43 (1978).

24. D. C. Dean, J. F. Barr, J. W. Freytag, and B. G. Hudson, *J. Biol. Chem.* **258**, 590 (1983).

25. J. W. Freytag, M. Ohno, and B. G. Hudson, *Biochem. Biophys. Res. Commun.* **72**, 796 (1976).

26. P. D. Benya, S. R. Padilla, and M. E. Nimni, *Biochemistry* **16**, 865 (1977).

27. U. Labermeier and M. C. Kenney, *Arch. Bichem. Biophys.* **213**, 50 (1982).

28. J. F. Woessner, *Arch. Biochem. Biophys.* **93**, 440 (1961).

29. R. S. Adelstein and W. M. Kuehl, *Biochemistry* **9**, 1355 (1970).

30. R.-G. Woodbury, M. Everitt, Y. Sanada, N. Katunuma, D. Lagunoff, and H. Neurath, *Proc. Natl. Acad. Sci. U.S.* **75**, 5311 (1978).

31. H. Sage, E. Crouch, and P. Bornstein, *Biochemistry* **18**, 5433 (1979).

32. H. Sage and P. Bornstein, in *Methods in Enzymology*, Vol. 82, L. W. Cunningham and D. W. Fredericksen (eds.) Academic Press, New York, 1982, pp. 96–127.

33. J. H. Elder, R. A. Pickett, J. Hampton, and R. A. Lerner, *J. Biol. Chem.* **252**, 6510 (1977).

34. H. Sage, P. Pritzl, and P. Bornstein, *Collagen Rel. Res.* **1**, 3 (1981).

35. S. E. Zweig and S. J. Singer, *Biochem. Biophys. Res. Commun.* **88**, 1147 (1979).

36. D. R. Tolan, J. M. Lambert, G. Boileau, T. G. Fanning, J. W. Kenny, A. Vassos, and R. R. Traut, *Analyt. Biochem.* **103**, 101 (1980).

37. W. E. Brown and G. C. Howard, *Anal. Bioch.* **101**, 294 (1980).

C

USE OF THE EHS TUMOR AS A MODEL FOR STUDYING BASEMENT MEMBRANE SYNTHESIS IN NORMAL AND DIABETIC MICE

DAVID H. ROHRBACH

Department of Cellular and Molecular Biology, University of Texas Health Science Center, San Antonio, Texas

STEVEN R. LEDBETTER, CLAYTON W. WAGNER, ELIZABETH A. HORIGAN, JOHN R. HASSELL, AND GEORGE R. MARTIN

Laboratory of Developmental Biology and Anomalies, National Institute of Dental Research, National Institutes of Health, Bethesda, Maryland

1. INTRODUCTION

Several transplantable animal tumors produce basement membrane and are good sources for isolating its components. These include type IV collagen, laminin, entactin, nidogen, and heparan sulfate proteoglycan. Antibodies prepared against proteins and proteoglycans prepared from the EHS tumor, a murine tumor, react with basement membranes in normal tissues. These observations and biochemical comparisons suggest that similar components exist in normal basement membranes. Type IV collagen is the major structural support for the basement membrane while the heparan sulfate proteoglycan forms a filtration barrier in the basement membrane. The glycoproteins, laminin, entactin, fibronectin, and nidogen, are involved in cell–matrix interaction as well as in other functions.

Basement membranes are thickened several-fold in diabetes yet appear to be more porous to the passage of macromolecules. Studies on tumor tissue grown in diabetic animals and on tissue from patients with diabetes suggest that the amount of heparan sulfate proteoglycan component is reduced in diabetes. A reduction in proteoglycan levels may impair the filtration function of basement membranes in tissues. Changes in the structure and/or function of such basement membrane components may induce a compensatory synthesis of more components. Methods are described for isolating basement membrane components from tumor tissue and for studying their form and function.

Many studies indicate that the basement membranes in certain anatomical sites become thickened in individuals who have had diabetes for many years (1–7). This change is associated with and may be a contributing factor to diverse degenerative changes in the tissues, including kidney failure, loss of vision, and blood vessel disease. More thickening is observed in the glomeruli and capillaries where the greatest flux of fluids occurs. In diabetes basement membranes, which are usually an efficient barrier to the passage of proteins (8–10), may be more permeable than normal (11–14). Since basement membranes are extracellular structures, changes in their appearance and function would be expected to arise from alterations in their composition or in their components. The thickening of basement membranes in diabetes at sites of high fluid flow may represent an induced synthesis of basement membrane components in an attempt to compensate for a functional defect such as a change in its permeability barrier (15, 16).

Basement membranes are minute (70–200 nm) structures, not readily separated from other tissue elements, which underlie epithelial cells and surround peripheral nerves, muscle fibers, smooth muscle cells, and fat cells. They contain a unique complement of macromolecules including type IV collagen, glycoproteins such as laminin and entactin, and a heparan sulfate proteoglycan (Table 1). These components are not solubilized without denaturing solvents or exposure to proteolytic enzymes. Further, basement membranes are long-lived and turn over at a slow rate (17–22). For these reasons it is difficult to

TABLE 1. Basement Membrane Components

Component	Molecular Weight	Composition	Source
Type IV collagen	450,000	pro α1(IV) (Mr = 185,000) pro α2(IV) (Mr = 170,000)	Kidney, aorta Placenta, EHS tumor, cultured cells
Laminin	1×10^6	A chain (Mr = 400,000)	EHS tumor, placenta
		B chain (Mr = 200,000)	Cultured cells
Heparan sulfate Proteoglycan	~750,000	Protein core (Mr = 400,000)	EHS tumor, kidney
		Glycosaminoglycans (Mr = 65,000)	Cultured cells
Entactin	150,000	Single chain	Cultured cells, EHS tumor
Nidogen	100,000	Single chain	EHS tumor
Fibronectin	440,000	Two chains (Mr = 220,000)	Serum, cultured cells

obtain basement membrane in quantity from normal tissue, isolate their constituent macromolecules in native form, or study their biosynthesis. Instead, a variety of other systems which actively produce basement membrane have been employed. These include fetal-associated membranes such as the parietal yolk sac (23–28) and the amnion (29, 30), cultured cells (30–36), and certain tumors (37–41). In this chapter we will discuss the basement membrane components produced by the EHS tumor (38), a transplantable murine tumor, which represents a good source of soluble, basement-membrane-specific products including type IV collagen, laminin, entactin, nidogen, and heparan sulfate proteoglycan. We will discuss the procedures used to isolate these materials, their structures, functions, and possible alterations in disease.

1.1.   Tumors as Models for Studying Basement Membranes

Pierce and associates showed that certain mouse tumors produced substantial amounts of basement membrane (24, 37, 42–44). These were parietal yolk sac carcinomas derived from teratocarcinomas and adapted for transplantation both as solid tumors and ascites forms, as well as for growth in culture. The tumor cells were found to deposit a matrix indistinguishable in its appearance from authentic basement membranes. The matrix material produced by the tumor cells in culture was isolated and used to prepare antibodies. These antibodies reacted with the matrix produced by the tumor cells but more significantly with Reichert's membrane and with basement membrane in kidney, testis, and other sites. These studies thus demonstrated a close similarity between the basement membranes produced by tumors and normal tissues and suggested that tumors could be used as a model for studying basement membranes.

1.2.   Basement Membrane Produced by the EHS Tumor

Histological studies have shown the EHS (Engelbreth–Holm–Swarm) tumor to contain clusters of cells separated by a homogeneous, nonfibrillar matrix (45, 46 and Fig. 1). Indeed, at one time it was thought to be a cartilagenous tumor (45, 46). However, subsequent chemical studies (38) showed that the tumor lacked type II collagen, a cartilage-specific protein, and instead contained type IV collagen, the characteristic collagen of basement membranes. Subsequently, laminin, a basement-membrane-specific glycoprotein (47) was isolated from the tumor and one of the chains of laminin was isolated from teratocarcinoma cells (48). As discussed below, heparan sulfate was found in kidney basement membranes, and we isolated a large heparan sulfate proteoglycan (49) from the tumor. Specific antibodies were prepared against these macromolecules and were found to react with the matrix in the tumor as well as with the basement membranes in normal tissues (47, 49–52). Such studies suggest that basement membranes, whether produced by normal or transformed cells, contain components in common, including type IV collagen, laminin, and the heparan sulfate proteoglycan.

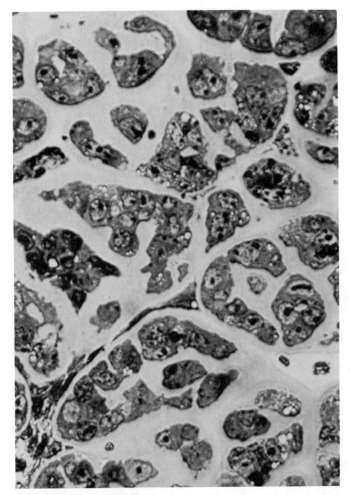

FIGURE 1.   Appearance of the EHS tumor. Tumor cells are surrounded by a homogeneous matrix that has been shown to contain basement membrane components. Taken from ref. 38 with permission.

The advantage of the EHS tumor is that it produces basement membrane rapidly and contains no other extracellular matrix components. In addition, the components of its basement membrane are readily solubilized. The EHS tumor grows to 5–7 g in an intramuscular or subcutaneous site in a variety of mouse strains and has little effect on the health of the host. In contrast, parietal yolk sac (PYS) cells show little host range and are highly malignant. Their obligatory host, 129 J mice, die before the tumor reaches much more than a gram in size (unpublished observations). However, unlike the PYS cells, the EHS tumor cells have not been adapted to extended cell culture, although it is possible to prepare organ cultures and isolate cells for brief *in vitro* studies as described below. Rat yolk sac tumors have also been identified (39–41) which produce basement-membrane-specific molecules.

2.   COMPONENTS OF BASEMENT MEMBRANE

2.1.   Type IV Collagen

It has been known for many years that basement membranes are collagenous structures (reviewed in ref. 22). Kefalides (53) showed that they contained a unique collagen species which he designated type IV. Type IV collagen comprises about 10 percent of the protein in the EHS tumor (38, 51, 54). Like other collagens, it is a helical molecule and contains two distinct chains, the pro $\alpha 1(IV)$ and pro $\alpha 2(IV)$ chains (33, 55). Following synthesis, the protein does not undergo appreciable proteolytic processing and the secreted form is deposited (54–56). In tissues, type IV collagen is found in the basement membrane as a fine mesh work (57–62) best visualized after treatment of tissue sections with plasmin (58). The collagen molecules are believed to be arranged in an open network with like ends in apposition (57, 63) and cross-linked together with disulfide bonds (54, 64) as well as cross-links formed by lysine-derived aldehydes (65). This network of type IV collagen provides a stable support for epithelial cells and also a high degree of elasticity. The openness of the structure would also facilitate the passage of fluids.

Due to cross-linking, type IV collagen resists extraction even in EHS tumor (54, 64). If the tumor is grown in mice made lathyritic with β-aminopropionitrile, native molecules can be extracted with aqueous solvents containing a reducing agent such as dithiothreitol.

2.2.   Glycoproteins

Basement membranes contain several glycoproteins, including fibronectin, laminin and entactin (reviewed in ref. 52). Fibronectin (Mr = 440,000) is in the basement membranes of developing tissues and may be present in smaller amounts in mature tissue (66–69), although it is often lost on maturation. Since fibronectin is generally considered to be a product of fibroblastic cells, the fibronectin associated with basement membranes is probably produced by stromal cells beneath the basement membrane or accumulated from the blood (11, 70). Fibronectin binds to type IV collagen (71) as well as to stromal collagens (72–74), to cell surfaces (75, 76), and to glycosaminoglycans (75–77). It has been implicated in the formation of the basement membrane (78) and may also serve to link this structure to underlying tissue and cells (61). It is not present in very significant amounts in the EHS tumor (unpublished observations).

Laminin (Mr = 10^6) is a basement-membrane-specific glycoprotein first isolated from the EHS tumor where it comprises 20–25 percent of the protein (47, and Fig. 2), Subsequently, it was found to be produced by epithelial and endothelial cells and by various tumor cells (27, 28, 32, 39, 40, 48, 50, 77, 79–83). In tissues it is observed only in basement membranes (47, 50, 60–62, 84–86) and does not occur in appreciable amounts in serum ($\leq$ 50 ng/

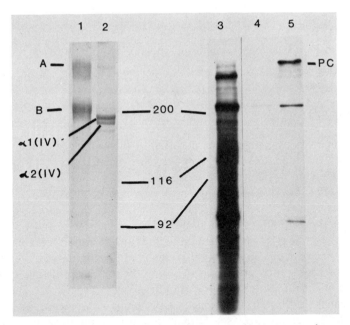

FIGURE 2. Polyacrylamide gel electrophoresis (5 percent) of basement membrane components purified from the EHS tumor. Laminin (lane 1) contains one A chain (Mr = 400,000) and three B chains (Mr = 200,000) that are connected by disulfide bonds. Type IV collagen (lane 2) contains two chains: α1 (IV) (Mr = 185,000) and α2 (IV), (Mr = 170,000). Basement membrane components produced by EHS tumor cells in culture and labeled with [^{35}S]methionine are visualized on a 4–10 percent gradient gel (lane 3). The heparan sulfate proteoglycan protein core, immunoprecipitated from EHS cell cultures labeled with [^{35}S]methionine, is a Mr = 400,000 protein (lane 4). Lane 5 is a preimmune serum control. Markers indicate molecular weight standards.

mL). Laminin binds to type IV collagen but not to other collagen types (79, 87), to heparin (88) and heparan sulfate proteoglycan (87, 89, 90), and to an integral cell membrane protein (Mr = 67,000), which appears to be the laminin receptor (91–93). Laminin is not readily extracted from normal tissues, although it has been obtained from these sources (94, 95). Laminin serves as an attachment protein and is utilized by cells in contact with or surrounded by basement membrane including epithelial and endothelial cells (79, 96), metastatic tumor cells (97, 98), and neuronal cells (82, 83, 99). It can also promote cell growth and migration (99–102). The interaction of laminin with cells is probably dependent on the cells exhibiting the receptor protein (Mr = 67,000), whereas its distribution in tissues maybe determined by its affinity for type IV collagen and heparan sulfate proteoglycan.

Entactin (Mr = 165,000) (103–105) and nidogen (Mr = 100,000) (106) are specific components of all basement membranes including that produced by the EHS tumor (unpublished observations). Although its function is not well defined, entactin is present in the basement membrane in close association with the surface of endothelial cells and may participate in cell–matrix inter-actions (104, 107, 108). Nidogen was also isolated from the EHS tumor (106). It appears to be a basement-membrane-specific protein and tends to self-ag-gregate, suggesting that it could function in the formation of the matrix.

2.3. Proteoglycans

Basement membranes contain heparan sulfate as their major glycosaminoglycan (49, 109–113). Heparan sulfate proteoglycans isolated from the EHS tumor (49) are larger (Mr $= 10^6$) than those isolated from glomeruli (Mr $= 120,000$) (112, 113) (Fig. 3). Heparan sulfate proteoglycans comprise about 1 percent of the proteins in the EHS tumor. The major species of heparan sulfate pro-teoglycan in the EHS tumor contains about 50 percent protein and 4–6 heparan sulfate glycosaminoglycans attached through a linkage region containing xylose bound to serine residues on the core protein (114). Preliminary studies indicate that this proteoglycan is processed to a slightly smaller proteoglycan with a lower proportion of protein to glycosaminoglycan (115, 116). The smaller proteoglycan is readily extracted from the EHS tumor with aqueous salt solutions, whereas the larger form resists extraction and requires denaturing solvents such as urea or guanidine (116). Antibodies prepared against these proteoglycans from the EHS tumor are directed against the protein portion of the molecule (117) and react with all authentic basement membranes including those in the kidney glomerulus (Fig. 3). It is possible that proteoglycans in basement mem-branes arise from a single precursor and the differences observed in size occur due to degradation of the proteoglycan. It should be noted that heparan-sulfate-containing molecules occur in many other tissues (see, e.g., ref. 118) but antibodies prepared against the basement membrane heparan sulfate proteoglycan react only with basement membranes. Presumably the protein core of other heparan sulfate proteoglycans must be distinct.

It has been shown that the basement membrane serves as a molecular filter preventing the passage of proteins, particularly negatively charged macro-molecules (8–10). The regularly arrayed anionic-charged groups (109, 119–121) which were shown in the kidney to be heparan sulfate (109, 120) are considered to be responsible for the filtration. Removal of the heparan sulfate groups from the kidney glomeruli by treating the tissue with heparitinase or with nitrous acid increased their permeability to protein (120, 122). In addition, studies on kidney tissue from rats with the nephrotic syndrome, induced by administration of the aminonucleoside of puromycin, have shown a depletion of anionic groups in glomerular basement membranes (123, 124). Immuno-histology of such tissue showed that glomerular basement membrane contained laminin and type IV collagen but lacked the heparan sulfate proteoglycan (124). These studies further indicate that loss of the basement membrane pro-teoglycan in the kidney is related to the increased passage of protein.

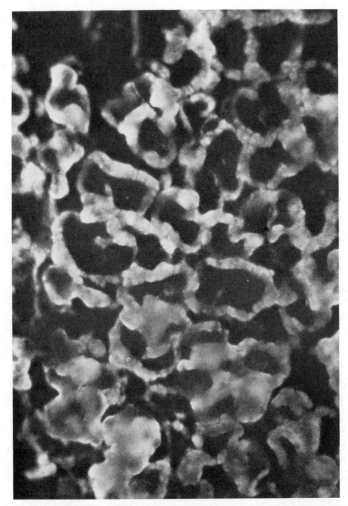

FIGURE 3. Indirect immunofluorescence of the EHS tumor with antibodies against the heparan sulfate proteoglycan. The extracellular matrix is intensely stained, whereas the tumor cells do not stain. Antibodies against laminin and type IV collagen (not shown) also localize to the extracellular matrix of the EHS tumor.

3. ORGANIZATION OF COMPONENTS IN THE BASEMENT MEMBRANE

As noted above, type IV collagen, laminin, entactin, nidogen, and heparan sulfate proteoglycan are found in all basement membranes so far studied (106, 108, 125). Functionally, type IV collagen serves as the major structural element of the basement membrane, forming a highly cross-linked network. Presumably the other components of the basement membrane may be bound to type IV collagen, although specific binding has only been shown with laminin and fibronectin (71, 76, 77, 87, 90, 126). The binding of these glycoproteins depends on the conformation of the collagen. Laminin requires a native type IV structure (87, 90) and fibronectin (71–74) binds better to a linear, nonhelical sequence. Heparan sulfate binds to both laminin and fibronectin (76, 77, 87–89) and could be fixed to the basement membrane in a ternary complex. Immunohistology shows that all components occur together in the basement membrane, and each therefore must be integrated into the structure (125). On the other hand these are very large molecules whose dimensions exceed the width of the basement membrane, and each could reach from the network of type IV collagen to adjacent cell surfaces. The anionic groups of the proteoglycan often appear to be distributed along the surfaces of the basement membrane. Possibly the protein portion of the proteoglycan is bound to the lamina densa and then electrostatic repulsion causes the sulfated glycosaminoglycan chains to separate from one another.

4. BASEMENT MEMBRANE PRODUCED BY DIABETIC EHS TUMOR CELLS

Several studies have shown increased amounts or an increased synthesis of type IV collagen in glomeruli from diabetic animals (127–130). This is expected given the thickening observed in the basement membranes at these sites. However, recent studies have established that the synthesis of the proteoglycan is reduced in diabetes and that there is an inverse relationship between heparan sulfate proteoglycan levels and serum glucose levels in diabetes (131–135).

We have used EHS tumor tissue grown in diabetic mice to study the effect of diabetes on various basement membrane components (131). In our studies mice are injected intramuscularly with tumor cells and three days later made diabetic by the injection of streptozotocin. This regimen obviates direct damage to the tumor cells by the streptozotocin but allows the tumor to grow under diabetic conditions. The animals administered streptozotocin show a wide range of blood glucose, probably resulting from variation in the extent of damage to the pancreas. In general, we define as diabetic those animals with blood glucose in excess of 250 mg/dL. These animals have low levels of insulin with hyperglycemia and survive for 3–4 weeks with tumor.

Tumor tissue grown in mice with this form of diabetes was assayed after 2–3 weeks. Tumor produced by intramuscular injection of the cells shows the same growth rate in normal and diabetic animals with similar levels of protein. In contrast, the amount of heparan sulfate proteoglycan in the diabetic tissue is reduced by as much as 80 percent (131). The proteoglycan that is produced appears to be very similar or even identical to the normal proteoglycan in size, charge, and the length of its glycosaminoglycan chains (131, 132).

We have also studied the basement membrane produced by EHS tumor tissue grown in genetically (db/db) diabetic mice (132). The mice, homozygous for the db gene, have relatively normal levels of blood glucose until 3 months of age and then develop hyperglycemia in the presence of high levels of insulin. These animals also show reduced amounts of heparan sulfate proteoglycan whereas laminin and type IV collagen levels are similar to control values.

Since the heparan sulfate proteoglycan is important for creating a permeability barrier in the basement membrane, it is not surprising that in diabetes the basement membranes may be more porous at times than normal. We have proposed that there is increased synthesis of basement membrane components to compensate for the increased permeability. However, the basement membrane deposited may still lack adequate amounts of the proteoglycan (Fig. 4). If synthesis exceeds normal turnover, a thickened, yet defective basement membrane could develop which would eventually lead to the degenerative changes seen in the tissues. Since this would be a compensatory change, the tissues through which the greatest filtration of fluid as well as those with a high osmotic pressure would be expected to show the greatest changes. Further studies are needed to evaluate these theories and to identify the site of action of insulin and the roles of hyperglycemia and nonenzymatic glycoslyation of proteins in causing basement membrane alterations.

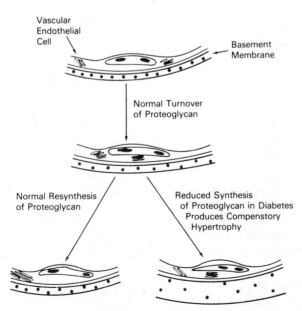

FIGURE 4. Proposed mechanism to account for the thickening of basement membranes in diabetes.

5. METHODS OF PROCEDURE

5.1. Maintenance of the EHS Tumor

The EHS tumor is maintained by implantation of the tumor into C57BL mice 6–8 weeks of age. Tumor tissue is excised after cervical dislocation of the animal. The tumor tissue is washed in sterile phosphate-buffered saline (PBS), dispersed by passage through a syringe and allowed to settle by gravity. The supernatant fraction is removed and more PBS added. The process is repeated two to three times until the supernatant solution is no longer colored from blood products. Tumor is passed to new hosts by intramuscular injection of 0.5 mL of the dispersed tissue into one hind limb of each mouse. After 3 weeks of growth, the tumor will generally be 3–5 g and is suitable for harvesting, further passage, and/or experimental manipulation.

5.2. Organ Culture

Tumors are harvested, dispersed by passage through a 0.85-mm^2 metal screen and washed with minimum essential media. Tumor tissue is pelleted by centrifugation at 1000 rpm and the supernatant fluid is decanted. The tissue is then aliquoted into 15-mL sterile conical centrifuge tubes using 0.3 g of tumor tissue per tube in 5 mL of medium. Waymouth's 752/1 medium formulated with $MgCl_2$ replacing $MgSO_4$, and without glucose and proline, is the standard medium used in these organ cultures. Glucose at 0.5, 1, 3, or 5 g/L is subsequently added sterilely. Other additives, such as hormones, serum, or tissue extracts, are also added sterilely. Unless otherwise stated, culture medium includes 75 μg/mL ascorbic acid, 2 mM L-glutamine, 0.5 mg/mL Lincocin (GIBCO), and 10 mM HEPES buffer, pH 7.4. The tubes are then incubated on a rocker platform at 37°C for the desired time. Tissue is separated from the medium by centrifugation for 15 min at 3000 rpm at 4°C. Medium and tissue are processed separately.

5.3. Cell Culture

Freshly harvested tumor (5 g) is passed through a stainless steel mesh, as described above, and 2.5 g of this tissue is added to 25 mL of Ca^{2+}–Mg^{2+}-free Hanks' solution containing 30 mM HEPES, pH 7.4. The tissue is gently dispersed with a pipette, centrifuged at 500 rpm for 3 min, and the supernatant is discarded. The tissue pellet is resuspended in 25 mL of Hanks' solution that contains 2.4 percent Dispase (Worthington) and incubated at 37°C for 45 min with gentle rocking. Following this incubation, any remaining clumps of cells are dispersed by reflux pipetting and 25 mL of medium (NCTC 109 containing 10 percent FCS) added. The cells are collected by centrifugation at 1000 rpm for 5 min. The cell pellet is then resuspended in 20 mL of fresh medium and passed through a 75 M mesh Nitex filter. The cells are collected by centrifugation, resuspended in fresh medium, and plated at 4×10^6 cells per 35-mm dish. The cells will attach within 2–3 hr but do not flatten, even after several days in culture.

5.4. Radiolabeling Matrix Components

Matrix macromolecules can be radiolabeled *in vivo* by intraperitoneal injection with radiolabeled precursors including [^{35}S] sulfate, [^{3}H] proline, [^{3}H] glucosamine, or [^{35}S] methionine. Tumor tissue harvested 18 hr after injection of isotope contains essentially no unincorporated isotope. Matrix molecules produced by EHS cells in cell or organ culture can also be radiolabeled. Under these conditions, considerable unincorporated isotope remains in the tissue, or cell layer, even after extensive incubation, and dialysis or chromatography is required before measuring unincorporated radioactivity.

5.5. Preparation of Type IV Collagen and Laminin

Detailed procedures have been published describing the isolation of type IV collagen (54) and laminin (47, 136, 137) from the EHS tumor. The procedure for isolating laminin is shown in Figure 5. In brief, laminin is readily extracted

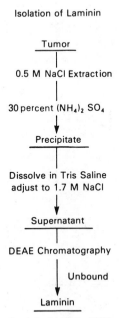

Isolation of Laminin

Tumor

0.5 M NaCl Extraction

30 percent (NH$_4$)$_2$ SO$_4$

Precipitate

Dissolve in Tris Saline
adjust to 1.7 M NaCl

Supernatant

DEAE Chromatography

Unbound

Laminin

FIGURE 5. Procedure for isolating laminin from the EHS tumor. Tumor tissue harvested from normal animals is homogenized in 20 percent NaCl and centrifuged to remove soluble proteins. Laminin is extracted with 0.5 *M* NaCl, 0.05 *M* Tris-HCl, pH 7.4, and purified by differential precipitation and by chromatographic methods.

from the EHS tumor with aqueous solvents. Purification is achieved by precipitation with ammonium sulfate and chromatography on a column of DEAE cellulose which removes some impurities. Laminin prepared in this fashion is substantially homogenous and biologically active. More highly purified preparations can be obtained by molecular sieve chromatography (47, 79) and chromatography on heparin (88) or *Griffonia Simplicifonia I* lectin columns (138).

Type IV collagen is largely insoluble due to cross-linking. Animals bearing the tumor are fed the lathyrogen β-aminoproprionitrile (0.2 percent) in the diet to increase its extraction. The tissue is extracted sequentially with salt and guanidine to remove laminin (Fig. 6). The type IV collagen is then solubilized by a reducing agent (54, 64). Chromatography on a column of DEAE cellulose removes some of the impurities including proteoglycans.

5.6. Extraction of Proteoglycans

Tumor tissue, or cultured cells are extracted with 2 mL/g tissue of a guanidine–detergent–inhibitor solution (4 *M* guanidine-HCl, 2 percent CHAPS, 0.05 *M* Tris-HCl, pH 6.8, 0.1 *M* 6-aminohexanoic acid, 0.020 *M* EDTA, 0.008 *M N-*

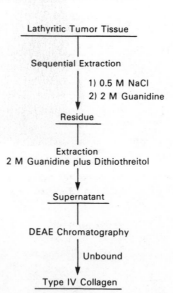

FIGURE 6.   Procedure for isolating type IV collagen from the EHS tumor. The tumor is grown in mice fed diet containing 0.2 percent β-aminoproprionitrile to block cross-linking by lysyl oxidase. The tumor is washed with 20 percent NaCl and the residue extracted with 0.5 *M* NaCl to remove laminin and other soluble components. Type IV collagen is solubilized with 1 *M* guanidine plus dithiothreitol. The collagen is purified by differential salt precipitation and chromatography.

ethylmaleimide and 0.005 PMSF) with stirring overnight at 4°C (Fig. 7). Alternatively, the tissue can be extracted in 6 M urea (4 mL/g tissue) containing protease inhibitors and detergent (Fig. 5). Unincorporated radioactivity is removed by chromatography on Sephadex G-25 equilibrated with the extracting solvent at pH 6.8, or by dialysis against 0.05 M Tris-HCl, pH 7.2, containing 0.85 percent NaCl and 2 mM sodium sulfate. These extracts will contain proteoglycans, laminin, and newly synthesized and uncross-linked collagen.

5.7. Biochemical Analysis

Extracted proteoglycans and glycosaminoglycans are fractionated according to density by centrifugation in cesium chloride (Fig. 5). Samples in 4 M guanidine-hydrochloride are adjusted to contain 0.5 g of cesium chloride per gram of fluid extract and centrifuged at 40,000 rpm in a 50-TI rotor for 68 hr at 10–12°C. Most of the proteoglycans appear in the bottom of the gradient and glycoproteins in the top.

Proteoglycans can also be separated from glycoproteins by DEAE Sephacel column chromatography (139 and Fig.5). Guanidine extracts are dialyzed three times against 10 volume changes of 7 M urea, 1 percent Triton X-100, 0.15 N NaCl, 0.05 M Tris-HCl, pH 6.8. Urea extracts can be used directly. The

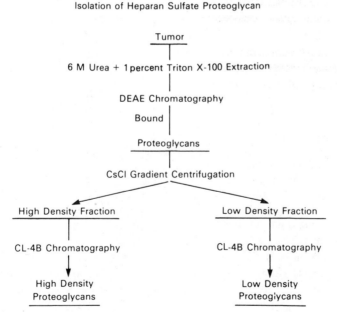

FIGURE 7. Procedures for isolation of high- and low-density forms of heparan sulfate proteoglycan. Saline extracts primarily the high-density form, which can be separated from glycoproteins by centrifugation and chromatography on DEAE-Sephacel. The low-density proteoglycan is extracted from the residue with concentrated urea or guanidine and purified by analogous procedures.

sample is applied to a DEAE-Sephacel column and eluted with a linear salt gradient of $0.15–0.75\,M$ NaCl. Under these conditions most proteins will pass through the column and the proteoglycans will elute within the salt gradient.

Proteoglycans of different sizes can be separated by molecular seive column chromatography in $4\,M$ guanidine-hydrochloride. The glycosaminoglycans of the basement membrane proteoglycans, are prepared from tumor extracts or from purified proteoglycans by digestion of the material with papain (1 mg/mL) in $1.0\,M$ sodium acetate, pH 6.5, at 60°C overnight.

REFERENCES

1. M. G. Farquhar, J. Hopper, Jr., and H. D. Moon, *Am. J. Pathol.* **35**, 721–753 (1959).

2. J. M. Bloodworth, Jr., R. L. Engerman, and K. L. Powers, *Diabetes* **18**, 455–458 (1969).

3. J. R. Williamson, N. J. Vogler, and C. Kilo, *Diabetes* **18**, 567–578 (1969).

4. R. Osterby, in *Vascular and Neurological Changes in Early Diabetes*, R. A. Camerini-Davalos and H. S. Cole (eds.), American Press, New York, 1973, pp. 323–332.

5. P. J. Beisswenger and R. G. Spiro, *Diabetes* **22**, 180–193 (1973).

6. M. D. Siperstein, *Western J. Med.* **121**, 404–412 (1974).

7. P. C. Johnson, *Lancet* **2**, 932–933 (1981).

8. J. P. Caulfield and M. G. Farquhar, *J. Cell Biol.* **63**, 883–903 (1974).

9. M. G. Farquhar, *Kidney Int.* **8**, 197–211 (1975).

10. G. B. Ryan and M. J. Karnovsky, *Kidney Int.* **9**, 36–45 (1976).

11. A. Martinez-Hernandez and P. S. Amenta, *Lab Invest.* **48**, 656–676 (1983).

12. N. Ashton, *British J. Ophthal.* **58**, 344–366 (1974).

13. A. E. Renold, D. H. Mintz, W. A. Muller, G. F. Cahill, "Diabetes Mellitus," in *The Metabolic Bases of Inherited Diseases*, J. B. Stanbury, J. B. Wyngaarden, and D. S. Frederickson (eds.), McGraw-Hill, New York, 1978, pp. 79–109.

14. B. J. Carrie and B. D. Myers, *Kidney Int.* **17**, 669–676 (1980).

15. D. H. Rohrbach and G. R. Martin, *Annal. N.Y. Acad. Sci.* **401**, 203–211 (1982).

16. G. R. Martin, D. H. Rohrbach, V. P. Terranova, and L. A. Liotta, "Structure, Function and Pathology of Basement Membranes," in *Connective Tissue Diseases*, International Academy of Pathology Monograph 24., B. M. Wagner, R. Fleischmajer, and N. Kaufman, (eds.), pp. 16–30, 1983.

17. M. P. Cohen and M. Surma, *J. Biol. Chem.* **255**, 1767–1770 (1980).

18. M. P. Cohen, M. L. Surma, V. Y. Wu, *Am. J. Physiology* **242**, F385–F389 (1982).

19. G. W. Laurie, C. P. Leblond, I. Cournil, and G. R. Martin, *J. Histochem. Cytochem.* **228**, 1267–1274 (1980).

20. F. Walker, *J. Pathol.* **110**, 233–239 (1973).

21. R. B. Price and R. G. Spiro, *J. Biol. Chem.* **252**, 8597–8602 (1977).

22. N. A. Kefalides, R. Alper, and C. C. Clark, *Int. Rev. Cytol.* **61**, 167–228 (1979).

23. C. C. Clark, E. A. Tomichek, T. R. Koszalka, R. R. Minor, N. A. Kefalides, *J. Biol. Chem.* **250**, 5259–5267 (1975).

24. A. Martinez-Hernandez, P. K. Nakane, and G. B. Pierce, Jr., *Am. J. Pathol.* **76**, 549–560 (1974).

25. E. D. Adamson and S. E. Ayers, *Cell* **16**, 953–965 (1979).

26. C. C. Clark, E. A. Tomichek, T. R. Kozalka, R. R. Minor, and N. A. Kefalides, *J. Biol. Chem.* **250**, 5259–5267 (1975).

27. G. W. Laurie, C. P. Leblond, and G. R. Martin, *J. Histochem. Cytochem.* **30**, 983–990 (1982).

28. G. W. Laurie, C. P. Leblond, G. R. Martin, and M. H. Silver, *J. Histochem. Cytochem.* **30**, 991–998 (1982).

29. J. M. Foidart, K. Tryggvason, P. Gehron Robey, L. A. Liotta, and G. R. Martin, *Collagen Res.* **1**, 137–150 (1981).

30. E. Crouch and P. Bornstein, *J. Biol. Chem.* **254**, 4197–4204 (1979).

31. K. Alitalo, J. A. Vaheri, T. Krieg, and R. Timpl, *Eur. J. Biochem.* **109**, 247–255 (1980).

32. B. L. M. Hogan, A. R. Cooper, and M. Kurkinen, *Dev. Biol.* **80**, 289–300 (1980).

33. E. Crouch, H. Sage, and P. Bornstein, *Proc. Natl. Acad. Sci. USA* **77**, 745–749 (1980).

34. D. H. Rohrbach, P. Russell, and R. L. Church, *Cur. Eye Res.* **1**, 267–273 (1981).

35. D. K. MacCallum, J. H. Lillie, L. J. Scaletta, J. C. Occhino, W. G. Frederick, and S. R. Ledbetter, *Exp. Cell Res.* **139**, 1–14 (1982).

36. A. E. Chung, I. L. Freeman, and J. E. Braginski, *Biochem. Biophys. Res. Comm.* **79**, 859–867 (1977).

37. G. B. Pierce, "Epithelial Basement Membrane: Origin, Development and Role in Disease," in *Chemistry and Molelcular Biology of the Intracellular Matrix*, E. A. Balaz (ed.), Academic Press, New York, 1970, pp. 471–506.

38. R. W. Orkin, P. Gehron, E. B. McGoodwin, G. R. Martin, T. Valentine, and R. Swarm, *J. Exp. Med.* **145**, 204–220 (1977).

39. A. Martinez-Hernandez, E. Miller, I. Damjanov, and S. Gay, *Lab Invest.* **47**, 247–257 (1982).

40. U. Wewer, R. Albrechtsen, and E. Ruoslahti, *Cancer Res.* **41**, 1518–1524 (1981).

41. U. Wewer, *Dev. Biol.* **93**, 416–421 (1982).

42. G. B. Pierce, A. R. Midgley, S. Sri Ram, and J. D. Feldman, *Am. J. Pathol.* **41**, 549–566 (1962).

43. G. B. Pierce and J. D. Feldman, *J. Exp. Med.* **117**, 339–348 (1963).

44. G. B. Pierce, A. Jones, N. G. Orfanakis, P. K. Nakane, and L. Lustig, *Differentiation* **23**, 60–72 (1982).

45. R. L. Swarm, *J. Natl. Canc. Inst.* **31**, 953–975 (1963).

46. R. L. Swarm, J. N. Correa, J. R. Andrews, and E. Miller, *J. Natl. Canc. Inst.* **33**, 657–672 (1964).

47. R. Timpl, H. Rohde, P. G. Robey, S. I. Rennard, J. M. Foidart, and G. R. Martin, *J. Biol. Chem.* **254**, 9933–9937 (1979).

48. A. E. Chung, R. Jaffe, I. L. Freeman, J. P. Vergnes, J. E. Braginski, and B. Carlin, *Cell* **16**, 277–287 (1979).

49. J. R. Hassell, P. G. Robey, H. J. Barrach, J. Wilczek, S. I. Rennard, and G. R. Martin, *Proc. Natl. Acad. Sci. USA* **77**, 4494–4498 (1980).

50. J. M. Foidart, E. W. Bere, M. Yaar, S. I. Rennard, M. Guillino, G. R. Martin, and S. I. Katz, *Lab Invest.* **42**, 336–342 (1980).

51. R. Timpl, G. R. Martin, P. Bruckner, G. Wick, and H. Weidemann, *Eur. J. Biochem.* **84**, 43–52 (1978).

52. R. Timpl and G. R. Martin, "Components of Basement Membranes," in *Immunochemistry of the Extracellular Matrix, Vol II: Applications*, H. Furthmayr (ed.), CRC Press, Boca Raton, Florida, 1982, pp. 119–150.

53. N. A. Kefalides, *Biochem. Biophys. Res. Commun.* **45**, 226–234 (1971).

54. H. K. Kleinman, M. L. McGarvey, L. A. Liotta, P. G. Robey, K. Tryggvason, and G. R. Martin, *Biochemistry* **24**, 6188–6193 (1982).

55. K. Tryggvason, P. Gehron-Robey, and G. R. Martin, *Biochem.* **19**, 1284–1289 (1980).

56. R. R. Minor, C. C. Clark, E. L. Straus, T. R. Koszalka, R. L. Brent, and N. A. Kefalides, *J. Biol. Chem.* **251**, 1789–1794 (1976).

57. R. Timpl, H. Wiedemann, V. van Delden, H. Furthmayr, and K. Kuhn, *Eur. J. Biochem.* **110**, 203–211 (1981).

58. S. Inoue, C. P. Leblond, and G. W. Laurie, *J. Cell Biol.* **97**, 1524–1537 (1983).

59. H. Yaoita, J. M. Foidart, and S. I. Katz, *J. Invest. Dermatol.* **70**, 191–193 (1978).

60. P. Monaghan, M. J. Warburton, N. Perusinghe, and P. S. Rudland, *Proc. Natl. Acad. Sci. USA* **80**, 3344–3348 (1983).

61. G. W. Laurie, C. P. Leblond, and G. R. Martin, *J. Cell Biol.* **95**, 340–344 (1982).

62. P. J. Courtoy, R. Timpl, and M. G. Farquhar, *J. Histochem. Cytochem.* **30**, 874–886 (1982).

63. R. Timpl, I. Oberbäumer, H. Furthmayr, and K. Kuehn, "Macromolecular Organization of Type IV Collagen," in *New Trends in Basement Membrane Research*, K. Kuehn, H. Schoene, and R. Timpl (eds.), Raven Press, New York, 1982, pp. 57–67.

64. M. W. Karakashian, P. Dehm, T. S. Gramling, and E. C. Leroy, *Coll. Rel. Res. Clin. Exp.* **2**, 3–17 (1982).

65. M. L. Tanzer and N. A. Kefalides, *Biochem. Biophys. Res. Commun.* **51**, 775–780 (1973).

66. S. Stenman and A. Vaheri, *J. Exp. Med.* **147**, 1054–1064 (1978).

67. B. W. Mayer, E. D. Hay, and R. O. Hynes, *Dev. Biol.* **82**, 267–286 (1981).

68. I. Thesleff, H. J. Barrach, J. M. Foidart, A. Vaheri, R. M. Pratt, and G. R. Martin, *Develop. Biol.* **81**, 182–192 (1981).

69. I. Thesleff, S. Stenman, A. Vaheri, and R. Timpl, *Develop. Biol.* **70**, 116–126 (1979).

70. E. Oh, M. Pierschbacher, and E. Ruoslahti, *Proc. Natl. Acad. Sci. USA* **78**, 3218–3221 (1981).

71. W. Dessau, B. C. Adelmann, R. Timpl, and G. R. Martin, *Biochem. J.* **169**, 55–59 (1978).

72. E. Engvall, E. Ruoslahti, and E. J. Miller, *J. Exp. Med.* **147**, 1584–1595 (1978).

73. F. Jilek and H. Hormann, *Hoppe-Seyler's Z. Physiol. Chem.* **359**, 247–250 (1978).

74. H. K. Kleinman, E. B. McGoodwin, G. R. Martin, R. J. Klebe, P. P. Fietzek, and D. E. Woodley, *J. Biol. Chem.* **253**, 5642–5646 (1978).

75. K. M. Yamada and K. Olden, *Nature* **275**, 179–184 (1978).

76. E. Ruoslahti, E. Engvall, and E. G. Hayman, *Coll. Res.* **1**, 95–128 (1981).

77. K. M. Yamada, *Ann. Rev. Biochem.* **52**, 761–800 (1983).

78. A. G. Brownell, C. C. Bessem, and H. C. Slavkin, *Proc. Natl. Acad. Sci. USA* **78**, 3711–3715 (1981).

79. V. P. Terranova, D. H. Rohrbach, and G. R. Martin, *Cell* **22**, 719–726 (1980).

80. S. Sakashita and E. Ruoslahti, *Arch. Biochem. Biophys.* **205**, 283–290 (1980).

81. I. Leivo, K. Alitalo, L. Risteli, A. Vaheri, R. Timpl, and J. Wartiovaara, *Exp. Cell. Res.* **137**, 15–23 (1982).

82. K. Alitalo, M. Kurkinen, I. Virtanen, K. Mellström, and A. Vahari, *J. Cell Biochem.* **18**, 25–35 (1982).

83. S. L. Palm and L. T. Furcht, *J. Cell Biol.* **96**, 1218–1226 (1983).

84. G. W. Laurie, C. P. Leblond, and G. R. Martin, *Am. J. Anat.* **167**, 71–82 (1983).

85. H. Rohde, G. Wick, and R. Timpl, *Eur. J. Biochem.* **102**, 195–201 (1979).

86. J. R. Sanes, *J. Cell Biol.* **93**, 442–451 (1982).

87. D. E. Woodley, C. N. Rao, J. R. Hassell, L. A. Liotta, G. R. Martin, and H. K. Kleinman, *Biochim. Biophys. Acta* **761**, 278 (1983).

88. S. Sakashita, E. Engvall, and E. Ruoslahti, *FEBS Lett.* **116**, 243–246 (1980).

89. M. Del Rosso, R. Cappelletti, M. Viti, S. Vannvechi, and V. Chiarugi, *Biochem. J.* **199**, 699–704 (1981).

90. H. K. Kleinman, M. L. McGarvey, J. R. Hassell, and G. R. Martin, *Biochem.* **22**, 4969–4974 (1983).

91. C. N. Rao, S. H. Barsky, V. P. Terranova, and L. A. Liotta, *Biochem. Biophys. Res. Commun.* **111**, 804–808 (1983).

92. H. Lesot, V. Kühl, and K. von der Mark, *EMBO J.* **2**, 861–865 (1983).

93. H. C. Malinoff and M. S. Wicha, *J. Cell Biol.* **96**, 1475–1479 (1983).

94. M. Ohno, A. Martinez-Hernandez, and N. A. Kefalides, *Biochem. Biophys. Res. Comm.* **112**, 1091–1098 (1983).

95. U. Wewer, R. Albrechtsen, M. Manthorpe, S. Varon, E. Engvall, and E. Ruoslahti, *J. Biol. Chem.* **258**, 12654–12660 (1983).

96. P. H. Burrill, I. Bernardini, H. K. Kleinman, and H. Kretchmer, *J. Supramolec. Struc. Cellul. Biochem.* **16**, 385–392 (1981).

97. V. P. Terranova, L. A. Liotta, R. Russo, and G. R. Martin, *Cancer Res.* **42**, 2265–2269 (1982).

98. I. Vlodavsky and D. Gospodarowicz, *Nature* **289**, 304–306 (1981).

99. M. L. McGarvey, A. Baron-van Evercooren, M. Dubois-Dalq, and H. K. Kleinman, unpublished.

100. J. B. McCarthy, S. L. Palm, and L. T. Furcht, *J. Cell Biol.* **97**, 772–777 (1983).

101. A. Rizzino, V. P. Terranova, D. H. Rohrbach, C. Crowly, and H. Rizzino, *J. Supramolec. Struct.* **13**, 243–253 (1980).

102. H. K. Kleinman, R. J. Klebe, and G. R. Martin, *J. Cell Biol.* **88**, 473–485 (1981).

103. B. Carlin, R. Jaffe, B. Bender, and A. E. Chung, *J. Biol. Chem.* **256**, 5209–5214 (1981).

104. B. L. Bender, R. Jaffe, B. Carlin, and A. E. Chung, *Am. J. Pathol.* **103**, 419–426 (1981).

105. B. L. M. Hogan, A. Taylor, M. Kurkinen, and J. R. Couchman, *J. Cell Biol.* **95**, 197–204 (1982).

106. R. Timpl, M. Dziadek, S. Fujiwara, H. Nowack, and G. Wick, *Eur. J. Biochem.*, in press.

107. S. Semoff, B. L. M. Hogan, and C. R. Hopkins, *EMBO J.* **1**, 1171–1175 (1982).

108. G. W. Laurie, C. P. Leblond, S. Inoue, G. R. Martin, and A. Chung, unpublished.

109. Y. S. Kanwar and M. G. Farquhar, *Proc. Natl. Acad. Sci. USA* **76**, 1303–1307 (1979).

110. D. M. Brown, A. F. Michael, and T. R. Oegema, *Biochem. Biophys. Acta* **674**, 96–104 (1981).

111. M. P. Cohen, V.-Y. Wu, and M. L. Surma, *Biochim. Biophys. Acta* **678**, 322–328 (1981).

112. Y. S. Kanwar, V. C. Hascall, and M. G. Farquhar, *J. Cell Biol.* **90**, 527–532 (1981).

113. J. Stow, E. F. Glasgow, C. J. Handley, and V. C. Hascall, *Arch. Biochem. Biophys.* **225**, 950–957 (1983).

114. S. Ledbetter, J. R. Hassell, and G. R. Martin, *J. Cell Biol.* **95**, 129a (1982).

115. B. Tyree, S. Ledbetter, and J. R. Hassell, *J. Cell Biol.* **97**, 230a (1983).

116. J. R. Hassell, W. C. Leyshon, S. Ledbetter, B. Tyree, and H. K. Kleinman, unpublished.

117. S. Ledbetter, J. R. Hassell, E. Horigan, B. Tyree, and G. R. Martin, "Identification of the Core Protein to a Heparan Sulfate Proteoglycan from Basement Membrane, in *Proceeding of the 7th International Symposium on Glycoconjugates*, Lund-Ronneby, Sweden, 1983, pp. 396.

118. A. Oldberg, K. Kjellen, and M. Höök, *J. Biol. Chem.* **254**, 8505–8510 (1979).

119. J. P. Caulfield and M. G. Farquhar, *Proc. Natl. Acad. Sci. USA* **73**, 1646–1650 (1976).

120. Y. S. Kanwar and M. G. Farquhar, *J. Cell Biol.* **81**, 137–153 (1979).

121. B. M. Brenner, T. H. Hostetter, and H. D. Humes, *N. Engl. J. Med.* **298**, 826–833 (1978).

122. Y. S. Kanwar, A. Linker, and M. G. Farquhar, *J. Cell Biol.* **86**, 688–693 (1980).

123. J. P. Caulfield and M. G. Farquhar, *J. Exp. Med.* **142**, 61–88 (1975).

124. L. A. Mynderse, J. R. Hassell, H. K. Kleinman, G. R. Martin, and A. Martinez-Hernandez, *Lab. Invest.* **48**, 292–302 (1983).

125. G. W. Laurie, C. P. Leblond, and G. R. Martin, *J. Cell Biol.* **95**, 340–344 (1982).

126. V. P. Terranova, C. N. Rao, T. Kalebic, I. M. Margulies, and L. Liotta, *Proc. Natl. Acad. Sci. USA* **80**, 444–448 (1983).

127. M. E. Grant, R. Harwood, and I. F. Williams, *J. Physiol. (London)* **257**, 56P–57P (1976).

128. N. A. Kefalides, "Biochemistry of Vascular Disease in Diabetes Mellitus," in *Proceeding of the IX Congress of the International Diabetes Federation*, J. S. Bajaj, (ed.), Excerpta Medica, Amsterdam, 1976, pp. 575–587.

129. M. P. Cohen and A. Khalifa, *Biochim. Biophys. Acta* **500**, 395–404 (1977).

130. M. P. Cohen, A. Dasmahapatra, and V. Y. Wu, *Nephron* **27**, 146–151 (1981).

131. D. H. Rohrbach, C. W. Wagner, V. Star, G. R. Martin, K. B. Brown, and J. W. Yoon, *J. Biol. Chem.* **258**, 11672–11677 (1983).

132. D. H. Rohrbach, J. R. Hassell, H. K. Kleinman, and G. R. Martin, *Diabetes* **31**, 185–188 (1982).

133. M. P. Cohen and M. L. Surma, *J. Lab. Clin. Med.* **98**, 715–722 (1981).

134. T. Pihlajaniemi, R. Myllylä, K. I. Kivirikko, and K. Tryggvason, *J. Biol. Chem.* **257**, 14914–14920 (1982).

135. N. Parthasarathy and R. Spiro, *Diabetes* **31**, 738–741 (1982).

136. R. Timpl, H. Rohde, L. Risteli, U. Ott, P. Gehron Robey, and G. R. Martin, "Laminin," in *Methods in Enzymology*, Vol. 82, L. W. Cunningham and D. W. Fredericksen (eds.), 1982, pp. 831–838.

137. S. R. Ledbetter, H. K. Kleinman, J. R. Hassell, and G. R. Martin, "Methods for the Isolation of Laminin," in *Methods in Cell Biology*, D. Barnes and G. Sato (eds.), in press.

138. S. Shibata, B. P. Peters, D. D. Roberts, I. J. Goldstein, and L. A. Liotta, *FEBS Lett.* **142**, 194–198 (1982).

139. C. A. Antonopoulos, I. Axelsson, D. Heinegård, and S. Gardell, *Biochim. Biophys. Acta* **338**, 108–119 (1974).

D

IMMUNOELECTROPHORETIC DETECTION OF INSULIN

**KEIJI KAKITA, KEITH O'CONNELL,
AND M. ALAN PERMUTT**

*Washington University School of Medicine, Department of Medicine,
St. Louis, Missouri*

1. INTRODUCTION

Analysis of DNA, RNA, or protein after electrophoresis and transfer to filters has become an accepted method for detection of specific molecules within crude extracts. This method has been very useful for proteins because it combines the high resolution of polyacrylamide gel electrophoresis with the specificity of immunodetection. This chapter describes an immunoelectrophoretic method for identification of insulin in pancreatic extracts or in serum. The method involves essentially four steps as outlined in Figure 1: (i) Polyacrylamide gel electrophoresis on a basic (pH 8.9) 12.5 percent acrylamide gel for 4 hr, is followed immediately by (ii) electrophoretic transfer in Tris-glycine buffer for 4 hr to nitrocellulose filters; (iii) photoaffinity coupling of the insulin to the filters is followed by immunodetection with anti-insulin antibody and [^{125}I]protein A, which binds to the antibody; (iv) The last step is autoradiography.

2. METHODS

2.1. Polyacrylamide Gel Electrophoresis

2.1.1. PROCEDURE

A slab gel apparatus (Bio-Rad or similar product) is used according to the manufacturer's directions.

2.1.2. SOLUTIONS FOR ORNSTEIN AND DAVIS (1) NONDENATURING GELS

1. Solution A: 1.5 M Tris-Cl, pH 8.8; 18.6 g Tris in 80 mL H$_2$O. Titrate. Raise volume to 100 mL.

2. Solution B: 0.5 M Tris-Cl, pH 6.8; 6.055 g Tris in 80 mL H$_2$O. Titrate. Raise volume to 100 mL.

3. Solution C: Acrylamide 50 percent acrylamide/1.33 percent bis; 50 g acrylamide/1.33 g bis. Dissolve in 100 mL H$_2$O. Filter.

4. Solution D: Acrylamide 20 percent acrylamide/5 percent bis; 20 g acrylamide, 5 g bis dissolved in 100 mL H$_2$O. Filter.

5. Solution E: Riboflavin 0.04 percent in H$_2$O. Dissolve 40 g in 100 mL H$_2$O. Store in dark bottle.

6. Solution F: TEMED (Sigma Chemical Company, St. Louis, MO).

7. Solution G: 10 percent ammonium persulfate; 100 mg/mL in H$_2$O. Dissolve fresh. Keep on ice.

8. Solution H: Sample buffer—5×. Mix 25 mL glycerin, 25 mL solution I. Add 10 mg bromophenol blue.

9. Solution I: Electrode buffer—5× solution—24 mM Tris/192 mM glycine, pH 8.9. 3 g Tris, 14.4 g glycine dissolved in 1 L H$_2$O. Check pH. Should be pH 8.9.

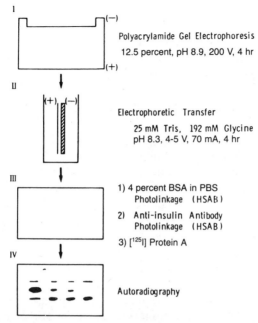

Polyacrylamide Gel Electrophoresis

12.5 percent, pH 8.9, 200 V, 4 hr

Electrophoretic Transfer

25 mM Tris, 192 mM Glycine
pH 8.3, 4-5 V, 70 mA, 4 hr

1) 4 percent BSA in PBS
   Photolinkage (HSAB)

2) Anti-insulin Antibody
   Photolinkage (HSAB)

3) [^{125}I] Protein A

Autoradiography

FIGURE 1. Immunoelectrophoretic detection of insulin. (I) Polyacrylamide gel electrophoresis, (II) electrophoretic transfer to the nitrocellulose filters, (III) photoaffinity coupling of insulin to the filter followed by immunodetection, and (IV) autoradiography.

Separating Gel		10 percent	12.5 percent	15 percent	20 percent
Mix:	Soln. A	4 mL	5 mL	6 mL	8 mL
	Soln. C	5 mL	5 mL	5 mL	5 mL
	Soln. F	6 μL	6 μL	6 μL	6 μL
	Soln. G	160 μL	160 μL	160 μL	160 μL

Raise volume to 20 mL with H_2O.
Mix. Deaerate 3 min. Pour.

Stacking gel		2.5 percent
Mix:	Soln. B	1 mL
	Soln. D	1 mL
	Soln. E	1 mL
	Soln. F	4.6 μL
	H_2O	5 mL

Must irradiate with long wave UV to polymerize.

2.1.3. PREPARATION OF SAMPLES

Sera: The easiest way is to immunoprecipitate with fivefold excess of anti-insulin antibody. For each different antisera conditions need to be optimized for quantitative precipitation of insulins. We normally work with samples containing a total of 50–75 ng of insulin in a volume of approximately 6 mL. We first add 50 μL of guinea pig antibovine insulin serum and mix over a 3-day period at 4°C.

Add second antibody—goat anti-guinea pig serum, 12.5 μL/tube and incubate overnight. Mix. Next day add additional 125 μL/tube. Mix. Incubate overnight. Next day, centrifuge at 2000 rpm for 30 min, 40°C. Wash pellets with cold PBS and recentrifuge as before. Begin extraction of pellets with acid-EtOH. (Acid-EtOH: 375 mL EtOH 95 percent, 7.5 mL HCl, and 145 mL H_2O.). Extract two to three overnights with 500 μL each. Lyophilize acid extracts. Reconstitute residue in 25 to 30 μL solution H, 1X.

2.1.4. ELECTROPHORESIS

Use current of 100 V until the dye reaches the separating gel, then increase current to 200 V. Run until dye front is within 1 cm of the bottom of the gel.

2.2. Electrophoretic Transfer

When gel electrophoresis is finished, remove gel from between glass plates. Place gel into E.C. electroblot apparatus (E.C. Apparatus Corporation, St. Petersburg, FL) as shown (Fig. 1 and E.C. directions), wrapped in Whatman 3 MM with presoaked nitrocellulose (0.45 μm, Schleicher and Schuell, Inc., NH). Place into tank with 6 L 192 mM glycine, 24 mM Tris, pH 8.3, (NaN_3 to final concentration 0.02 percent is optional).

Connect two electrode ends on apparatus to assure that there is tight contact between gel and nitrocellulose.

Connect electrodes with power supply. Electroblot 4 hr with current running at 70 mA approximately (6–9 V), per centimeter.

Turn on pump to circulate buffer.

After 4 hr turn off power supply.

Remove gel and nitrocellulose.

Air dry nitrocellulose 15 min. Mark date and lanes on blot.

Store nitrocellulose overnight 4°C in a Seal-N-Save (Sears) bag.

2.3. Photoaffinity Linkage and Immunodetection

2.3.1. LINKAGE

Incubate filter 1 hr at 40°C in 4 percent bovine serum albumin (BSA) in 10 mM phosphate buffered saline (PBS), pH 7.5, without agitation. Wash blot in a Seal-N-Save (Sears) three times for 5 min total in 10 mL each 10 mM PBS to remove excess BSA. Force liquid out with glass rod.

In cold room in dark add to tube with 9.8 mL 10 mM PBS 200 μL 25 mM HSAB (N-hydroxysuccinimidyl-p-azidobenzoate (Pierce Chemical, Agent 21560). Dissolve 3.3 mg in 500 μL dimethyl sulfoxide (DMSO) and empty into a Seal-N-Save bag containing nitrocellulose. Swish for 3 min to aid in dispersion of cross-linking reagent. Irradiate with a long-wave UV lamp for 10 min at a distance of approximately 7–10 in., making sure that there are no bubbles between light path and nitrocellulose. The UV lamp (principle wave length 366 nm) is obtained from Black Ray B100 A Ultraviolet Products Inc., (California).

After 10 min, add 200 μL 1.5 M Tris-Cl, pH 8.8, to bag and mix to stop reaction. Move to lab in light. Remove solution from bag as before. Wash four times over 10-min period with 10 mL each 10 mM PBS.

2.3.2. IMMUNOPRECIPITATION

Add 10 mL antibody solution, 10^5 dilution of guinea pig anti-bovine insulin sera in 5 percent BSA in PBS. Seal bag. Incubate 3 hr 37°C with agitation. Wash as previously described and repeat coupling.

After washing thoroughly, incubate 1 hr at 30°C in protein A (Pharmacia).

Dilute 1 mL aliquot of protein A in 10 mL with 5 percent BSA in PSB. (The amount of radioactivity added has varied in the past from 14 μCi total to approximately 1 μCi total depending upon success in the iodination procedure. The lower level of radioactivity is preferable. It gives equally good sensitivity, and perhaps better, because background is reduced—it is preferable to store the protein A in 1 mL aliquots of approximately 3 mCi at −20°C.

After incubation, discard radioactivity. Wash blot in a 9 × 9 pie dish for 30 min in 10 mL/blot, 1 percent Triton X-100 in PBS. Agitate frequently. Rinse blot in dish three to four times with distilled water, air dry, and expose film 16–24 hr.

2.3.3. IODINATION OF PROTEIN A

1. Reagents
    (a) 0.5 M PO$_4$pH 7.5.
    (b) 10 mM PBS pH 7.5.
    (c) Protein A (Pharmacia) 4 mg/mL in 0.05 M P.B. Stored at −80°C in 50 and 25 μL aliquots.
    (d) Chloramine-T (Sigma): 15 mg in 5 mL 0.05 M of P.B. on day of use.
    (e) Sodium metabisulfite: 35 mg in 10 mL 0.05 M of P.B. on day of use.
    (f) Trasylol (Mobay Chemical Corporation).
    (g) KI:10 mg in 10 mL H$_2$O stable if covered with aluminum foil.

(h)   5 percent BSA in PBS.

(j) ^{125}I usually 1 mCi/10 μL (Amersham).

2.   Columns

(a)   Sephadex G-25 Resin (Sigma): Swell 5 gm in H_2O. Remove fines. Pack column in PBS, 19.6 cm high in 10 mL glass pipettes ($r = 0.4$ cm)

(b)   Sephadex G-200 (Sigma): Swell 5 gm in H_2O. Pack column in PBS. Dimensions $r = 0.75 \times 45.5$ cm approximately 80 cm^3.

3.   Iodination reaction

(a)   Mix 50 μL of 0.5 M PB.

(b)   5 μL (or 10 μL) ^{125}I 0.5 mCi (or 1 mCi).

(c)   25 μL chloramine-T in siliconized tube or isotope vial.

(d)   12.5 μL protein A. 50 ng (or 25 μl to 100 ng) when using 1 mCi of ^{125}I.

(e)   Mix on a Vortex mixer 10 sec.

(f)   Add 100 μL sodium metabisulfite.

(g)   200 μL Trasylol

(h)   100 μL KI.

(i)   Place on Sephadex G-25 column.

4.   Collect fractions immediately into siliconized tubes:

(a)   Tube 1: 33 drops/tube.

(b)   Tube 2: 22 drops/tube.

(c)   Tubes 3–20: 11 drops/tubes.

Tubes 3–17 should contain 1 mL each 5 percent BSA in PBS. Keep on ice after fraction is collected. Count 10 μL aliquot for 30 sec. Then pool tubes, usually fractions 6–10 or 11.

Mix a little bromphenol blue (BPB) in with fractions before applying. Apply to Sephadex G-200 column. Gravity flow. Start collecting 50-drop fractions when blue dye is ready to come out.

Count 50 μL for 30 sec. Pool first enriched 30 sec fractions and count. Determine mCi/mL. Dilute to 3–8 mCi/mL with BSA/PBS. Freeze in 1 mL aliquots. Store at −20°C.

3.   COMMENTS

3.1.   Sensitivity, Specificity, and Limits of Detection

To detect insulin in pancreatic extracts after electrophoresis we evaluated previously described methods (2–5) but encountered a number of problems.

In general, the methods were for proteins larger than 20,000 MW and were not suitable for detection of proinsulin and insulin, which are considerably smaller (MW 9000 and 6000, respectively) and more soluble. Recovery was initially monitored with bovine insulin and proinsulin (6). After electrophoresis of [^{125}I]bovine insulin and transfer from the gel to nitrocellulose filters, recovery was evaluated. Transfer by simple diffusion required 24–48 hr and yielded approximately 20 percent recovery. Electrophoretic transfer in Tris-glycine buffer yielded quantitative recovery on nitrocellulose filters in 4 hr. Addition of SDS and urea lowered recovery to between 38–49 percent.

Following electrophoretic transfer of insulin to nitrocellulose filters, the filters were dried and treated with anti-insulin antibody and iodinated Staph A protein. Nonspecific binding to the filters was often unacceptably high, but could be minimized by washing extensively. The insulin was progressively washed from the filters, however. When nitrocellulose filters were adsorbed with 4 percent BSA and insulin subsequently photoaffinity cross-linked the recovery was quantitative.

The limit of detection of insulin could be greatly enhanced by treating the filter-bound insulin antibody complex a second and third time with anti-insulin antibody and [^{125}I]protein A (6). As little as 10 ng of bovine insulin could be detected with three anti-insulin antibody and [^{125}I] iodinated protein A treatments. Analysis of autoradiographs of [^{125}I] Staph A protein bound provided a quantitative measure of the insulin applied if the gels were not overloaded with protein (less than 1 μg) and the film was not overexposed. This relationship could be optimized by altering exposure time according to the amount of insulin analyzed so that the radioactivity on the filter is within the linear detection range of the X-ray film (7).

One of the advantages of the immunoelectrophoretic analysis is that large numbers of samples can be analyzed. Older methods required electrophoresis followed by slicing the gels into multiple pieces, extracting each gel, and performing radioimmunoassay on each gel slice extract. With the present method multiple samples can be analyzed on a single gel, and the resolution is far better than column chromatographic separation of insulin. The method takes 2 days total for electrophoresis, electroblotting, and immunodetection, and 5–15 hr for autoradiography. The system is very sensitive since as little as 10 ng of insulin present in a concentration of 1 part in 1000 cell proteins could be detected.

3.2. Assessment of the Two Rodent Insulins in Pancreatic Extracts

The immunoelectrophoretic method was used to separate and quantitate rodent insulins I and II in growth hormone tumor-bearing hyperinsulinemic rats (8). These rats were found to contain 5-6 times more insulin I than II compared to control nontumor-bearing rats with 1.5 times more I (ref. 8 and Fig. 2). Furthermore, when rat islets were incubated in high glucose (16 mM), insulin I appeared to be synthesized 5–6 times more than insulin II. These findings suggested that conditions which stimulate insulin biosynthesis in the rat produced

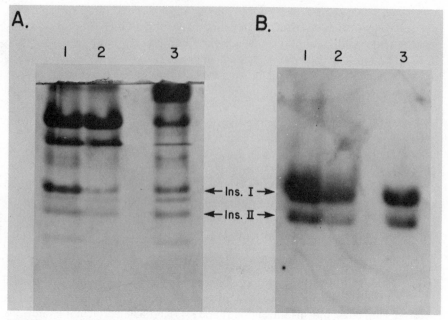

FIGURE 2.   Electrophoresis of pancreatic extracts on polyacrylamide gels. (A) Coomassie blue staining patterns of electrophoresed pancreatic extracts. Lane 1: Growth hormone tumor bearing Wistar-Furth rat; lane 2: Normal Wistar–Furth rat pancreatic extract; lane 3: Normal Sprague–Dawley pancreatic extract. (B) Immunoelectrophoretic detection of rat insulin I and II. The gel from (A) was treated with anti-insulin antibody and then with [^{125}I]-labeled protein A and an autoradiograph was obtained. Ins. = insulin.

a preferential synthesis of insulin I. Analysis of the relative proportion of the two insulins in the pancreas of inbred strains of mice also indicated that insulin I predominated (9). These experiments were done utilizing bovine insulin as a standard.

Quantitative recovery of the two rat insulins was recently evaluated when we obtained purified rat insulin I and II in microgram quantities from D. Steiner (Chicago, IL). Recovery of the two rodent insulins was analyzed following staining and immunodetection. Equal amounts of rat insulin I and II were electrophoresed and then either stained by the silver staining method (10) or Coomassie blue (11). Silver staining was more sensitive with as little as 200 ng insulin readily detected, but the proportions of I and II were very variable. Coomassie blue staining (at least 1 μg of insulin) consistently yielded approximately 50 percent less insulin II than I on repeated analysis (Fig. 3). Immunoelectrophoretic detection of equal amounts of the two rodent insulins again showed a surprising result. The recovery of rat insulin II was approximately 50 percent less than that of insulin I (Fig. 4). This suggests that all of our previous estimates are off by 50 percent. This correction would indicate that the rodent insulins are present in approximately equal quantities in the un-

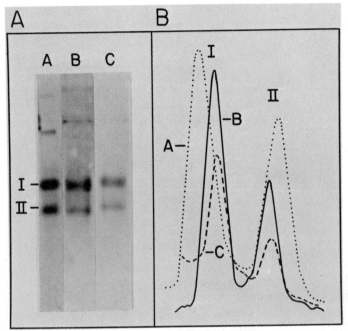

FIGURE 3. Recovery of purified rat insulin I and II by electrophoresis and staining with Coomassie blue. (A) Equal quantities of rat insulin I and II (5 μg) were electrophoresed on three separate gels as indicated. These gels were stained with Coomassie blue. (B) Densitometric tracings of the gels in (A.) The ratio of insulin I to II in lane 1 was 1.8, lane 2, 1.6, and lane 3, 1.9. The recovery of insulin II relative to I was on the average 57 percent.

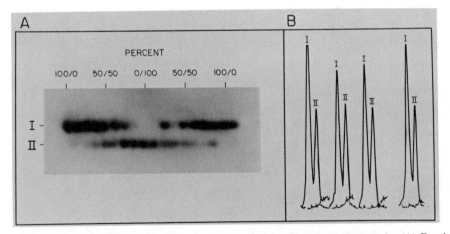

FIGURE 4. Recovery of purified rat insulin I and II by immunoelectrophoresis. (A) Equal amounts of rat insulin I and II were analyzed alone or in a 50:50 mixture as indicated. (B) Following immunodetection, the autoradiographs were scanned repeatedly in the area of the gel containing a 50:50 mixture of the insulin.

stimulated state (12–15), and that insulin I is at most two- to threefold elevated in hyperinsulinemic rodents as compared to what was originally reported (8, 9).

Quantitation of rodent insulins is further complicated by the overlap between proinsulin and the more basic insulin I. Coelectrophoresis of bovine proinsulin with rat pancreatic extracts showed that the leading edge of bovine proinsulin slightly overlapped the rat insulin I band. For this reason in hyperinsulinemic animals, rat insulin I may be mixed with an increased amount of proinsulin or proinsulin intermediates which are more acidic than proinsulin. This may be responsible for the high ratio of rodent insulin I to II in the hyperinsulinemic conditions previously reported (8, 9). D. Steiner found equal amounts of rat insulin I and II in pregnant hyperinsulinemic rats by high-pressure liquid chromatography (personal communication).

3.3. Analysis of Serum

Since plasma insulin in the fasted state is usually less than 1 ng/mL, we have been evaluating 10 mL samples of serum after glucose or tolbutamide stimulation. The insulin is quantitatively removed by immunoprecipitation which serves to partially purify it from 1 part in 10^7 to approximately 1 in 10^4 serum proteins. Then 100 μg of anti-insulin antibody precipitates aliquots are subjected to immunoelectrophoresis. One major band has been identified in all samples (about 50), which comigrates with bovine insulin, and one minor more basic immunoreactive protein (10–20 percent), which has not been identified. This minor immunoreactive insulin peptide is more acidic than proinsulin and could well be a proinsulin intermediate such as arginyl insulin. We have no human proinsulin intermediate standards at the present time and have not chemically identified this minor component. This immunoelectrophoretic method should ultimately be useful for screening large numbers of human sera for variant insulins (16).

REFERENCES

1. B. J. Davis, *Ann. N.Y. Acad. Sci.* **121**, 404–427 (1964).
2. R. T. M. J. Vaessen, J. Kreike, and G. S. P. Groot, *FEBS Lett.* **124**, 193–196 (1981).
3. H. Towbin, T. Staehelin, and J. Gordon, *Natl. Acad. Sci. USA* **76**, 4350–454 (1979).
4. J. Renart, J. Reiser, and G. R. Stark, *Proc. Natl. Acad. Sci. USA* **76**, 3116–3120 (1979).
5. J. Symington, M. Green, and K. Brackmann, *Proc. Natl. Acad. Sci. USA* **78**, 177–181 (1981).
6. K. Kakita, K. O'Connell, and M. A. Permutt, *Diabetes* **31**, 648–652 (1982).
7. R. A. Laskey and A. D. Mills, *Eur. J. Biochem.* **56**, 335–341 (1975).
8. K. Kakita, S. Giddings, and M. A. Permutt, *Proc. Natl. Acad. Sci. USA* **79**, 2803–2807, 1982.
9. K. Kakita, K. O'Connell, and M. A. Permutt, *Diabetes* **31**, 841–845 (1982).

10. C. R. Merril, D. Goldman, S. Sedman, and M. Ebert, *Science* **211**, 1437–38 (1981).

11. U. K. Laemli, *Nature (London)* **227**, 680–85 (1970).

12. J. L. Clark and D. F. Steiner, *Proc. Natl. Acad. Sci. USA* **62**, 278–85 (1969).

13. T. Tanese, N. R. Lazarus, S. Devrim, and L. Recant, *J. Clin. Invest.* **49**, 1394–1404 (1970).

14. L. B. Rall, R. L. Pictet, and W. J. Rutter, *Endocrinology* **105**, 835–41 (1979).

15. N. Itoh, K. Nose, and H. Okamoto, *Eur. J. Biochem.* **97**, 1–9 (1979).

16. S. Shoelson, M. Haneda, P. Blix, A. Nanjo, T. Sanke, K. Inouye, D. Steiner, A. Rubenstein, and H. Tager, *Nature* **302**, 540–43 (1983).

VI

HORMONE SYNTHESIS AND DEGRADATION

A

IN VITRO BIOLOGICAL CHARACTERIZATION OF IODINATED INSULIN PREPARATIONS

OLE SONNE

Institute of Physiology, University of Aarhus, Universitetsparken, Aarhus, Denmark

1. INTRODUCTION

Preparations of insulin iodinated with ^{125}I are widely used as tracers for insulin in radioimmunoassays and in *in vivo* and *in vitro* biological experiments. Iodination of insulin results in a mixture of unlabeled insulin and different isomers of monoiodinated and diiodinated insulins depending on the degree of iodination, method, pH, and so forth. In biological experiments, whether performed *in vivo* or *in vitro*, the labeled insulin used should ideally possess the same biological properties as native insulin in order to be a valid tracer. Monoiodoinsulin is biologically active as first shown by Freychet et al. (1), but the potency will depend on the tyrosine residue substituted. Thus, we have previously shown that in the rat adipocyte [Tyr^{A19}-^{125}I]monoiodoinsulin possesses a reduced binding affinity and potency compared to native insulin (2–5) and that the B26 isomer has an increased affinity and potency (4–5).

The iodination, isolation, and purification of the monoiodinated isomers are described in Vol IB, VI A by Welinder et al. In the present chapter details are given about the characterization of the biological properties of monoiodinated insulin preparations. The major emphasis is put on the isolated rat adipocyte system, as this allows the investigator to test for both affinity (cf. section 2) and biological potency (cf. section 3).

Chemicals and labware mentioned in the following sections are presently in use in our laboratory. This does not exclude the successful use of similar items obtained from other sources.

2. RECEPTOR BINDING AFFINITY

2.1. Theory

Experimentally, it is easier to assess the binding affinity of a $[^{125}I]$monoiodo-insulin preparation relative to that of a standard tracer preparation (cf. 2.1.2) than to determine the absolute binding affinity (cf. 2.1.1).

The isotherm for the binding at steady state of a ligand to one single class of independent receptors can be described by the following equation:

$$\frac{B}{F} = \frac{[RI]}{[I]} + \left(\frac{B}{F}\right)_{nonsp} = \frac{R_0}{K_d + [I]} + \left(\frac{B}{F}\right)_{nonsp} \tag{1}$$

where B/F is the bound/free ratio for the total binding, [RI] is the concentration of receptor insulin complex, [I] the concentration of unbound insulin (which is close to the total concentration, as usually not more than 3 percent is bound), R_0 the total number of receptors, K_d the dissociation constant, and $(B/F)_{nonsp}$ the bound/free ratio for nonspecifically bound insulin, that is, the binding of $[^{125}I]$monoiodoinsulin in the presence of a saturating concentration (1 μM) of unlabeled insulin (cf. 2.4.1.1).

2.1.1. ABSOLUTE BINDING AFFINITY

Determination of the absolute binding affinity of an insulin preparation can be performed by comparing the ability of several different concentrations of the test substance and a standard insulin preparation to displace tracer insulin from receptors. The determination of the concentrations is, therefore, the crucial point in this assay, and sufficient amounts of the material should be available allowing the measurement of UV absorbance, nitrogen contents, or amino acid analysis. The concentrations of standards and test substances should be performed using the same method in order to avoid any systematic bias, and the presence of iodotyrosine residues should not influence the result. Determination with radioimmunoassay may not be without problems as 7 out of 10 guinea pig anti-human insulin sera tested exhibited a higher binding of $[Tyr^{A14}-^{125}I]$monoiodoinsulin than of $[Tyr^{A19}-^{125}I]$monoiodoinsulin (3).

2.1.2. Relative Binding Affinity

In these experiments it is possible to use concentrations as low as 10–20 pM, which is much less than the apparent K_d for the binding (about 1 nM). For [I] $<< K_d$, that is, at trace concentration Equation (1) can be simplified to

$$\frac{[RI]}{[I]} = \frac{B}{F} - \left(\frac{B}{F}\right)_{nonsp} = \frac{R_0}{K_d} = R_0 \times K_a \qquad (2)$$

where K_a is the association constant for the binding. When experiments are carried out on the same pool of cells, R_0 will remain the same in all tubes, and therefore, the B/F value for the receptor binding (total binding minus nonspecific binding) will be directly proportional to the affinity of the tracer.

Even when the cells have more than one class of receptors, this comparison will be valid as long as the insulin concentration used is small compared to the K_d for the class of receptors with the highest affinity (lowest K_d).

2.2. Buffers

In all incubations we use the same Krebs–Ringer salt solution, buffered with HEPES [4-(2-hydroxyethyl)-1-piperazineethanesulfonic acid] and fortified with different concentrations of bovine serum albumin and bacitracin.

2.2.1. Stock Solutions

2.2.1.1. Mixed Salt Solution 10X Concentrated
76.74 g NaCl (this and other inorganic chemicals of analytical grade).
3.51 g KCl.
3.06 g $MgSO_4 \cdot 7H_2$).
3.63 g $CaCl_2 \cdot 2H_2O$.

Bring to 1000 mL with distilled water. Should be stored at 4°C.

2.2.1.1. HEPES-Phosphate Solution 10X Concentrated
23.80 g HEPES (Sigma).
3.42 g $NaH_2PO_4 \cdot H_2O$.

Adjust to pH 7.6 with NaOH and bring to 1000 mL with distilled water. Should be stored at 4°C.

2.2.1.3. Bovine Serum Albumin
100 g bovine serum albumin, fraction V (Sigma, cat. no. A4503).
500 mL distilled water.

When dissolved (perhaps overnight at 4°C) this solution is divided and put into two dialysis tubings (Servapor 29 mm or Visking 27/32) that have been presoaked in cold water. Dialyze each tube with magnetic stirring against five changes of 5 L each of distilled water at 4°C, taking 12 hr for each change. Then adjust the pH to 7.6 with NaOH and the volume to 1000 mL (i.e., final concentration 10 percent w/v). The solution is filtered through the following sequence of filters: Whatman 41, Whatman 42 ashless filter papers, Millipore filter type SM (5-μm pore size), and Millipore filter type AA (0.8-μm pore size). Please note that this is not sufficient to sterilize the albumin solution, and it should therefore be stored at −20°C, aliquoted in, for example, 20 mL scintillation vials.

2.2.2. COLLAGENASE BUFFER FOR ADIPOCYTE ISOLATION

For isolation of rat adipocytes (cf. 2.3.1) make a mixture of the following:
   45 vol distilled water.
   10 vol mixed salts solution 10X (2.2.1.1).
   10 vol HEPES-phosphate solution 10X (2.2.1.2).
   35 vol Albumin 10 percent w/v (2.2.1.3).

Glucose to a final concentration of 0.55 mM (0.1 g/L) and crude collagenase from *Cl. histolyticum* (Worthington type I) to a final concentration of 0.5 g/L. Adjust pH to 7.6 at 20°C. This will give pH 7.4 at 37°C. Should be stored at −20°C in 3 mL aliquots.

2.2.3. WASHING BUFFER

The buffer used for washing the cells is made up as follows:
   7 vol distilled water.
   1 vol mixed salts solution 10X (2.2.1.1).
   1 vol HEPES-phosphate solution 10X (2.2.1.2).
   1 vol albumin 10 percent w/v (2.2.1.3).

Adjust pH to 7.6 at 20°C. This will give pH 7.4 at 37°C. If using other temperatures, the pH should be adjusted accordingly.

2.2.4. INCUBATION BUFFER

The final incubation buffer for binding experiments is made up as follows:
   3 vol distilled water.
   1 vol mixed salts solution 10X (2.2.1.1).
   1 vol HEPES-phosphate solution 10X (2.2.1.2).
   5 vol albumin 10 percent w/v (2.2.1.3).

Bacitracin to a final concentration of 0.35 mM (0.5 g/L). Adjust pH to 7.6 at 20°C. This will give pH 7.4 at 37°C. If using other temperatures, the pH should be adjusted accordingly.

The ionic composition of this buffer is (in millimolar concentrations) Na$^+$, 140; K$^+$, 4.7; Ca^{2+}, 2.5; Mg^{2+}, 1.25; phosphate, 2.5; SO$_4^{2-}$, 1.25; HEPES 10; remaining anions as Cl$^-$.

2.3. Cells

Different types of cells can be used in binding studies. We are mainly working with isolated rat adipocytes (cf. 2.3.1), but isolated rat hepatocytes (cf. 2.3.2), cultured human lymphocytes of the IM-9 line (cf.2.3.3), and colon carcinoma cells of the HT-29 line (cf. 2.3.4) have also been employed (5).

2.3.1. ISOLATED RAT ADIPOCYTES

The isolation of adipocytes (6) follows the principles originally given by Rodbell (7). The epididymal and perirenal fat pads from a male rat weighing 140— 200 g and fed *ad libitum* are removed and transferred to a 30 mL plastic beaker (60 × 27 mm inside diameter) with a smooth and even bottom (NUNC, Kampstrup, Denmark, cat. no. 536455). the casting bump in the bottom may have to be removed. Three milliters of prewarmed collagenase buffer (2.2.2) is added together with a 5 × 15-mm Teflon-coated stir bar. The tissue may be minced using scissors, but the mincing should be quite course leaving not less than 2–3-mm cubes. The vial is incubated with magnetic stirring in a 37°C water bath (water bath 01T443 with a MA6VS magnetic stirrer, both from HETO, Birkerød, Denmark. This setup allows the simultaneous stirring of six beakers, each with two "standard" fat pads). Use the minimum speed which will disintegrate the tissue in 60 min but incubate only for 45 min, that is, until the tissue is about 90 percent disintegrated (depending on the batch of collagenase) and carefully center the stir bar. It is important to use the minimal mechanical treatment as possible. In case shaking has to be used instead of stirring, it is usually necessary to use about 100 cpm and again use the minimal mechanical treatment releasing the cells in about 60 min with 0.5 g/L collagenase.

The cell suspension is diluted with a few milliters of washing buffer (2.2.3) and filtered through an approximately 300 μm nylon mesh (Polyman, PES300, Schweizerische Seidengazefabrik AG, Zürich) into polyethylene centrifuge tubes (Minisorp 100 × 15-mm tubes, NUNC, cat. no. 468608). Allow the cells (from two to three rats per tube) to float for about 1 min and remove the infranatant, including sedimented debris, using a 12-cm long 14-gauge needle. Add 10 mL washing buffer and turn the tube *gently*, wait and remove the infranatant. Repeat this procedure three times. Add another wash using the incubation buffer (2.2.4) and aspirate the infranatant.

The packed-cell volume in this concentrated cell suspension is now measured (should be 40–45 percent v/v). Shake the suspension gently by hand, fill a capillary tube, seal, and centrifuge for 1 min in a hematocrit centrifuge. The trapped extracellular buffer will be about 4 percent of the volume of packed cells. Dilute the cells with incubation buffer (2.2.4) to the required cell concentration in terms of packed-cell volume.

2.3.2. ISOLATED RAT HEPATOCYTES

Rat hepatocytes can be isolated by *in vitro* perfusion of a rat liver through the portal vein (8) first with a 37°C Ca^{2+}-free buffer (9) followed by a Ca^{2+}-containing buffer with 0.5 g/L collagenase (10, 11). Filter of the cell suspension through a 56 μm nylon mesh and wash at 1 *g* twice followed by purification on a linear gradient (1.005–1.110 kg/L) of Percoll (Pharmacia, Uppsala, Sweden) (12). Details are given in the quoted references and in refs. 4, 13, and 14.

2.3.3. CULTURED HUMAN LYMPHOCYTES OF THE IM-9 LINE

These cells grow in suspension in RPMI 1640 medium supplemented with either 5 percent fetal calf serum or 10 percent newborn cal serum (Flow Laboratories). Details are given elsewhere (15, 16).

2.3.4. CULTURED HUMAN COLON CARCINOMA CELLS OF THE HT-29 LINE

These cells (17) are dependent on attachment to the flasks or dishes and can be grown in Dulbecco's modification of Eagle's medium fortified with 10 percent fetal calf serum. When transferring, they have to be trypsinized (please consult a handbook in tissue culture techniques or ref. 18). Two days prior to the binding experiment the culture is trypsinized, the cells washed, filtered through a sterile nylon mesh (56 μm), and $3-4 \times 10^5$ cells seeded in each well on a 24-well multidish plate (culture area 1.9 cm^2; Nunclon Delta, NUNC (5).

2.4. Incubation

As the apparent binding affinity of insulin varies with pH (19) and temperature (20), and as the receptor ligand interaction in some cell types cannot be regarded as a simple reversible reaction (16, 21, 22), it is important to use standardized incubation conditions and have a knowledge about which parameters will be included in the measured binding data. Generally, we incubate at physiological pH and temperature and therefore include the receptor binding and all subsequent cellular events.

2.4.1. INCUBATION OF ISOLATED RAT ADIPOCYTES

The adipocytes are incubated in polyethylene centrifuge tubes (cf. 2.3.1) in a final volume of 0.5 mL in the incubation buffer (2.2.4) with the tracer and test substances added in volumes not less than 50 μL. Typically we use four replicates each with the following:

  100 μL tracer diluted in incubation buffer (2.2.4).

  100 μl test substance diluted in incubation buffer (2.2.4).

  300 μL adipocytes 8.3 percent v/v.

This will give a final cell concentration of 5 percent v/v. Incubate in a shaking water bath at 37°C and 80–100 cpm for 45 min.

The incubation is stopped by the addition of 9 mL of 0.15 M NaCl at 10°C followed by 1.4 mL of silicone oil (0.99 kg/L, 200 centistokes) and centrifugation for 40 sec at $\sim$ 1000 g_{max}. The cells will now float as a pellet on top of the silicone oil and the diluted unbound ligand will remain beneath the oil layer. Do not handle more tubes than can be centrifuged within 30 sec after the addition of the saline. The cells can be transferred to γ-counting vials by adsorption to a brushlet formed by bending one-eight of a pipe cleaner 180° and held by forceps. More tedious and expensive is to aspirate the cells into a disposable pipette tip with cut tip so it is wide bored.

An alternative method is to transfer 400 μL to 0.55 mL microfuge tubes (Milian, Switzerland) containing ∼0.1 mL of the silicone oil and centrifuging for 1 min in a Beckman microfuge. The cells are isolated by cutting the tube through the oil layer (23).

2.4.1.1. Nonspecific Binding. Insulin readily adsorbs to glass, plastic, and to cell surfaces. The first is prevented by including albumin in solutions containing insulin, and the latter is a minor problem if the tracer is of a high quality. The nonspecific binding is characterized by a high capacity and a low affinity. Thus, it is directly proportional to the concentration of free insulin (cf. Eq. 1, Section 2.1.). Therefore, when a high concentration of unlabeled insulin, for example, 1 μM (= $10^3 \times K_d$ and approximately 10^5 times the tracer concentration) is added along with the [^{125}I]monoiodoinsulin, the receptors will be saturated with unlabeled insulin, and the observed B/F will then represent (B/F)$_{nonsp}$, the nonspecific binding.

All binding experiments should be corrected for nonspecific binding measured in parallel incubates. To these otherwise identical tubes add 10 μL of 100 μM native insulin dissolved in 0.01 M HCl. As the binding affinity for the nonspecific binding is very low, the nonspecifically bound insulin will quickly dissociate even at low temperatures in contrast to the specifically receptor-bound insulin. Therefore, the nonspecific binding is reduced to very low levels when the incubation is stopped by the NaCl–oil floatation technique (cf. Sections 2.4.1, first alternative, and 2.4.1.2).

2.4.1.2.   *Determination of Relative Binding Affinities.* When the relative affinity of different isomers of [^{125}I]monoiodoinsulins is determined, we incubate 100 μL isomer diluted in incubation buffer (2.2.4) and 400 μL adipocytes 6.3 percent v/v, and further as described in Section 2.4.1.

Each isomer is applied in two concentrations, for example, 5000 and 10,000 cpm/tube corresponding to approximately 5 and 10 pM depending on the specific activity and the counting efficiency. According to Equation (1) these should give the same B/F if [I] $<< K_d$, and, if so, the affinity of the different isomers will be directly proportional to the specific B/F [= (B/F)$_{total}$ − (B/F)$_{nonsp}$]. For this reason this assay is relatively insensitive to minor differences in the specific activity.

For [Tyr^{A14}-^{125}I]monoiodoinsulin prepared as described in ref. 3, the B/F should be about 0.02 and the nonspecific binding about 2 percent of this, that is, (B/F)$_{nonsp}$ = 0.0004 using the NaCl–oil floatation technique (cf. Section 2.4.1, first alternative). The binding per unit cell volume will, however, vary with the cell size, which is a function of the rat weight (= age) (6). Previously, we have found [Tyr^{A14}-^{127}I]monoiodoinsulin to possess the same affinity as native insulin (Fig. 1; Section 2.4.1.3; ref. 2). Therefore, we have in Table 1 related the affinities for the three other isomers to that of A14, although the above connection only has been experimentally established for the rat adipocyte

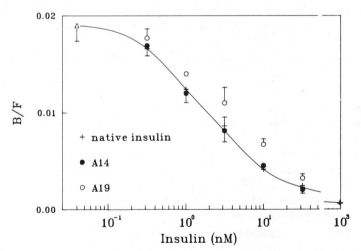

FIGURE 1.   Determination of the absolute binding affinity of [Tyr^{A14}-^{127}I]monoiodoinsulin and [Tyr^{A19}-^{127}I]monoiodoinsulin. Isolated adipocytes were incubated as described in sections 2.4.1 and 2.4.1.3 with 40 pM [Tyr^{A14}-^{125}I]monoiodoinsulin alone (△) or plus insulin (+), [Tyr^{A14}-^{127}I]monoiodoinsulin (●), or the corresponding A19 isomer (○). The iodoinsulin preparations were iodinated with the lactoperoxidase method and purified by disc polyacrylamide gel electrophoresis. The concentrations of the insulin standard and the two [^{127}I]monoiodoinsulins were determined by the UV absorbance and the protein concentration assay according to Lowry. Bars represent SD when exceeding the size of the symbol, n = 4. Further details are given in ref. 2, from which the figure has been modified.

TABLE 1.   Relative Binding Affinity of the Four
Isomers of [^{125}I]monoiodoinsulin to Different Cell
Types

	A14	A19	B16	B26
Rat adipocytes	1	0.6	1.1	1.8
Rat hepatocytes	1	0.7	1.2	1.0
IM-9	1	0.8	1.8	2.3
HT-29	1	0.9	1.4	2.1

The cells were incubated as described in Section 2.4 using a
concentration of [^{125}I]monoiodoinsulin of 10 pM. For each cell
type the binding affinities for the A19, B16, and B26 isomers
are expressed as a fraction of that found for the A14 isomer
(cf. 2.1.2), although the latter experimentally only has been
determined to be indistinguishable from that of native insulin
in the rat adipocyte (2). Modified from ref. 5.

(2–5). It should, however, be stressed that this is not necessarily the case
when the monoiodoinsulins are prepared by methods other than disc gel electrophoresis and ion exchange chromatography (2, 3). Thus, when prepared by
reversed-phase high-performance liquid chromatography as described in Vol.
IB, VI A by Welinder et al., the binding affinity may be reduced by about 40
percent compared to tracers purified with low-pressure methods (24).

2.4.1.3.   Determination of Absolute Binding Affinities.   In this case the
composition of the incubate is as depicted in Section 2.4.1. Tracer is 10 pM
[Tyr^{A14}-^{125}I]monoiodoinsulin. As concentrations in the nanomolar range are
required, the test substance will be native insulin standards or insulin isomers
iodinated with ^{127}I and purified to monoiodinated insulins. The iodinated samples
should be applied in concentrations covering the steep slope of the binding
curve (cf. Fig. 1) and the concentration of standards and test substances preferably be determined with the same method (cf .2.1.1).

The concentration of insulin giving half maximal binding of the tracer (=
ED$_{50}$ = apparent K_d) should be in the range 1–3 nM when measured as described.
In the isolated rat adipocyte we found [Tyr^{A14}-^{127}I]monoiodoinsulin to possess
the same affinity as native insulin (Fig. 1 and ref. 2).

2.4.1.4.   Insulin Degradation.   All binding experiments should include an
assessment of the insulin degradation. The simplest is to determine the ^{125}I
solubility in trichloroacetic acid. Although this method underestimates the
actual size of the degradation (25), it is convenient and sufficient for the
present purpose. After transfer of the cell pellet, aspirate the oil, and to small
centrifuge tubes transfer 0.3 mL of the infranatant. Add 5–10 µg carrier
protein [0.1 mL 10 percent w/v albumin (2.2.1.3)] and 2 mL ice-cold 0.75 M

trichloroacetic acid. Centrifuge for 5 min and count the pellet and supernatant. The increment in the soluble fraction should, if it originates only from the receptor-mediated degradation (i.e., the unavoidable turnover of insulin molecules on its receptor), be about 8 percent for the A14 isomer (21). As the tracer should be prepared with less than 2 percent acid-soluble activity, the total solubility should not exceed 10 percent when incubated as outlined in Section 2.4.1.

2.4.2. INCUBATION OF ISOLATED RAT HEPATOCYTES

The hepatocytes are incubated in a final concentration of 10^5 cells/mL essentially as described for adipocytes (cf. 2.4.1). The incubation is stopped by transferring 400 μL aliquots to 0.55-mL microfuge tubes containing approximately 0.1 mL of a mixture of di-*n*-butyl phthalate and dinonyl phthalate (3:1) (BDH Chemicals Ltd., Poole, England) followed by centrifugation for 1 min in a Beckman microfuge. This oil will have a density (1.03 kg/L) between that of the cells (1.07 kg/L) and the buffer. The cells are isolated by cutting the tube through the oil layer (26). This procedure can also be used for other cell types with a density higher than that of the buffer.

2.4.3. INCUBATION OF IM-9 LYMPHOCYTES

The lymphocytes are incubated in a final concentration of 10^6 cells/mL as described for hepatocytes (cf. 2.4.2).

2.4.4. INCUBATION OF HT-29 COLON CARCINOMA CELLS

On the day of the experiment cells are washed with the incubation buffer (2.2.4), and for each point six wells are incubated for 120 min at 37°C with [^{125}I]monoiodoinsulin alone or plus test substances in a final volume of 0.5 mL. The incubation is stopped by removing the incubation medium, washing the cells twice with 2 mL of ice-cold 0.15 *M* NaCl, and finally dissolving the bound ^{125}I activity in 1 mL 0.5 *M* NaOH for 6 hr at 80°C. The NaOH is transferred to counting vials and the wells washed with another milliliter of NaOH which is pooled with the initial extracts. The number of cells is determined by counting the nuclei in a hemocytometer after treatment of one well with 0.2 mL of 1.2 m*M* crystal violet in 30 m*M* citric acid (27). This procedure can also be used for other plated cells in culture.

2.5. Artifacts and Trouble Shooting

In the following discussion some of the most commonly occurring troubles in connection with the isolated adipocyte system are listed, together with the most likely explanations for these.

2.5.1. FEW CELLS

1. *Bad Collagenase (cf. 2.3.1).* If only few cells are released from the tissue despite a vigorous shaking/stirring and a prolonged (60–70 min) incubation, try another batch of collagenase.

2. *Too Little Mechanical Action.* Although it is never advisable to suggest the use of more vigorous stirring/shaking, it can of course be possible that the treatment is slightly too gentle. If an increased speed of shaking/stirring releases more intact cells without increasing the cell lysis, this is acceptable (see also Section 3.5.2).

2.5.2. OIL IN THE CELL SUSPENSION

1. *Too Much Mechanical Action.* Rough treatment of the cells will cause cell lysis resulting in free oil floating on top of the cells. This can occur because of too vigorous shaking/stirring during the collagenase treatment or too vigorous centrifugation during the washing. We use only 1 *g* during the washing for the same reason.

2. *Unacceptable Plasticware.* Some types of plastic as well as unsiliconized glassware cause cell lysis. We do not know what the ideal plastic surface characteristics should be, but the charge distribution may be of importance. Usually cells accept most laboratory plasticware, pipette tips, and tubes but where possible polyethylene or polypropylene are preferred to polystyrene.

3. *Cold Buffers.* The lower the buffer temperature the more fragile the cells. Therefore, when placing the tissue in the collagenase buffer and when washing and diluting the cells, use buffer with a temperature not less than 25°C.

2.5.3. LARGE STANDARD DEVIATIONS

The SD on the B/F value should not be more than 10 percent of the mean. If larger than this, it might be because of one of the following conditions:

1. *Cell Lysis.* Too much mechanical action or unacceptable plasticware (see 2.5.2). The diameter of the adipocytes is about 60 μm. Therefore, make sure that the bore in, for instance, the disposable pipette tips is wide enough. Alternatively, cut the tips. Cell lysis can also be induced by stopping the incubation with saline which is too cold. A temperature of 10°C is a compromise temperature being reasonably acceptable for the cells if added gently and at the same time causing so slow a dissociation of the receptor-bound insulin that this error will be negligible.

2. *Foam Formation.* Due to the high concentration of proteins and peptides, foam can be formed if the saline is splashed into the tubes. This foam

may layer at the interphase between oil and buffer and become a hindrance for the cells' penetration of the oil or go to the top trapping unbound ^{125}I radioactivity.

3. *Too Few Cells.* Not only the difference in densities between cells, oil, and buffer but also the geometry determine the phase distribution. Thus, when less than 20 μL packed-cell volume is incubated, the variation on the cell recovery increases. Perhaps it can be of some help to use an oil with a viscosity of only 50 centistokes. Cell recovery can be measured by adding a few μCi of [U-^{14}C]-D-glucose to the collagenase buffer (2.2.2). The adipocytes will then be [^{14}C] labeled in their central fat vacuole. After centrifugation through the oil phase, the cell pellet is counted in a β spectrometer in scintillation fluid. The [^{14}C] radioactivity will be directly proportional with the amount of cells. This can also be used to correct for differences in cell recovery due to differences in the incubation conditions (19, 22).

4. *Too Many Tubes Are Handled at a Time.* When the saline is added, the binding reaction is changed to a net dissociation process as the free concentration of insulin is diluted about 20 times, although slow at the low temperature.

5. *Too Warm Saline.* If the temperature of the saline is considerably higher than 10°C, the dissociation of receptor-bound insulin is enhanced.

2.5.4. SCATTERED CELLS

If the adipocytes do not coalesce on top of the oil, it is a symptom of cell lysis (see 2.5.2).

2.5.5. LARGE AMOUNTS OF CELLULAR MATERIAL AT THE INTERPHASE BETWEEN BUFFER AND OIL

1. It cannot be avoided completely, but a large amount is a symptom on cell lysis (see 2.5.2).
2. The viscosity of the oil is too large or the density too low.

2.5.6. CELLS WILL NOT ADSORB TO THE PIPE CLEANER

This is a symptom of cell lysis (see 2.5.2).

2.5.7. HIGH INSULIN DEGRADATION

Isolated rat adipocytes release proteolytic activity into the incubation medium, and this activity can be inhibited by different peptides (21). A high degradation is another symptom of unhealthy cells (see 2.5.2), or the unavoidable extracellular proteolysis has not been inhibited by the use of 5 percent w/v albumin and 0.35 m*M* bacitracin (16, 21) (cf. Section 2.2.4).

2.5.8.   RIGHTWARD SHIFT OF THE DISPLACEMENT CURVE

1.   Erroneous insulin dilutions.
2.   High insulin degradation (cf. 2.5.7).
3.   The collagenase is not washed off the cells (cf. 2.3.1).
4.   The pH is in the acid range (19).

2.5.9.   LEFTWARD SHIFT OF THE DISPLACEMENT CURVE

1.   Erroneous insulin dilutions.
2.   The temperature is below 37°C.
3.   The pH is in the alkaline range (19).

3.   BIOLOGICAL POTENCY

3.1.   Theory

In principle, any insulin-sensitive biological process can be used. The assay should be specific, easy to perform for a large number of samples, have a high precision and accuracy, and be insensitive to the presence of ^{125}I from iodinated insulins.

We use the insulin-induced conversion of [U-^{14}C]-D-glucose to lipids in isolated rat adipocytes (7, 21, 28, 29). At low extracellular concentrations of glucose, the intracellular glucose concentration will be much smaller than the K_m for the key enzymes catalyzing this process and, therefore, the rate of lipid formation will reflect the rate of transmembranal glucose transport. The latter being insulin-sensitive showing a 10 to 20 fold increase when the insulin concentration is increased from 10 to 500 pM, the steep slope being from 20 to 100 pM (Fig. 2) (for further details, please consult Chapter C, Part II, by Gliemann). In this assay it is possible to determine the potency when the concentration of the sample is known or vice versa.

3.1.1.   ABSOLUTE BIOLOGICAL POTENCY

When determining the absolute biological potency of an insulin preparation, the ability of the test substance and of the standard insulin preparation to stimulate the lipogenesis from [^{14}C]-D-glucose must be compared in several different concentrations within the same experiment. The determination of the concentrations is, therefore, the crucial point in this assay (see Section 2.1.1).

3.1.2.   RELATIVE BIOLOGICAL POTENCY

When information about the concentrations of the samples are unavailable (this will be the case for tracers, i.e., [^{125}I]monoiodoinsulins), it is still possible

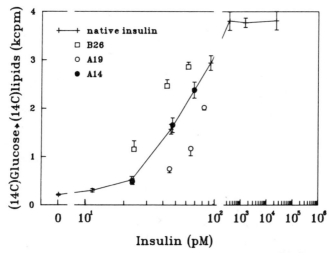

FIGURE 2. Determination of the relative biological potency of [Tyr^{B26}-^{125}I]monoiodoinsulin and [Tyr^{A19}-^{125}I]monoiodoinsulin. Isolated adipocytes were incubated as described in Section 3.4 with native insulin (+), [Tyr^{A14}-^{125}I]monoiodoinsulin (●), or the corresponding A19 (O) or B26 (□) isomers. Since both the concentration and the potency cannot be determined in the same assay, the potency of the A14 isomer has been assumed to be identical with that of native insulin (cf. 3.1.2). Therefore, the experimental points for A14 are superimposed on the standard curve for native insulin. The concentration of the other isomers are calculated from the [^{125}I] activity assuming the three isomers to possess the same specific activity (cf. 3.1.2). Bars represent SD when exceeding the size of the symbol. Redrawn from ref. 5.

to determine the relative biological potency of these preparations if certain assumptions are valid. Thus, we have previously shown that the A14 isomer is equipotent with native insulin. This was shown in experiments using [Tyr^{A14}-^{127}I]monoiodoinsulin, the concentration of which was determined in parallel to that of native insulin using both optical density and protein concentration determinations according to Lowry (2). Based on this assumption, the specific activity of the A14 isomer can be calculated. The second assumption is that the specific activity of the [^{125}I]monoiodoinsulin isomers is identical when prepared under the same iodination conditions. This is, however, only the case if the procedures of purification separate equally well all monoiodo isomers from diiodinated insulin [which will contribute more to the ^{125}I activity than to the bioactivity (30)] and from unlabeled insulin and bioactive derivatives of this, for example, desamidoinsulin (which will only contribute to the bioactivity). Based on this assumption, the potencies of the other isomers can be calculated from the standard curve and the specific activity (5). It should be mentioned, however, that recent results using determination of eight stable amino acids with an amino acid analyzer to assess the concentrations have revealed that the A14 isomer has a potency of about 120 percent of that of native insulin (31). Also that it has only been demonstrated that the A14 isomer is (close to being?) equipotent with insulin when the monoiodoinsulin isomer is isolated by disc gel electrophoresis or ion exchange chromatography (2, 3).

When isolated by reversed-phase high-performance liquid chromatography as described in Vol IB, VI A by Welinder et al., the potency may be reduced by about 40 pecent (Sonne, Welinder, and Linde, unpublished observation).

3.2. Buffer

In the bioassay we use Krebs–Ringer HEPES buffer with 1 percent w/v bovine serum albumin (i.e., corresponding to washing buffer, Section 2.2.3) fortified with 12 μM D-glucose (for the rationale of this, please consult Chapter C, Part II, by Gliemann).

3.3 Cells

Rat adipocytes are isolated as described in Section 2.3.1, except that the buffer used for wash and incubation is as described in Section 3.2.

3.4. Incubation

The adipocytes are incubated in 20 mL polyethylene scintillation vials in a final volume of 1.0 mL with isotope and standards or samples added in volumes not less than 50 μL. Typically, we use four replicates each with the following:

100 μL [U-^{14}C]-D-glucose containing 1.85 kBq (= 0.05 μCi).

100 μL buffer or insulin standard or sample.

800 μL adipocytes 0.63 percent v/v.

This will give a final cell concentration of 0.5 percent v/v. Incubate in a shaking water bath at 37°C for 2 hr.

The incubation is stopped by the addition of 5 mL scintillation fluid of the following composition: 5.5 g Permablend III (PPO and bis-MSB, 91:9) (Packard) and 1 L toluene (technical grade). The vials are corked and left overnight at 4°C to complete the lipid extraction and phase separation. Next day 1.0 mL of the upper phase is transferred to minivials and counted in a liquid scintillation counter set with a narrow ^{14}C window.

The following experimental points are needed:

1. *Blanks.* For each concentration of [^{125}I]monoiodoinsulin and one set without [^{125}I]monoiodoinsulin add scintillation fluid before cells. The ^{125}I activity should be hydrophilic and remain in the water (lower) phase. If present in the organic phase, the energy spectrum of ^{125}I corresponds more to that of ^{3}H than to ^{14}C, therefore the narrow window.

2. *Basal.* No insulin present.

3. *Standards.* We use a standard curve consisting of 240 M, 15 M, 3.75 nM and four concentrations by 1 + 1 dilution from 1.0 nM. This will in the incubate give final concentrations one-tenth of these.

4. *Samples.*   Each sample should be included in two or three different concentrations, giving an incorporation of glucose into lipids corresponding to the steep slope of the standard curve.

5. *Total.*   100 μL [U-^{14}C]-D-glucose plus any scintillation fluid miscible with this amount of water. When the other data are compared with this total value, lack of substrate present during the incubation can be excluded.

3.5. Artifacts and Trouble Shooting

In this section some of the most commonly occurring troubles and possible explanations for these are listed.

3.5.1. FEW CELLS

Bad collagenase (see Sections 2.3.1 and 2.5).

3.5.2. HIGH BASALS

1. *Insulin Contamination of Buffers or Solutions.*   If incubated with an excess of anti-insulin antibody, the basal should be brought down.

2. *Collagenase.*   Some batches of collagenase will result in cells with a high basal glucose uptake. Before buying collagenase, several batches should be tested for their ability to (i) release cells in a resonable time and amount (cf. 2.3.1) and (ii) release cells with a low basal and high insulin-stimulated glucose uptake resulting in a steep standard curve. Usually the maximally stimulated value is the same for the different batches, whereas the basal value varies. Choose the lowest basal.

3. *Bovine Serum Albumin.*   Some brands and some batches contain factors other than insulin (cannot be inhibited with anti-insulin antibodies) which increase the glucose incorporation. Such activity can be reduced by treatment of the albumin preparation with trypsin (32).

4. *The Mechanics.*   Vega and Kono (33) observed that the basal (but not the insulin-stimulated) glucose transport decreases when the adipocytes are preincubated at 37°c in the presence of glucose for 30 min. Upon vigorous shaking or centrifugation the basal rate would go again. We have not observed this, perhaps because our cells have received the gentle handling. However, it is worth trying to introduce a restoration period.

5. *Too High Glucose Concentration.*   If the glucose concentration is too high, the enzymes will be rate limiting and not the insulin-sensitive trans-membranal transport (cf. 3.1).

6. *Alkaline pH.*   For unknown reasons an alkaline pH will increase the basal but not the maximally stimulated glucose uptake (19).

3.5.3.   Rightward Shift of the Standard Curve

1. *High Insulin Degradation.*   The cells isolated are lysing, releasing proteolytic enzymes into the medium. This can be because of a too harsh mechanical treatment, or the cells do not like the plastic used (cf. 2.5). Try to be more gentle. Try another kind of plastic. Try to increase the albumin concentration to 5 percent w/v. This will partly protect in both cases but is only a "cure of the symptoms not the disease". This degradation can be detected by adding [^{125}I]monoiodoinsulin in parallel incubations and measuring the solubility of the ^{125}I in trichloroacetic acid (cf. 2.4.1.4).

3. *The Collagenase Is Not Washed Off the Cells.*   As the collagenase in addition contains proteolytic enzymes, it is important to wash the adipocytes carefully (cf. 2.3.1) but gently (cf. this section).

4. *Acid pH (19).*

3.5.4.   LEFTWARD SHIFT OF THE STANDARD CURVE

1. *Erroneous Insulin Dilutions.*

2. *Lack of Substrate.*   Compare the ^{14}C radioactivity in the samples with the maximally stimulating insulin concentration (remember that only one-fifth the volume have been counted) with the total ^{14}C activity added (cf. 3.4). Too long incubation or too high cell concentration.

3. *Alkaline pH (19)*

REFERENCES

1. P. Freychet, J. Roth, and D. M. Neville, Jr., *Biochem. Biophys. Res. Commun.* **43**, 400 (1971).

2. J. Gliemann, O. Sonne, S. Linde, and B. Hansen, *Biochem. Biophys. Res. Commun.* **87**, 1183 (1979).

3. S. Linde, B. Hansen, O. Sonne, J. J. Holst, and J. Gliemann, *Diabetes* **30**, 1 (1981).

4. S. Linde, O. Sonne, B. Hansen, and J. Gliemann, *Hoppe-Seyler's Z. Physiol. Chem.* **362**, 573 (1981).

5. O. Sonne, S. Linde, T. R. Larsen, and J. Gliemann, *Hoppe-Seyler's Z. Physiol. Chem.* **364**, 101 (1983).

6. J. E. Foley, A. L. Laursen, O. Sonne, and J. Gliemann, *Diabetologia* **19**, 234 (1980).

7. M. Rodbell, *J. Biol. Chem.* **239**, 375 (1964).

8. M. N. Berry and D. S. Friend, *Exp. Cell Biol.* **43**, 507 (1969).

9. P. O. Seglen, *Exp. Cell Res.* **74**, 450 (1972).

10. P. O. Seglen, *Exp. Cell Res.* **76**, 25 (1973).

11. P. O. Seglen, *Exp. Cell Res.* **82**, 391 (1973).

12. H. Pertoft, K. Rubin, L. Kjellén, T. C. Laurent, and B. Klingeborn, *Exp. Cell Res.* **110**, 449 (1977).

13. P. O. Seglen, in *Cell Populations*, E. Reid (ed.), Ellis Horwood Ltd., Chichester, 1979, chapter B-1.

14. H. Pertoft, M. Hirtenstein, and L. Kågedal, in *Cell Populations*, E. Reid (ed), Ellis Horwood Ltd., Chichester, 1979, chapter B-4.

15. P. De Meyts, in *Methods in Receptor Research*, M. Blecher (ed.), Marcel Dekker, New York, 1976, pp. 303–311.

16. O. Sonne and J. Gliemann, *J. Biol. Chem* **255**, 7449 (1980).

17. J. Fogh and G. Trempe, in *Human Tumor Cells in Vitro*, J. Fogh (ed.), Plenum Press, New York, 1975, chapter 5.

18. Flow Laboratories, catalogue, section 1.

19. O. Sonne, J. Gliemann, and S. Linde, *J. Biol. Chem.* **256**, 6250 (1981).

20. M. Waelbroeck, E. van Obberghen, and P. De Meyts, *J. Biol. Chem.* **254**, 7736 (1979).

21. J. Gliemann and O. Sonne, *J. Biol. Chem.* **253**, 7857 (1978).

22. O. Sonne and J. Gliemann, *Mol. Cell. Endocrinol.* **31**, 315 (1983).

23. J. Gliemann, K. Østerlind, J. Vinten, and S. Gammeltoft, *Biochim. Biophys. Acta* **286**, 1 (1972).

24. B. S. Welinder, S. Linde, B. Hansen, and O. Sonne, *J. Chromatogr.*, unpublished.

25. J. S. Brush, O. Sonne, and J. Gliemann, *Biochim. Biophys. Acta* **757**, 269 (1983).

26. P. A. Andreasen, B. P. Schaumburg, K. Østerlind, J. Vinten, S. Gammeltoft, and J. Gliemann, *Anal. Biochem.* **59**, 610 (1974).

27. R. J. Bonney, J. E. Becker, P. R. Walker, and V. R. Potter, *In vitro* **9**, 399 (1974).

28. J. Gliemann, *Diabetologia* **3**, 382 (1967).

29. A. J. Moody, M. A. Stan, M. Stan, and J. Gliemann, *Horm. Metab. Res.* **6**, 12 (1974).

30. B. P. Maceda, S. Linde, O. Sonne, and J. Gliemann, *Diabetes* **31**, 634 (1982).

31. K. H. Jørgensen, A. J. Moody, and M. C. Christensen, in *Eleventh Congress of the International Diabetes Federation*, Excerpta Medica International Congress Series, Vol. 577, K. G. M. M. Alberti, T. Ogada, J. A. Aluoch, and E. N. Mngola (eds.), Excerpta Medica, Amsterdam, 1982, p. 173, abstract P16.

32. J. E. Jordan and T. Kono, *Anal. Biochem* **104**, 192 (1980).

33. F. V. Vega and T. Kono, *Arch. Biochem. Biophys.* **192**, 120 (1979).

INDEX